T0343382

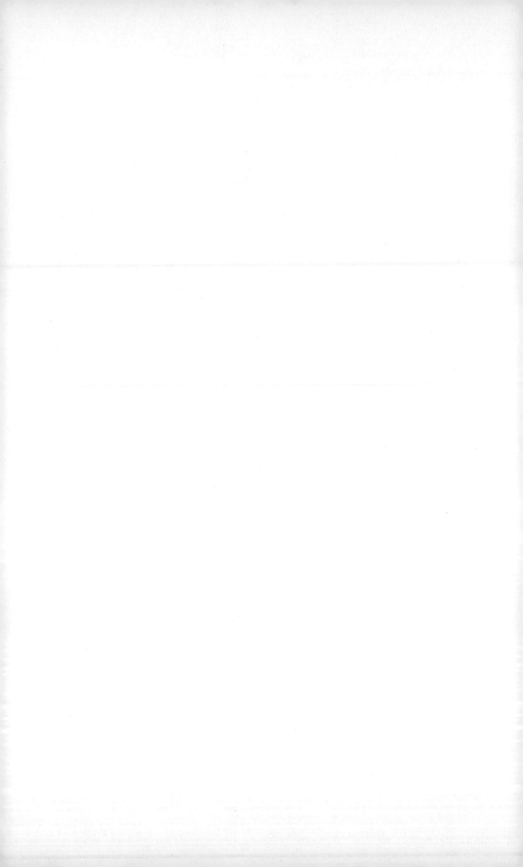

2012
YEAR BOOK OF
EMERGENCY MEDICINE®

The 2012 Year Book Series

Year Book of Anesthesiology and Pain Management™: Drs Chestnut, Abram, Black, Gravlee, Lien, Mathru, and Roizen

Year Book of Cardiology®: Drs Gersh, Cheitlin, Elliott, Gold, Graham, and Thourani

Year Book of Critical Care Medicine®: Drs Dries, Zanotti-Cavazzoni, Latenser, Martinez, Rincon, and Zwank

Year Book of Dermatology and Dermatologic Surgery™: Dr Del Rosso

Year Book of Diagnostic Radiology®: Drs Elster, Abbara, Oestreich, Offiah, Rosado de Christenson, Stephens, and Strickland

Year Book of Emergency Medicine®: Drs Hamilton, Bruno, Handly, Minczak, Mullin, Quintana, and Ramoska

Year Book of Endocrinology®: Drs Schott, Apovian, Clarke, Eugster, Ludlam, Meikle, Oetjen, Schteingart, and Toth

Year Book of Gastroenterology™: Drs Talley, DeVault, Harnois, Murray, Pearson, Philcox, Picco, and Smith

Year Book of Hand and Upper Limb Surgery®: Drs Yao and Steinmann

Year Book of Medicine®: Drs Barker, Garrick, Gersh, Khardori, LeRoith, Panush, Talley, and Thigpen

Year Book of Neonatal and Perinatal Medicine®: Drs Fanaroff, Benitz, Donn, Neu, Papile, Polin, and Van Marter

Year Book of Neurology and Neurosurgery®: Drs Klimo, Minagar, Breningstall, Gandhi, House, Kevill, Liu, Mazia, Panagariya, Ragel, Riesenburger, Shafazand, Uhm, and Yang

Year Book of Obstetrics, Gynecology, and Women's Health®: Drs Dungan and Shulman

Year Book of Oncology®: Drs Arceci, Bauer, Chiorean, Gordon, Lawton, Murphy, Thigpen, and Tsao

Year Book of Ophthalmology®: Drs Rapuano, Cohen, Flanders, Hammersmith, Milman, Myers, Nagra, Nelson, Penne, Pyfer, Sergott, Shields, Talekar, and Vander

Year Book of Orthopedics®: Drs Morrey, Huddleston, Swiontkowski, and Trigg

Year Book of Otolaryngology-Head and Neck Surgery®: Drs Sindwani, Balough, Franco, Gapany, and Mitchell

Year Book of Pathology and Laboratory Medicine®: Drs Raab and Bissell

Year Book of Pediatrics®: Dr Stockman

Year Book of Plastic and Aesthetic Surgery™: Drs Miller, Gosman, Gurtner, Gutowski, Ruberg, Salisbury, and Smith

Year Book of Psychiatry and Applied Mental Health®: Drs Talbott, Ballenger, Buckley, Frances, Krupnick, and Mack

Year Book of Pulmonary Disease®: Drs Barker, Jones, Maurer, Spradley, Tanoue, and Willsie

Year Book of Sports Medicine®: Drs Shephard, Cantu, Feldman, Galea, Jankowski, Janssen, Lebrun, and Nieman

Year Book of Surgery®: Drs Copeland, Behrns, Daly, Eberlein, Fahey, Huber, Klodell, Mozingo, and Pruett

Year Book of Urology®: Drs Andriole and Coplen

Year Book of Vascular Surgery®: Drs Moneta, Gillespie, Starnes, and Watkins

2012

The Year Book of EMERGENCY MEDICINE®

Editor-in-Chief
Richard J. Hamilton, MD
Professor and Chair, Department of Emergency Medicine, Drexel University College of Medicine, Philadelphia, Pennsylvania

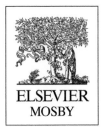

ELSEVIER
MOSBY

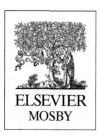

ELSEVIER
MOSBY

Vice President, Continuity: Kimberly Murphy
Editor: Yonah Korngold
Production Supervisor, Electronic Year Books: Donna M. Skelton
Electronic Article Manager: Emily Ogle
Illustrations and Permissions Coordinator: Dawn Vohsen

2012 EDITION
Copyright 2012, Mosby, Inc. All rights reserved.

No part of this publication may be reproduced, stored in a retrieval system, or transmitted, in any form or by any means, electronic, mechanical, photocopying, recording, or otherwise, without prior written permission from the publisher.

Permission to photocopy or reproduce solely for internal or personal use is permitted for libraries or other users registered with the Copyright Clearance Center, provided that the base fee of $35.00 per chapter is paid directly to the Copyright Clearance Center, 21 Congress Street, Salem, MA 01970. This consent does not extend to other kinds of copying, such as copying for general distribution, for advertising or promotional purposes, for creating new collected works, or for resale.

Printed and bound by CPI Group (UK) Ltd, Croydon, CR0 4YY
Composition by TNQ Books and Journals Pvt Ltd, India
Transferred to Digital Print 2012

Editorial Office:
Elsevier
1600 John F. Kennedy Blvd.
Suite 1800
Philadelphia, PA 19103-2899

International Standard Serial Number: 0271-7964
International Standard Book Number: 978-0-323-08878-7

Associate Editors

Eric C. Bruno, MD, FAAEM
Attending Emergency Physician, Middle Tennessee Emergency Physicians, Middle Tennessee Medical Center and Baptist Hospital, Murfreesboro and Nashville, Tennessee

Neal B. Handly, MD, MSc, MS
Associate Professor of Emergency Medicine, Associate Research Director, Department of Emergency Medicine, Drexel University College of Medicine, Philadelphia, Pennsylvania

Bohdan M. Minczak, MS, MD, PhD
Assistant Professor of Emergency Medicine, EMS Division Head, EMS Fellowship Director, Department of Emergency Medicine, Drexel University College of Medicine; Philadelphia, Pennsylvania

Daniel K. Mullin, MD
Assistant Professor of Emergency Medicine, Director of Continuing Medical Education, Department of Emergency Medicine, Drexel University College of Medicine, Philadelphia, Pennsylvania

Eileen C. Quintana, MD, MPH
Assistant Professor of Emergency Medicine and Pediatrics, Department of Emergency Medicine, Drexel University College of Medicine; St. Christopher's Hospital for Children, Philadelphia, Pennsylvania

Edward A. Ramoska, MD, MPH
Clinical Associate Professor of Emergency Medicine, Program Director, Emergency Medicine, Department of Emergency Medicine, Drexel University College of Medicine, Philadelphia, Pennsylvania

Associate Editors

Eric C. Bruno, MD, FAAEM

Neal B. Handly, MD, MSc, MS

Bohdan M. Minczak, MS, MD, PhD

Daniel K. Nishijima, MD

Edward A. Ramoska, MD, MPH

Table of Contents

Journals Represented

Journals represented in this YEAR BOOK are listed below.
Academic Emergency Medicine
Acta Anaesthesiologica Scandinavica
Acta Oto-Laryngologica
Air Medical Journal
American Heart Journal
American Journal of Cardiology
American Journal of Emergency Medicine
American Journal of Medicine
American Journal of Public Health
American Journal of Surgery
American Journal of Transplantation
Anaesthesia
Annals of Emergency Medicine
Annals of Surgery
Annals of Thoracic Surgery
Archives of Internal Medicine
Archives of Pediatrics & Adolescent Medicine
Archives of Surgery
British Journal of Anaesthesia
British Journal of Sports Medicine
British Medical Journal
Burns
Canadian Journal of Emergency Medicine
Cancer Epidemiology, Biomarkers & Prevention
Circulation
Clinical Chemistry
Clinical Pediatrics
Clinical Pediatrics (Philadelphia)
Clinical Toxicology
Clinical Toxicology (Philadelphia)
Contraception
Critical Care
Critical Care Medicine
Europace
European Heart Journal
European Journal of Paediatric Neurology
Gastrointestinal Endoscopy
Heart
Injury
Intensive Care Medicine
International Journal of Cardiology
International Journal of Sports Medicine
Journal of Cardiothoracic and Vascular Anesthesia
Journal of Clinical Endocrinology & Metabolism
Journal of Clinical Microbiology

Journal of Clinical Neuroscience
Journal of Emergency Medicine
Journal of Laryngology and Otology
Journal of Pain
Journal of Pediatric Gastroenterology and Nutrition
Journal of Pediatric Surgery
Journal of Periodontology
Journal of Stroke and Cerebrovascular Diseases
Journal of the American College of Cardiology
Journal of Trauma
Journal of Vascular Surgery
Lancet
Medical Care
Medicine and Science in Sports and Exercise
Nature
Nephrology Dialysis Transplantation
New England Journal of Medicine
Pediatric Dermatology
Pediatric Emergency Care
Pediatric Infectious Disease Journal
Pediatrics
Prehospital Emergency Care
Skeletal Radiology
Stroke
Surgery
Thrombosis Research
Transfusion
World Journal of Surgery

STANDARD ABBREVIATIONS

The following terms are abbreviated in this edition: acquired immunodeficiency syndrome (AIDS), central nervous system (CNS), cardiopulmonary resuscitation (CPR), cerebrospinal fluid (CSF), computed tomography (CT), deoxyribonucleic acid (DNA), electrocardiography (ECG), emergency department (ED), emergency medical services (EMS), human immunodeficiency virus (HIV), health maintenance organization (HMO), intensive care unit (ICU), intramuscular (IM), intravenous (IV), magnetic resonance (MR) imaging (MRI), ribonucleic acid (RNA), ultrasound (US), and ultraviolet (UV).

NOTE

The YEAR BOOK OF EMERGENCY MEDICINE® is a literature survey service providing abstracts of articles published in the professional literature. Every effort is made to assure the accuracy of the information presented in these pages. Neither the editors nor the publisher of the YEAR BOOK OF EMERGENCY MEDICINE® can be responsible for errors in the original materials. The editors' comments are their own opinions. Mention of specific products within this publication does not constitute endorsement.

To facilitate the use of the YEAR BOOK OF EMERGENCY MEDICINE® as a reference tool, all illustrations and tables included in this publication are now identified as they appear in the original article. This change is meant to help the reader recognize that any illustration or table appearing in the YEAR BOOK OF EMERGENCY MEDICINE® may be only one of many in the original article. For this reason, figure and table numbers will often appear to be out of sequence within the YEAR BOOK OF EMERGENCY MEDICINE®.

1 Trauma

Evaluation

Assessing the Feasibility of the American College of Surgeons' Benchmarks for the Triage of Trauma Patients
Mohan D, Rosengart MR, Farris C, et al (Univ of Pittsburgh, PA)
Arch Surg 146:786-792, 2011

Objective.—To test the feasibility of accomplishing the American College of Surgeons Committee on Trauma benchmarks of less than 5% undertriage (treatment of patients with moderate to severe injuries at nontrauma centers [NTCs]) and less than 50% overtriage (transfer of patients with minor injuries to trauma centers [TCs]) given current practice patterns by describing transfer patterns for patients taken initially to NTCs and estimating volume shifts and potential lives saved if full implementation were to occur.

Design, Setting, and Patients.—Retrospective cohort study of adult trauma patients initially evaluated at NTCs in Pennsylvania (between April 1, 2001, and March 31, 2005). We used published estimates of mortality risk reduction associated with treatment at TCs.

Main Outcome Measures.—Undertriage and overtriage rates, estimated patient volume shifts, and number of lives saved.

Results.—A total of 93 880 adult trauma patients were initially evaluated at NTCs in Pennsylvania between 2001 and 2005. Undertriage was 69%; overtriage was 53%. Achieving less than 5% undertriage would require the transfer of 18 945 patients per year, a 5-fold increase from current practice (3650 transfers per year). Given an absolute mortality risk reduction of 1.9% for patients with moderate to severe injuries treated at TCs, this change in practice would save 99 potential lives per year or would require 191 transfers per year to save 1 potential life.

Conclusions.—Given current practice patterns, American College of Surgeons Committee on Trauma recommendations for the regionalization of trauma patients may not be feasible. To achieve 5% undertriage, TCs must increase their capacity 5-fold, physicians at NTCs must increase their capacity to discriminate between moderate to severe and other injuries, or the guidelines must be modified.

▶ Picture yourself at a nontrauma center emergency department (ED). A patient suffering from traumatic injury arrives and you begin your evaluation and treatment. Once you decide that the injuries will require further care in a hospital, you need to decide if that care needs to be done at a trauma center or if your hospital can adequately care for this patient.

The American College of Surgeons Committee on Trauma (ACS-COT) has established transfer criteria based on injury severity (commonly measured with the injury severity score [ISS]). To ensure optimal outcomes for patients, ACS-COT set a maximum undertriage level at 5% (keeping patients at non-trauma centers when they need to be transferred) and a maximum overtriage level of 50% (transferring patients to trauma centers who could be managed at nontrauma centers). Undertriage might put patients at risk for unnecessary mortality and morbidity, especially if the nontrauma center does not regularly care for these patients. Clearly overtriage can be costly to the trauma center (not including the cost of the transfer) because of increased workload that is somewhat unpredictable, but also there may be risk of under- or uninsured patients being transferred.

Over the course of the study (2001–2005), it was found that there was about 53% overtriage and about 70% undertriage. Limitations of the study come into play here—first, patients transferred or sent directly home from the nontrauma center ED were not counted in this study. Instead, only patients already admitted to in-patient status at the nontrauma center were considered for transfer. Second, the authors used ISS as the tool to describe injury severity. Yet ISS from the nontrauma center was not available to the authors. Instead, they converted ICD-9 diagnostic codes to ISS. Regardless of the validity of that generated score, often the information describing the injury is not completely known in the early phase of trauma resuscitation, so it is likely not going to explain the thinking of physicians when making decisions about transfer.

But if we accept that the ISS can be used to assess the transfer decision, there were still problems using the ACS-COT transfer criteria, as there was some overlap between the ISS values of those who should have been and those who were not transferred. This suggested that inherent in a desired increase of transfers to trauma centers of those with higher level of injuries would come an increase in the level of overtriage that would create a significant burden on the trauma center.

How physicians determine who does need a trauma center admission is likely to be more complicated than just the ISS. Additionally, nontrauma centers may have the expertise to handle some types of trauma, and this expertise can be hospital and date/time specific when certain physicians are on call.

The authors were unable to comment on the outcomes of these triage decisions; they lacked morbidity information, and they were unable to link the information for the patients who were transferred from the nontrauma center to the trauma center. We need to know a lot more to provide cost and clinically effective care.

N. B. Handly, MD, MSc, MS

Effect of the Modified Glasgow Coma Scale Score Criteria for Mild Traumatic Brain Injury on Mortality Prediction: Comparing Classic and Modified Glasgow Coma Scale Score Model Scores of 13

Mena JH, Sanchez AI, Rubiano AM, et al (Univ of Pittsburgh, PA; Neiva Univ Hosp, Colombia; et al)

J Trauma 71:1185-1193, 2011

Background.—The Glasgow Coma Scale (GCS) classifies traumatic brain injuries (TBIs) as mild (14—15), moderate (9—13), or severe (3—8). The Advanced Trauma Life Support modified this classification so that a GCS score of 13 is categorized as mild TBI. We investigated the effect of this modification on mortality prediction, comparing patients with a GCS score of 13 classified as moderate TBI (classic model) to patients with GCS score of 13 classified as mild TBI (modified model).

Methods.—We selected adult TBI patients from the Pennsylvania Outcome Study database. Logistic regressions adjusting for age, sex, cause, severity, trauma center level, comorbidities, and isolated TBI were performed. A second evaluation included the time trend of mortality. A third evaluation also included hypothermia, hypotension, mechanical ventilation, screening for drugs, and severity of TBI. Discrimination of the models was evaluated using the area under receiver operating characteristic curve (AUC). Calibration was evaluated using the Hosmer-Lemershow goodness of fit test.

Results.—In the first evaluation, the AUCs were 0.922 (95% CI, 0.917—0.926) and 0.908 (95% CI, 0.903—0.912) for classic and modified models, respectively. Both models showed poor calibration ($p < 0.001$). In the third evaluation, the AUCs were 0.946 (95% CI, 0.943—0.949) and 0.938 (95% CI, 0.934—0.940) for the classic and modified models, respectively, with improvements in calibration ($p = 0.30$ and $p = 0.02$ for the classic and modified models, respectively).

Conclusion.—The lack of overlap between receiver operating characteristic curves of both models reveals a statistically significant difference in their ability to predict mortality. The classic model demonstrated better goodness of fit than the modified model. A GCS score of 13 classified as moderate TBI in a multivariate logistic regression model performed better than a GCS score of 13 classified as mild.

▶ Is the mortality outcome of a patient suffering from a traumatic brain injury (TBI) rated with a Glasgow Coma Scale (GCS) value of 13 more like that of a patient with a GCS value of 12 or 14? What is (are) the rationale for modifying the definitions of mild and moderate TBI based on GCS?

One might imagine that "mild," "moderate," and "severe" are terms that patients and families will understand better than presenting them the GCS value and how it is both derived and what is different at each value. Another reason for developing the boundary between mild and moderate is that in many institutions, mild injuries are handled by reduced service teams, and moderate injuries are managed by full trauma teams. This is not just the fact that our descriptors are important to team response but that there is a known increase in mortality with worsening GCS.

The authors chose to compare mortality rates for TBI victims admitted to trauma centers with each GCS value. Then they examined the rates of mortality based on 2 mild/moderate/severe grade systems of TBI based on GCS values: one in which values of 14 and 15 were considered mild and a second in which values of 13, 14, and 15 were considered mild.

By GCS alone (no grouping), it does appear that mortality risk for 13 is more like 12 than 14. When grouping with 13 included in the moderate group, the models that were generated better describe the risk of mortality.

Although it seems that the old model is better than one that puts 13 in the mild injury category, I am still concerned about the quality of work and its bearing on the conclusions. The sum of patients (as percentages) in the 2 grouping methods do not add to the same values (not that the severe group did not change between the 2 methods). The old grouping sum of mid and moderate injured patients is 78.3% and the sum with the new grouping of mild and moderate injured patients is 75.6%; the caption and figures in the original article are confusing.

The problem is interesting, the methods attempted seem appropriate, and the conclusions might be true, but the authors and editors could have done a better job presenting the work. The reader deserves better.

N. B. Handly, MD, MSc, MS

Over Reliance on Computed Tomography Imaging in Patients With Severe Abdominal Injury: Is the Delay Worth the Risk?

Neal MD, Peitzman AB, Forsythe RM, et al (Univ of Pittsburgh Med Ctr, PA)
J Trauma 70:278-284, 2011

Background.—Computed tomography (CT) has a high sensitivity and specificity for detecting abdominal injuries. Expeditious abdominal imaging in "quasi-stable" patients may prevent negative laparotomy. However, the significance of potential delay to laparotomy secondary to abdominal imaging remains unknown. We sought to analyze whether the use of abdominal CT (ABD CT) in patients with abdominal injury requiring laparotomy results in a significant delay and a higher risk of poor outcome.

Methods.—A retrospective analysis of data from the National Trauma Data Bank (version 7.1) was performed. Inclusion criteria were adult patients (age >14 years), a scene admission (nontransfer), hypotension on arrival (emergency department systolic blood pressure <90 mm Hg), an abdominal Abbreviated Injury Scale (AIS) score >3, and undergoing a laparotomy within 90 minutes of arrival. Patients with severe brain injury (head AIS score >3) were excluded. The independent mortality risk associated with a preoperative ABD CT was determined using logistic regression after controlling important confounders.

Result.—This cohort of patients (n = 3,218) was significantly injured with a median Injury Severity Score of 25 ([interquartile range, 16−34]). Patients who underwent ABD CT had similar Glasgow Coma Scale scores, a lower head AIS, longer time delays to the operating room, and a higher crude mortality (45% vs. 30%; $p = 0.001$). Logistic regression revealed that ABD CT was independently associated with more than a 70% higher risk of mortality (odds ratios, 1.71; 95% CI, 1.2–2.2; $p < 0.001$). When stratified by injury mechanism, intubation status and whether or not a head CT was performed, the mortality risk remained significantly increased for each subgroup. When the laparotomy was able to occur within 30 minutes of arrival, an ABD CT was independently associated with more than a sevenfold higher risk of mortality (odds ratios, 7.6; $p = 0.038$).

Conclusion.—Delay secondary to abdominal imaging in patients who require operative intervention results in an independent higher risk of mortality. ABD CT imaging is an important and useful tool after injury; however, these results suggest that delay caused by overreliance on ABD CT may result in poor outcome in specific patients. Clinicians who take care of critically injured patients should be aware of and understand these potential risks.

▶ Hypotensive trauma patients who stabilize with early interventions are identified as responders and pose a diagnostic dilemma for emergency physicians (EPs) and traumatologists. Where is the blood? and "Can this patient go to CT?" are inquiries that must be addressed during the initial management. The authors of this retrospective database review assessed the mortality risk associated with proceeding with diagnostic testing—specifically computed tomography— rather than going to surgical intervention. Using the laughable, but completely understandable, phrase "quasi-stable" and logistic regression statistics, they were able to demonstrate a 70% higher independent risk of mortality in those patients who receive abdominal CT rather than pushing on to the operating room (OR). Patients receiving the radiographic diagnostic testing (abdominal CT and/or head CT) had a 30-minute delay in transport to the OR more than 98% of the time. These precious minutes in a "quasi-stable" patient may be the difference. The intervention-responsive patient remains a "moving target." EPs must work directly with their trauma surgeons to determine whether the patient has stabilized enough for CT or transport to the OR is required.

A more relevant question is, "Are EPs and traumatologists overrelying on CT imaging in patients with significant injury mechanism, but no signs or symptoms of severe injury? Are observation and serial examinations worth the effort?"

E. C. Bruno, MD

Validation and Refinement of a Rule to Predict Emergency Intervention in Adult Trauma Patients

Haukoos JS, Byyny RL, Erickson C, et al (Denver Health Med Ctr, CO; et al)
Ann Emerg Med 58:164-171, 2011

Study Objective.—Trauma centers use "secondary triage" to determine the necessity of trauma surgeon involvement. A clinical decision rule, which includes penetrating injury, an initial systolic blood pressure less than 100 mm Hg, or an initial pulse rate greater than 100 beats/min, was developed to predict which trauma patients require emergency operative intervention or emergency procedural intervention (cricothyroidotomy or thoracotomy) in the emergency department. Our goal was to validate this rule in an adult trauma population and to compare it with the American College of Surgeons' major resuscitation criteria.

Methods.—We used Level I trauma center registry data from September 1, 1995, through November 30, 2008. Outcomes were confirmed with blinded abstractors. Sensitivity, specificity, and 95% confidence intervals (CIs) were calculated.

Results.—Our patient sample included 20,872 individuals. The median Injury Severity Score was 9 (interquartile range 4 to 16), 15.3% of patients had penetrating injuries, 13.5% had a systolic blood pressure less than 100 mm Hg, and 32.5% had a pulse rate greater than 100 beats/min. Emergency operative intervention or procedural intervention was required in 1,099 patients (5.3%; 95% CI 5.0% to 5.6%). The sensitivities and specificities of the rule and the major resuscitation criteria for predicting emergency operative intervention or emergency procedural intervention were 95.6% (95% CI 94.3% to 96.8%) and 56.1% (95% CI 55.4% to 56.8%) and 85.5% (95% CI 83.3% to 87.5%) and 80.9% (95% CI 80.3% to 81.4%), respectively.

Conclusion.—This new rule was more sensitive for predicting the need for emergency operative intervention or emergency procedural intervention directly compared with the American College of Surgeons' major resuscitation criteria, which may improve the effectiveness and efficiency of trauma triage.

▶ The American College of Surgeons (ACS) requires that a surgeon be in attendance on trauma patient arrival when 1 of 6 major resuscitation criteria is present. These criteria were not developed experimentally and have only been assessed by 1 previous study. Steele et al,[1] in 2007, found the sensitivity and specificity of using these criteria in adult trauma patients to be 82% and 76%, respectively. These same investigators developed another set of clinical decision rules (the Loma Linda rules) to predict emergency operative management and whether it would therefore be advantageous to have a surgeon present when an adult trauma patient arrives.

This study from Denver Health Medical Center seeks to validate the Loma Linda rules and to compare them with the ACS major resuscitation criteria. The ACS Committee on Trauma suggests that a 10% false-negative secondary triage rate (ie, undertriage) is unavoidable and a 50% false-positive secondary triage rate (ie, overtriage) is acceptable. This equates to a sensitivity of 90% and a specificity of 50%. These data show that the Loma Linda rules exceed these thresholds, whereas the ACS criteria are less sensitive but more specific. Moreover, the authors derived a refinement to the Loma Linda rules to include penetrating injury to the torso and less conservative physiologic criteria (ie, systolic blood pressure < 90 mm Hg and pulse rate > 110 beats/min). This modification resulted in a lower sensitivity, 89.7% (95% confidence interval [CI], 87.9% to 91.5%), and an improved specificity, 75.2% (95% CI, 74.6% to 75.8%) when compared with the original Loma Linda rules. This revision just barely meets the ACS suggested 10% undertriage rate, while dramatically improving the 50% overtriage rate. If the revised Loma Linda rules are further validated in larger studies, they may be quite useful for determining when it is most efficient and effective for an emergency physician to summon a surgeon to the bedside of a trauma patient.

E. A. Ramoska, MD, MPHE

Reference

1. Steele R, Gill M, Green SM, Parker T, Lam E, Coba V. Do the American College of Surgeons' "major resuscitation" trauma triage criteria predict emergency operative management? *Ann Emerg Med.* 2007;50:1-6.

Extremity Injury

An Evaluation of Two Tourniquet Systems for the Control of Prehospital Lower Limb Hemorrhage

Taylor DM, Vater GM, Parker PJ (Friarage Hosp, Northallerton, North Yorkshire; Royal Centre for Defence Medicine, Birmingham, UK)
J Trauma 71:591-595, 2011

Background.—Hemorrhage remains the main cause of preventable death on the modern battlefield. As Improvised Explosive Devices in Afghanistan become increasingly powerful, more proximal limb injuries occur. Significant concerns now exist about the ability of the windlass tourniquet to control distal hemorrhage after mid-thigh application. To evaluate the efficacy of the Combat Application Tourniquet (CAT) windlass tourniquet in comparison to the newer Emergency and Military Tourniquet (EMT) pneumatic tourniquet.

Methods.—Serving soldiers were recruited from a military orthopedic outpatient clinic. Participants' demographics, blood pressure, and body mass index were recorded. Doppler ultrasound was used to identify the popliteal pulses bilaterally. The CAT was randomly self-applied by the participant at mid-thigh level, and the presence or absence of the popliteal pulse on Doppler was recorded. The process was repeated on the contralateral leg with the CAT now applied by a trained researcher. Finally, the EMT tourniquet was applied to the first leg and popliteal pulse change Doppler recorded again.

Results.—A total of 25 patients were recruited with 1 participant excluded. The self-applied CAT occluded popliteal flow in only four subjects (16.6%). The CAT applied by a researcher occluded popliteal flow in two subjects (8.3%). The EMT prevented all popliteal flow in 18 subjects (75%). This was a statistically significant difference at $p < 0.001$ for CAT versus EMT.

Conclusion.—This study demonstrates that the CAT tourniquet is ineffective in controlling arterial blood flow when applied at mid-thigh level. The EMT was successful in a significantly larger number of participants.

▶ Understanding that hemorrhage is a leading cause of preventable death on the battlefield, numerous devices and techniques are available to attempt to gain hemorrhage control. American servicemen and servicewomen enter the theater of operations with a 1-handed Combat Application Tourniquet (CAT) to render self aid and buddy care. The authors of this project compared the effectiveness of the CAT with the pneumatic Emergency and Military Tourniquet (EMT) to halt life-threatening bleeding. They report that the EMT was markedly more effective (75% vs 16.6%) than the CAT to occlude the popliteal pulse when applied to the mid thigh. The difference is statistically significant, but there is more to the issue. Charged with providing all combatants with a self-administered tourniquet, the United States military chose the CAT, a cost-effective, mass produced, readily available, and virtually indestructible device that easily fits into a pocket or individual first aid kit. The costs and durability of the EMT may limit the use in the field, regardless of the statistically significant results. The pneumatic properties of the EMT raise concerns in the aeromedical transportation arena.

E. C. Bruno, MD

Head and Neck Injury

Cheerio, Laddie! Bidding Farewell to the Glasgow Coma Scale
Green SM (Loma Linda Univ Med Ctr and Children's Hosp, CA)
Ann Emerg Med 58:427-430, 2011

Background.—The Glasgow Coma Scale (GCS) was devised originally not for acute care but as a way to perform repeated bedside assessments and detect changes in states of consciousness and/or duration of coma. It was never designed to have numeric scores assigned to its elements or for the elements to be merged into a single value. However, the GCS is widely seen as the universal criterion for mental status assessment. It is a fundamental part of emergency medicine, out-of-hospital care, trauma surgery, and neurosurgery and a core component of trauma and life support courses used routinely for assessing patients with trauma or altered mental status. Its limitations, however, make it an unacceptable choice for acute care medicine.

Problems.—The GCS offers the advantages of face validity, wide acceptance, and established statistical associations with adverse neurologic outcomes, such as brain injury, neurosurgical intervention, and mortality. However, its drawbacks include a lack of reliability because it contains several subjective elements and repeatedly shows low interrater reliability. Reliability is also compromised in tracheally intubated patients who cannot respond verbally. In addition, clinicians do not consistently remember the GCS components and procedure, so its correct application is also at risk.

Predictions based on the GCS are only grossly accurate. The GCS is used in acute care settings to predict clinically important outcomes, but its prognostic value is weak, not allowing accurate outcome predictions for individual patients. Its sensitivity and specificity combinations are comparable to those of weather forecasters to predict rain.

The summation of the three scales is inherently unsound and was never the intended use. The likelihood that each gradation of each subscale has a similar magnitude of clinical importance is intuitively unlikely and has been refuted statistically. The summary score actually offers less prognostic information than its components.

Alternatives.—The GCS predicts mortality well at the extremes and poorly in its midrange. Some elements are highly predictive and some are just redundant or unneeded. Essentially equivalent test performance is shown for the individual subscales compared to the total in out-of-hospital or ED settings and in adults and children. The best performance of the three subscales has been posted by the 6-point motor component.

Even simpler scales have been proposed, including the AVPU and the ACDU 4-point scores. Three of the 6 points of the GCS motor score may define its total performance, and these have been collapsed into the Simplified Motor Scale or Test Responsiveness: Obeys, Localizes, or Less (TROLL). The Simplified Motor Scale/TROLL provides the same information as the GCS, is statistically derived, is simple, has been externally validated, and shows better interrater reliability.

Conclusions.—Clinicians continue to use the GCS despite compelling evidence that it is not reliable, is too complex, and offers little prognostic relevance over most of its range. Simple clinical judgment is likely to be as accurate. If a scale is needed, one that is easier to learn, use, and retain than the GCS should be selected, such as the Simplified Motor Scale/TROLL instrument (Fig 1).

▶ This is a really fabulous article, discussing many of the limitations to the Glasgow Coma Scale (GCS). In 1978, the original creators of the GCS, Teasdale and Jennett, said, "We have never recommended using the GCS alone, either as a means of monitoring coma, or to assess the severity of brain damage or predict outcome." Nevertheless, for decades afterward, clinicians worldwide have persisted in using the GCS for all of these things.

The GCS is not reliable because of its multiple subjective elements and has repeatedly demonstrated surprisingly low interrater reliability. In a 2004 study of independent attending emergency physician's GCS assessments, GCS scores were the same in only 38% and were 2 or more points apart in 33%. The GCS is not consistently remembered. A 1999 study found that only 48% of all clinicians and 56% of neurosurgeons correctly scored the GCS on a written clinical scenario. The GCS is only grossly predictive, and summing of the 3 scales is inherently unsound. The 13 possible GCS values (3–15) can include 120 combinations of its components. A GCS score of 4 predicts a mortality rate of 48% if calculated 1 + 1 + 2 for eye, verbal, and motor, a mortality of 27% if calculated 1 + 2 + 1, but a mortality rate of only 19% if calculated 2 + 1 + 1.

Glasgow Coma Score

Eye Opening
4-Spontaneous
3-To speech
2-To pain
1-None

Verbal Response
5-Oriented
4-Confused conversation
3-Inappropriate words
2-Incomprehensible sounds
1-None

Motor Response
6-Obeys commands
5-Localizes pain
4-Normal flexion (withdrawal)
3-Abnormal flexion (decorticate)
2-Extension (decerebrate)
1-None

Simplified Motor Scale*
Obeys commands
Localizes pain
Withdrawal to pain or less response

*Alternative name: TROLL
(Test Responsiveness: Obeys, Localizes,
or Less)

AVPU
A-Alert
V-Responds to verbal stimuli
P-Responds to painful stimuli
U-Unresponsive to all stimuli

ACDU
A-Alert
C-Confused
D-Drowsy
U-Unresponsive

FIGURE 1.—The GCS and selected simpler neurologic assessment scales. (Reprinted from Annals of Emergency Medicine, Green SM. Cheerio, laddie! bidding farewell to the glasgow coma scale. *Ann Emerg Med.* 2011;58:427-430. Copyright 2011, with permission the American College of Emergency Physicians.)

GCS predicts mortality well at its extremes (13–15 have good outcomes and 3–5 have poor outcomes) but poorly in its midrange. There are other much simpler scales physicians have tried that are easier to remember, are just as prognostic, and have been externally validated (see Fig 1). The author of this editorial makes a great case to completely abandon the GCS for either clinical judgment or more simplified scoring systems.

D. K. Mullin, MD

Computed Tomography Alone May Clear the Cervical Spine in Obtunded Blunt Trauma Patients: A Prospective Evaluation of a Revised Protocol
Como JJ, Leukhardt WH, Anderson JS, et al (MetroHealth Med Ctr, Cleveland, OH)
J Trauma 70:345-351, 2011

Background.—Cervical spine (CS) clearance in obtunded blunt trauma patients (OBTPs) remains controversial. When computed tomography (CT) of the CS is negative for injury, debate continues over the role of magnetic resonance imaging (MRI). Use of MRI in OBTPs is costly, time-consuming, and potentially dangerous. Our study evaluated the safety of a protocol to discontinue the cervical collar in OBTPs based on CT scan alone.

Methods.—A prospective study was performed from October 2006 to September 2008 at a regional Level I trauma center on OBTPs with gross movement of all extremities. After a CT of the CS was read as negative for injury, the CS was cleared and the collar was removed. Patients were then followed prospectively for related complications.

Results.—One hundred ninety-seven patient had their collars removed and CS cleared at a mean of 3.3 days. There were 144 males (73%), and the average age was 47.1 years. Sixty-two percent of patients were reexamined by a physician when no longer obtunded and found to have no CS signs or symptoms. Five patients (2.5%), when no longer obtunded, had persistent pain for which MRI CS was negative for injury. Coroner reports and autopsies were reviewed for missed spinal cord injuries in the 13% who died before reexamination. One of these patients had an autopsy report of an isolated CS ligamentous injury, deemed to be stable by our attending neurosurgeon. We followed up an additional 12% by phone or chart review, with no report of new onset neurologic deficit. The remaining 11% were lost to follow-up, but no patient contacted our hospital to report deterioration in function. One patient (0.5%) developed a minor CS decubitus ulceration.

Conclusion.—Removal of CS precautions in OBTPs with gross movement of all extremities is safe and efficacious if CT CS is negative for injury. Supplemental MRI CS is not needed in this patient population.

▶ The authors of this prospective study wanted to determine whether the routine use of cervical spine (CS) MRI was necessary in the obtunded blunt trauma patient (OBPT) with negative CT of the CS. The researchers took OBPTs with negative CS CTs and gross movement of all 4 extremities and removed the cervical collars, essentially clearing the patients. Following nearly 200 patients, they were unable to identify a significant, unstable CS injury in a patient with gross motor activity and a negative CS CT. The methods used had an inherent bias: using physician opinion of the patient's ability to describe the presence or absence of cervical spine findings to determine inclusion in the study. The article has limited application for the average emergency physician (EP), because the patients are admitted or transferred because of their concurrent head injury. However, extrapolation to patients who are transiently obtunded (ie, the alcohol-intoxicated patient who falls, is assaulted, or is involved in a motor vehicle crash) might have significant use. EPs likely have experienced intoxicated trauma patients who simply need their cervical collars removed so that they can roll onto their sides to "sleep it off." The improved comfort and subsequent behavior modification may decrease the need for sedatives and airway management.

E. C. Bruno, MD

Concussive symptoms in emergency department patients diagnosed with minor head injury

Cunningham J, Brison RJ, Pickett W (Queen's Univ, Kingston, Ontario, Canada)
J Emerg Med 40:262-266, 2011

Background.—Evidence-based protocols exist for Emergency Department (ED) patients diagnosed with minor head injury. These protocols focus on the need for acute intervention or in-hospital management. The frequency and nature of concussive symptoms experienced by patients discharged from the ED are not well understood.

Objectives.—To examine the prevalence and nature of concussive symptoms, up to 1 month post-presentation, among ED patients diagnosed with minor head injury.

Methods.—Eligible and consenting patients presenting to Kingston EDs with minor head injury (n = 94) were recruited for study. The Rivermead Post-Concussion Symptoms Questionnaire was administered at baseline and at 1 month post-injury to assess concussive symptoms. This analysis focused upon acute and ongoing symptoms.

Results.—Proportions of patients reporting concussive symptoms were 68/94 (72%) at baseline and 59/94 (63%) at follow-up. Seventeen percent of patients (18/102) were investigated with computed tomography scanning during their ED encounter. The prevalence of somatic symptoms declined between baseline and follow-up, whereas some cognitive and emotional symptoms persisted.

Conclusion.—The majority of patients who present to the ED with minor head injuries suffer from concussive symptoms that do not resolve quickly. This information should be incorporated into discharge planning for these patients.

▶ Patients routinely present to emergency departments after experiencing closed head injuries (CHI), the majority of which are deemed minor. Practice guidelines and protocols can guide the evaluation (CT or not) and management of the severe conditions. Guidance regarding the disposition and subsequent follow-up for those patients with concussive symptoms can be sporadic. The authors of this project provided a baseline and 30-day follow-up questionnaire as part of an ongoing CHI surveillance program. They discovered that more than half (63%) of the surveyed patients continued to have postconcussive symptoms, as defined by the World Health Organization's criteria, with the most frequent complaint being headache. Two major limitations exist: First, the patients are likely to be biased, because they are aware of the pending follow-up evaluation to assess their symptoms, which might otherwise have gone unnoticed. Second, the study only evaluated 94 patients, which is a small sample size, considering the number of patients with minor CHI that present to emergency departments.

E. C. Bruno, MD

Do Children With Blunt Head Trauma and Normal Cranial Computed Tomography Scan Results Require Hospitalization for Neurologic Observation?

Holmes JF, the TBI Study Group for the Pediatric Emergency Care Applied Research Network (Univ of California, Sacramento; et al)
Ann Emerg Med 58:315-322, 2011

Study Objective.—Children evaluated in the emergency department (ED) with minor blunt head trauma, defined by initial Glasgow Coma Scale (GCS) scores of 14 or 15, are frequently hospitalized despite normal cranial computed tomography (CT) scan results. We seek to identify the frequency of neurologic complications in children with minor blunt head trauma and normal ED CT scan results.

Methods.—We conducted a prospective, multicenter observational cohort study of children younger than 18 years with blunt head trauma (including isolated head or multisystem trauma) at 25 centers between 2004 and 2006. In this substudy, we analyzed individuals with initial GCS scores of 14 or 15 who had normal cranial CT scan results during ED evaluation. An abnormal imaging study result was defined by any intracranial hemorrhage, cerebral edema, pneumocephalus, or any skull fracture. Patients with normal CT scan results who were hospitalized were followed to determine neurologic outcomes; those discharged to home from the ED received telephone/mail follow-up to assess for subsequent neuroimaging, neurologic complications, or neurosurgical intervention.

Results.—Children (13,543) with GCS scores of 14 or 15 and normal ED CT scan results were enrolled, including 12,584 (93%) with GCS scores of 15 and 959 (7%) with GCS scores of 14. Of 13,543 patients, 2,485 (18%) were hospitalized, including 2,107 of 12,584 (17%) with GCS scores of 15 and 378 of 959 (39%) with GCS scores of 14. Of the 11,058 patients discharged home from the ED, successful telephone/mail follow-up was completed for 8,756 (79%), and medical record, continuous quality improvement, and morgue review was performed for the remaining patients. One hundred ninety-seven (2%) children received subsequent CT or magnetic resonance imaging (MRI); 5 (0.05%) had abnormal CT/MRI scan results and none (0%; 95% confidence interval [CI] 0% to 0.03%) received a neurosurgical intervention. Of the 2,485 hospitalized patients, 137 (6%) received subsequent CT or MRI; 16 (0.6%) had abnormal CT/MRI scan results and none (0%; 95% CI 0% to 0.2%) received a neurosurgical intervention. The negative predictive value for neurosurgical intervention for a child with an initial GCS score of 14 or 15 and a normal CT scan result was 100% (95% CI 99.97% to 100%).

Conclusion.—Children with blunt head trauma and initial ED GCS scores of 14 or 15 and normal cranial CT scan results are at very low risk for subsequent traumatic findings on neuroimaging and extremely low risk of needing neurosurgical intervention. Hospitalization of children with minor head trauma after normal CT scan results for neurologic observation is generally unnecessary.

▶ Disposition of pediatric patients with closed head injuries and ensuing abnormal head CT is generally straightforward. Patients with minor injuries (defined by Glasgow Coma Scores of 14 or 15) and a negative CT are a bit more nebulous of a proposition. The authors of this prospective, multicenter observational cohort study assessed whether admission for observation and potentially further imaging was a worthwhile endeavor. No patient in the discharge group or the observation group received neurosurgical intervention for complications related to the initial injury, making the negative predictive value of a negative CT 100%. The authors recommend outpatient observation for patients with minor head injuries, which seems reasonable.

Approximately 2% of the included patients (admitted and discharged) underwent secondary imaging (CT or MRI), but the clinical parameters that prompted the next test is not disclosed. In each cohort approximately 1% or less had an abnormality on follow-up imaging. This risk reiterates the importance of activity restrictions in patients with minor head injuries. If all patients were discharged to home, the responsibility for the follow-up and ordering of the second test will likely fall to the primary pediatrician. The emergency physician should confirm close follow-up with the primary doctor.

E. C. Bruno, MD

Factors Associated With Cervical Spine Injury in Children After Blunt Trauma
Leonard JC, for the Pediatric Emergency Care Applied Research Network (Washington Univ in St Louis School of Medicine, MO; et al)
Ann Emerg Med 58:145-155, 2011

Study Objective.—Cervical spine injuries in children are rare. However, immobilization and imaging for potential cervical spine injury after trauma are common and are associated with adverse effects. Risk factors for cervical spine injury have been developed to safely limit immobilization and radiography in adults, but not in children. The purpose of our study is to identify risk factors associated with cervical spine injury in children after blunt trauma.

Methods.—We conducted a case-control study of children younger than 16 years, presenting after blunt trauma, and who received cervical spine radiographs at 17 hospitals in the Pediatric Emergency Care Applied Research Network (PECARN) between January 2000 and December 2004. Cases were children with cervical spine injury. We created 3 control groups of children free of cervical spine injury: (1) random controls, (2) age and mechanism of injury-matched controls, and (3) for cases receiving out-of-hospital emergency medical services (EMS), age-matched controls who also received EMS care. We abstracted data from 3 sources: PECARN hospital, referring hospital, and out-of-hospital patient records. We performed multiple logistic regression analyses to identify predictors of cervical spine injury and calculated the model's sensitivity and specificity.

Results.—We reviewed 540 records of children with cervical spine injury and 1,060, 1,012, and 702 random, mechanism of injury, and EMS controls, respectively. In the analysis using random controls, we identified 8 factors associated with cervical spine injury: altered mental status, focal neurologic findings, neck pain, torticollis, substantial torso injury, conditions predisposing to cervical spine injury, diving, and high-risk motor vehicle crash. Having 1 or more factors was 98% (95% confidence interval 96% to 99%) sensitive and 26% (95% confidence interval 23% to 29%) specific for cervical spine injury. We identified similar risk factors in the other analyses.

Conclusion.—We identified an 8-variable model for cervical spine injury in children after blunt trauma that warrants prospective refinement and validation.

▶ Emergency physicians (EPs) hope for common sense tools to facilitate the practice of a very complicated segment of medicine. In the clinical situation of potential cervical spine injury in pediatric patients, deciding which patients require imaging is likely based on a combination of gestalt, experience, and extrapolation and application of the National Emergency X-Radiography Utilization Study criteria. Authors of this case-control study used the Pediatric Emergency Care Applied Research Network to determine which clinical elements predicted a significant cervical spine injury. The authors identified 8 variables (altered mental status, focal neurological deficits, complaint of neck pain, torticollis, substantial injury to the torso, predisposing condition, high-risk motor vehicle crash, and diving/axial loading injury) that were highly predictive of cervical spine injury but ultimately not all encompassing. EPs may use these factors to determine the need for imaging but should maintain suspicion on injury because the use of these variables do not reach 100% sensitivity.

E. C. Bruno, MD

Pain Control and Sedation

A Randomized Controlled Trial of Ketamine/Propofol Versus Propofol Alone for Emergency Department Procedural Sedation
David H, Shipp J (Univ of Missouri—Columbia)
Ann Emerg Med 57:435-441, 2011

Study Objective.—We compare the frequency of respiratory depression during emergency department procedural sedation with ketamine plus propofol versus propofol alone. Secondary outcomes are provider satisfaction, sedation quality, and total propofol dose.

Methods.—In this randomized, double-blind, placebo-controlled trial, healthy children and adults undergoing procedural sedation were pretreated with intravenous fentanyl and then randomized to receive either intravenous ketamine 0.5 mg/kg or placebo. In both groups, this procedure was immediately followed by intravenous propofol 1 mg/kg, with repeated doses of 0.5 mg/kg as needed to achieve and maintain sedation. Respiratory depression was defined according to any of 5 predefined markers. Provider satisfaction was scored on a 5-point scale, sedation quality with the Colorado Behavioral Numerical Pain Scale, and propofol dose according to the total number of milligrams of propofol administered.

Results.—The incidence of respiratory depression was similar between the ketamine/propofol (21/97; 22%) and propofol-alone (27/96; 28%) groups, difference 6% (95% confidence interval −6% to 18%). With ketamine/propofol compared with propofol alone, treating physicians and nurses were more satisfied, less propofol was administered, and there was a trend toward better sedation quality.

Conclusion.—Compared with procedural sedation with propofol alone, the combination of ketamine and propofol did not reduce the incidence of respiratory depression but resulted in greater provider satisfaction, less propofol administration, and perhaps better sedation quality.

▶ Emergency physicians charged with providing procedural sedation covet a medication (or combination of medications) that is safe, effective, and fleeting. Propofol continues to gain a foothold in the emergency department but can cause respiratory depression and hemodynamic instability. Recent literature has suggested that the addition of ketamine may attenuate the negative effects of propofol. In this randomized, double-blind, placebo-controlled trial that assessed respiratory depression in patients receiving propofol verses the combination of propofol and ketamine, the authors were primarily unable to distinguish a difference in respiratory depression in either group. Assessing secondary measures, the authors did find trends toward longer sedation and identified staff (physician and nursing) preference toward the medication cocktail. One potential systematic failure of the study relates to the premedication. As propofol does not provide analgesia, there should be a rigid protocol to regulate narcotic administration. Patients should have adequate pain control prior to the initiation of procedural sedation with propofol.

E. C. Bruno, MD

Analgesic Efficacy and Safety of the Diclofenac Epolamine Topical Patch 1.3% (DETP) in Minor Soft Tissue Injury

Kuehl K, Carr W, Yanchick J, et al (Oregon Health & Science Univ, Portland; Leslie Surgery, UK; Alpharma Pharmaceuticals, Bridgewater, NJ; et al)
Int J Sports Med 32:635-643, 2011

The diclofenac epolamine topical patch 1.3% was designed to deliver analgesic concentrations of diclofenac to an underlying soft tissue injury site, while limiting systemic exposure to diclofenac. This randomized, double-blind, placebo-controlled study evaluated the safety and efficacy of the diclofenac epolamine topical patch for the treatment of acute pain due to minor soft tissue injury. Patients (18—65 years, inclusive) with clinically significant minor soft tissue injuries (mild or moderate sprain, strain, or contusion) incurred within 7 days of study entry and having pain scores ≥ 5 on a Visual Analog Scale of 0—10 were enrolled. Patients were randomized to receive the diclofenac epolamine topical patch (n = 207) or placebo patch (n = 211) application twice daily for 14 days or until pain resolution. Patients recorded pain scores every 12 h at the time of patch removal using the Visual Analog Scale. Investigator-assessed global response to therapy was also evaluated. Safety data were collected throughout the study. Twice-daily treatment with diclofenac epolamine topical patch produced a statistically significant reduction in mean pain score relative to baseline by an additional 18.2% in the diclofenac epolamine topical patch group (0.435 ± 0.268) compared with the placebo group (0.532 ± 0.293) (p = 0.002; overall) beginning after application of the second patch. Consistent with this treatment effect, median time to pain resolution was shortened by 2 days in the diclofenac epolamine topical patch group relative to the placebo group (p = 0.007). These results were reinforced independently by investigators who reported treatment as good or excellent for 58% of diclofenac epolamine topical patch-treated patients compared with 49% in the placebo patch group (p = 0.008). The most common adverse events were treatment site related (n = 16, 7.9% diclofenac epolamine topical patch; n = 12, 5.8% placebo patch). Most (80%) patients reported tolerability as excellent or good. In conclusion, the diclofenac epolamine topical patch provides effective, rapid pain relief for the treatment of acute pain from minor soft tissue injury and appears generally safe and well tolerated.

▶ If nonsteroidal anti-inflammatory drugs (NSAIDs) are risky because of increased gastrointestinal bleeding or increased risk of cardiac injury, what choices do we have to provide adequate pain relief to our patients? Can we optimize drug delivery to tissues that need treatment without systemic exposure? Topical medications are one way to accomplish a more localized dosage, but a main complication is to get medications across the skin barrier.

In this study, the authors compared the efficacy and safety of diclofenac in topical patch form with a placebo topical patch for a cluster of common soft-tissue injuries (strains, sprains and contusions). A double-blind design was used with the placebo patch identical to the treatment patch but without diclofenac. The main efficacy variable was proportion decline in visual analog pain score. Although a useful score for assessing pain and comparing pre- and post-treatment, it has some limitations. The patches could not be applied to injuries with open wounds to minimize any systemic distribution.

Consider that treatment with a NSAID may be otherwise appropriate but that the risk of gastrointestinal bleeding or increased cardiac injury is not negligible. Effective topical medications may be a valuable solution.

N. B. Handly, MD, MSc, MS

Thoraco-Abdominal Injury

Appropriate Use of Emergency Department Thoracotomy: Implications for the Thoracic Surgeon

Mollberg NM, Glenn C, John J, et al (Mount Sinai Hosp and the Univ of Illinois at Chicago)

Ann Thorac Surg 92:455-461, 2011

Background.—Practice guidelines for the appropriate use of emergency department thoracotomy (EDT) according to current national resuscitative guidelines have been developed by the American College of Surgeons Committee on Trauma (ACS-COT) and published. At an urban level I trauma center we analyzed how closely these guidelines were followed and their ability to predict mortality.

Methods.—Between January 2003 and July 2010, 120 patients with penetrating thoracic trauma underwent EDT at Mount Sinai Hospital (MSH). Patients were separated based on adherence (group 1, n = 70) and nonadherence (group 2, n = 50) to current resuscitative guidelines, and group survival rates were determined. These 2 groups were analyzed based on outcome to determine the effect of a strict policy of adherence on survival.

Results.—Of EDTs performed during the study period, 41.7% (50/120) were considered outside current guidelines. Patients in group 2 were less likely to have traditional predictors of survival. There were 6 survivors in group 1 (8.7%), all of whom were neurologically intact; there were no neurologically intact survivors in group 2 ($p = 0.04$). The presence of a thoracic surgeon in the operating room (OR) was associated with increased survival ($p = 0.039$).

Conclusions.—A policy of strict adherence to EDT guidelines based on current national guidelines would have accounted for all potential survivors while avoiding the harmful exposure of health care personnel to blood-borne pathogens and the futile use of resources for trauma victims unable to benefit from them. Cardiothoracic surgeons should be familiar with current EDT guidelines because they are often asked to contribute their operative skills for those patients who survive to reach the OR.

▶ What are our brothers in the trauma surgical specialties thinking about emergency department thoracotomies (EDTs)? I thought the criteria for use were pretty well settled; however, the authors were able to review the results of 120 EDTs, of which about 40% were performed out of protocol.

The difference for those out of protocol was that the time without vitals was greater than 15 minutes. The fact that the EDT was performed outside of protocol may result from a number of causes: inconsistent protocols (some of the patients treated in the early part of the study may have been treated under different established policies); perhaps information from prehospital crews was unclear or not trusted by hospital staff; or perhaps the hospital staff felt the patient deserved "one more chance" for life. One could ask, "Is 16 minutes without vitals so much worse than 15 minutes without?" Every minute of delay is worse, but by how much?

One way to think about the decision to open a chest is as a cost-benefit analysis. How many medical resources are committed once the decision to perform EDT is made? What are the hazards to medical staff when performing EDT? Certainly an EDT is performed under less control and structure than one in an operating room (OR), so the chance of injury to staff is greater.

As a substudy, the authors reviewed cases in which a thoracic surgeon was present in the OR for survival to hospital discharge and for full neurological function at discharge. It appears that outcomes are better when a thoracic surgeon is present, but this conclusion is only an association at this time. The authors note that the thoracic surgeon was the only attending surgeon in a number of cases, so it is unclear whether it was the skill of the thoracic surgeon that made the difference. Operative reports do not show that the thoracic surgeon did anything distinctly different from the trauma surgeon.

I do not think that maintaining access to thoracic surgeons for the rare number of cases of post-EDT after penetrating injuries to the chest is practical in many cases. Down time has to be short, so the hospital must be close to injury occurrence. The duration from 911 call to declaration of the scene as safe may chew up available resuscitative opportunity before any care can be rendered. However, it might be difficult to determine signs of life at the scene unless reliable witnesses or prehospital providers are available to assess this.

N. B. Handly, MD, MSc, MS

Risk factors that predict mortality in patients with blunt chest wall trauma: A systematic review and meta-analysis
Battle CE, Hutchings H, Evans PA (Univ of Wales Swansea, Morriston, UK)
Injury 43:8-17, 2012

Background.—The risk factors for mortality following blunt chest wall trauma have neither been well established or summarised.

Objective.—To summarise the risk factors for mortality in blunt chest wall trauma patients based on available evidence in the literature.

Data Sources.—A systematic review of English and non-English articles using MEDLINE, EMBASE and the Cochrane Library from their introduction until May 2010. Additional studies were identified by hand-searching bibliographies and contacting relevant clinical experts. Grey literature was sought by searching abstracts from all Emergency Medicine conferences. Broad search terms and inclusion criteria were used to reduce the number of missed studies.

Study Selection.—A two step study selection process was used. All published and unpublished observational studies were included if they investigated estimates of association between a risk factor and mortality for blunt chest wall trauma patients.

Data Extraction.—A two step data extraction process using pre-defined data fields, including study quality indicators.

Study Appraisal and Synthesis.—Each study was appraised using a previously designed quality assessment tool and the STROBE checklist. Where sufficient data were available, odds ratios with 95% confidence intervals were calculated using Mantel–Haenszel method for the risk factors investigated. The I^2 statistic was calculated for combined studies in order to assess heterogeneity.

Results.—Age, number of rib fractures, presence of pre-existing disease and pneumonia were found to be related to mortality in 29 identified studies. Combined odds ratio of 1.98 (1.86–2.11, 95% CI), 2.02 (1.89–2.15, 95% CI), 2.43 (1.03–5.72, 95% CI) and 5.24 (3.51–7.82) for mortality were calculated for blunt chest wall trauma patients aged 65 years or more, with three or more rib fractures, pre-existing conditions and pneumonia respectively.

Conclusions.—The risk factors for mortality in patients sustaining blunt chest wall trauma were a patient age of 65 years or more, three or more rib fractures and the presence of pre-existing disease especially cardiopulmonary disease. The development of pneumonia post injury was also a significant risk factor for mortality. As a result of the variable quality in the studies, the results of the selected studies should be interpreted with caution.

▶ Citing a paucity of standard guidelines for the management of blunt thoracic trauma, the authors performed a meta-analysis of the pertinent literature to identify which clinical parameters prognosticated negative outcomes. Patients requiring emergent/urgent surgical intervention or mechanical ventilation were excluded. After sorting through over 4000 references, the authors whittled down to 29 suitable articles and were able to identify 3 separate risk factors that predict mortality in blunt chest trauma—age greater than 65, 3 or more rib fractures, and the presence of a pre-existing condition. While the cutoff of 65 years old was used, this age is not a rigid indicator, as included studies used younger benchmarks. The treating clinician should be aware that advancing age forecasts a worse outcome. The criterion of 3 fractures demonstrated a statistically significant increase in mortality, although some discrepancy was present. The authors referenced 4 studies in which the number of fractures was inconsequential. The presence of a pre-existing condition also predicted detrimental events. The included studies specifically identified congestive heart failure, but the authors extrapolated this link to all cardiopulmonary disorders. The authors suggest that patients lacking these findings are suitable for discharge, but the emergency physician must be vigilant for other reasons for admission or transfer, including anticoagulation, pain medication requirements, or concomitant injuries.

E. C. Bruno, MD

The ribs or not the ribs: which influences mortality?

Jones KM, Reed RL II, Luchette FA (Loyola Univ Med Ctr, Maywood, IL; Clarian Methodist Hosp and Indiana Univ, Indianapolis)
Am J Surg 202:598-604, 2011

Background.—The relative impact of rib fractures on mortality risk is unclear. This study examined the respective relationships between mortality and the number of fractured ribs, patient age, and severity of intrathoracic and extrathoracic injuries.

Methods.—The National Trauma Data Bank was queried, abstracting mortality, age, number of ribs fractured, associated intrathoracic and extrathoracic injury, and Abbreviated Injury Score codes.

Results.—Multivariate logistic regression indicated the strongest influence on mortality was severity of intrathoracic injury, followed by severity of extrathoracic injury, age 65 years or older, more than 5 ribs fractured, and age 46 to 65 years. The mortality rate for isolated rib fractures ranged from 1.8% to 3.2%.

Conclusions.—Mortality related to rib fractures is affected independently by severe intrathoracic injury, presence of extrathoracic injury, advanced age, and more than 5 fractured ribs. Patients with these conditions may benefit from a higher level of care (Figs 2 and 4, Table 1).

▶ Traumatic thoracic injury ranks second only to head injury as the leading cause of trauma-related death. Mortality rates related to rib fractures prior to this study are reported to range from 2% to 20%. This study, which was a retrospective analysis of data from the National Trauma Data Bank version 4.0 of more than 1 million patients, of which approximately 100 000 had 1 or more rib fracture, demonstrated several important facts. First, patients with isolated rib fractures—those without any other associated injuries—had a low mortality rate of 2% to 3% that did not depend on how many rib fractures there were. As

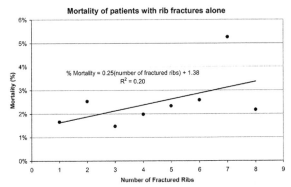

FIGURE 2.—Mortality rates for patients with rib fractures and no other injuries as a function of the number of fractured ribs. The relationship is statistically insignificant ($P = .31$). (Reprinted from The American Journal of Surgery, Jones KM, Reed RL II, Luchette FA. The ribs or not the ribs: which influences mortality? *Am J Surg.* 2011;202:598-604. Copyright © 2011, with permission from Elsevier.)

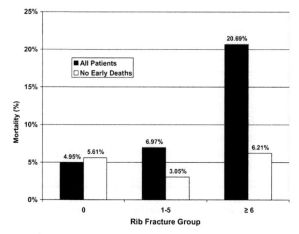

FIGURE 4.—Mortality rates by rib fracture groupings, comparing all injured patients (including deaths within 24 hours) with all injured patients with early deaths within the first 24 hours of emergency department presentation excluded. (Reprinted from The American Journal of Surgery, Jones KM, Reed RL II, Luchette FA. The ribs or not the ribs: which influences mortality? *Am J Surg.* 2011;202:598-604. Copyright © 2011, with permission from Elsevier.)

TABLE 1.—Total Cases and Mortality Rates of National Trauma Data Bank (Version 4.0) Cases with rib Fractures Classified by ICD-9 codes

Ribs Fractured, n	Cases, n (%)	Mortality Rate, %
1	26,882 (27.20)	6.18
2	15,194 (15.37)	6.34
3	10,399 (10.52)	6.70
4	6,874 (6.95)	8.23
5	4,096 (4.14)	9.24
6	2,694 (2.73)	10.89
7	1,667 (1.69)	13.57
8	3,139 (3.18)	30.51
Unspecified	27,891 (28.22)	14.05
Totals	98,836 (100.00)	9.78

you can see from Fig 2, patients with 1 to 8 rib fractures and no other injuries had no change in mortality rate. That said, the overall mortality rate did increase with each successive increase in the number of fractured ribs (see Table 1), so they are important when there are associated intrathoracic or extrathoracic injuries. Of particular importance is that the mortality rate drastically increases when there are more than 5 rib fractures (see Fig 4). Given the relatively high mortality rates of patients with rib fractures with other injuries, emergency physicians at nontrauma centers should strongly consider transferring these patients to their nearest trauma center, especially if there are 6 or more ribs fractured. If there is no other associated injury, patients with isolated rib fractures, regardless of number, could possibly be discharged or admitted for pain control.

D. K. Mullin, MD

Clinical Policy: Critical Issues in the Evaluation of Adult Patients Presenting to the Emergency Department With Acute Blunt Abdominal Trauma
ACEP Clinical Policies Committee; Clinical Policies Subcommittee on Acute Blunt Abdominal Trauma
Ann Emerg Med 43:278-290, 2004

Background.—The American College of Emergency Physicians (ACEP) developed a clinical policy regarding adult patients coming for emergency management of acute blunt abdominal trauma. Such trauma is a leading cause of morbidity, mortality, and intra-abdominal injuries in adults. However, the clinical assessment of such patients is controversial. Evidence-based recommendations were developed regarding the accuracies of computed tomography (CT), diagnostic peritoneal lavage, and focused abdominal sonography for trauma (FAST).

Methods.—The guidelines were developed for physicians working in hospital-based emergency departments and only applied to nonpregnant adults with blunt force injuries to the abdomen. A MEDLINE search included articles published in English between January 1966 and June 2002. All were separated into three classes based on study design, then graded on six dimensions: blinded versus nonblinded outcome assessment, blinded or randomized allocation, direct or indirect outcome measures, biases, external validity, and sufficient sample. The final grade was assigned using a predetermined formula. Three levels of recommendations were offered: A, generally accepted principles with a high degree of clinical certainty; B, moderate clinical certainty; and C, based on preliminary, inconclusive, or conflicting evidence, or panel consensus.

Evaluation.—The overall accuracy of abdominal CT is difficult to study because of constant changes in technology and in the criteria for doing surgery. CT can accurately assess the liver and spleen and identify hemoperitoneum but does not exclude bowel, pancreas, or diaphragm injuries (level B). CT interpretation relies heavily on the reader's experience.

Using oral contrast medium before CT scans allows one to identify extravasation of bowel contents, delineate mesentery, and distinguish opacified bowel from hematomas and pancreatic injury. Risks with oral contrast administration include vomiting, aspiration, and delayed diagnosis related to bowel transit time for the contrast medium. Oral contrast medium is not essential for assessing blunt abdominal trauma (level B).

The ultrasonographic technique FAST can visualize the right and left upper quadrants and the pouch of Douglas in the pelvis. Finding intraperitoneal fluid in a patient with blunt abdominal trauma clarifies whether laparotomy and further diagnostic studies are needed. FAST is useful as an initial screening examination (level B).

Diagnostic peritoneal lavage is a sensitive test for intraperitoneal blood and can be performed via open or closed technique with similar sensitivity, specificity, and complication rates. The closed technique is faster. A positive result for hemoperitoneum is obtained with aspiration of 5 to 10 mL of frank blood, red blood cell count of 100,000/mL in the effluent after abdominal lavage with 1 L of isotonic fluid, or white blood cell count over 500/mL in the effluent. Using Gram's stain and biochemical marker analysis on lavage fluid is nonspecific and insensitive for detecting intra-abdominal injury. Diagnostic peritoneal lavage cannot delineate extent of injury, has a complication rate of 1% to 2%, and may lead to nontherapeutic laparatomies (level B).

Conclusions.—Depending on the patient's hemodynamic stability, the best choices for blunt abdominal trauma assessment appear to be CT and FAST.

▶ This clinical policy focuses on issues pertaining to the radiographic evaluation of patients with blunt abdominal trauma. CT and ultrasound (U/S), specifically focused assessment with sonography in trauma (FAST), are the modalities addressed. The policy states that FAST is an acceptable modality when evaluating the hemodynamically unstable blunt abdominal trauma patient. A FAST examination will identify the presence or absence of intra-abdominal free fluid but may not satisfy the question of what type of free fluid is present (blood, ascites, etc). The FAST examination is brief, noninvasive, and safe and therefore should be an integral part of the initial trauma evaluation. Clinical decisions based on the U/S results should be a collaborative approach between the emergency physician and the trauma surgeon.

Additional imaging may be necessary to address the risks associated with blunt trauma, and CT is generally accepted as the more definitive modality. Although use of intravenous contrast is generally accepted as necessary to properly assess the intra-abdominal contents, oral contrast remains controversial. Emergency physicians are quite familiar with radiologists' reports that include the "lack of oral contrast limits the quality of images" disclaimer. This clinical policy states that with level B recommendations, oral contrast is unnecessary, even in the evaluation of suspected bowel injury.

The policy advises caution when discharging hemodynamically stable patients with blunt abdominal trauma and a negative CT. Based on limited trials addressing this specific question, level B recommendations state that stable patients with isolated injuries may be discharged. With advancing technology of the 64-slice CT scanners, more subtle injuries are likely to be discovered.

E. C. Bruno, MD

Miscellaneous

An assessment of the impact of pregnancy on trauma mortality
John PR, Shiozawa A, Haut ER, et al (The Johns Hopkins Hosp, Baltimore, MD) *ĆSurgery* 149:94-98, 2011

Background.—In the United States, trauma is the leading cause of maternal mortality and an important source of maternal morbidity. Few studies have compared outcomes in injured pregnant women to their nonpregnant counterparts. Some clinical literature regarding hormonal influences on outcomes after trauma suggests a survival advantage in premenopausal women with higher estrogen levels. Given this, as well as possible outcome differences as a result of physiologic changes that occur during pregnancy, we tested the hypothesis that pregnant women have different outcomes after trauma compared with similarly injured nonpregnant women in the same age groups.

Methods.—We used data derived from 1.46 million patients listed in The National Trauma Data Bank from 2001 to 2005, to query all injured patients between ages 12 and 49 years inclusive, and divided them into 2 comparison groups: nonpregnant and pregnant women. We compared differences in outcome after trauma between pregnant and nonpregnant women. Because the number of pregnant women was small in comparison to the number of nonpregnant women, multivariate analysis after 1:3 (pregnant:nonpregnant) matching was attempted.

Results.—Crude mortality rate comparisons and unadjusted logistic regression analyses both before and after matching data reveal lower mortality rates in pregnant women. Multivariate logistic regression analyses both before and after matching data also reveal lower mortality rates in pregnant women; but this is statistically significant ($P = .01$) only after matching data.

Conclusion.—Among women of similar age groups who are equivalently injured, those who are pregnant exhibit lower mortality. These findings suggest that hormonal and physiologic differences during the gestation period may play a role in outcomes following trauma in pregnant women (Tables 2 and 4).

▶ Emergency physicians are well aware that injury is the leading cause of mortality during the first 3 decades of life in both males and females. Additionally, in the United States, trauma is the leading cause of maternal mortality during pregnancy. Based on experimental animal models, some studies have shown that both increased levels of estrogen and progesterone confer a survival advantage in trauma and hemorrhagic shock. Because of these findings, the authors of this study wanted to determine if in fact this benefit may be passed onto pregnant women (who have elevated levels of endogenous estrogen and progesterone). This is the largest study of its kind, drawing data from the National Trauma Data Bank (1.46 million patients from 2001 to 2005), including 3763 pregnant women.

TABLE 2.—Unadjusted Mortality, Nonpregnant Women Versus Pregnant Women (Before and After Matching)

	Nonpregnant (%)	Pregnant (%)	Total (%)	P Value
Before matching				
Alive	208,700 (97.3)	3,719 (98.8)	212,419 (97.4)	<.001
Dead	5,694 (2.7)	44 (1.2)	5,738 (2.6)	
Total	214,394 (100)	3,763 (100)	218,157 (100)	
After matching				
Alive	10,989 (98.1)	3,694 (98.9)	14,683 (98.3)	.001
Dead	219 (2.0)	42 (1.1)	261 (1.8)	
Total	11,208 (100)	3,736 (100)	14,944 (100)	

TABLE 4.—Odds of Death for Pregnant Women Compared with Nonpregnant Women (After Matching)

	OR	CI	P Value
All patients			
Unadjusted logistic regression	0.57	0.41−0.80	.001
Multivariate logistic regression*	0.59	0.39−0.89	.01
Patient subgroups			
Severe injury (ISS ≥15)	0.89	0.56−1.43	.65
Severe head injury	0.65	0.24−1.75	.40
Severe abdominal injury	1.94	0.66−5.66	.23
Low blood pressure (systolic <90)	1.04	0.54−1.98	.91
Younger patients (age <25)	0.42	0.21−0.82	.01
Blunt injury	0.56	0.37−0.86	.008

*Variables: pregnant, insurance category, shock, comorbidity, mechanism and type of injury, year of admission.

See Tables 2 and 4, which demonstrate that before and after matched analysis, pregnant women had a statistically significant survival advantage after a traumatic injury. There was, however, a trend toward increased likelihood of death in pregnant patients with severe abdominal injury. We can only speculate about the reasons for the apparent survival pregnant patients have over matched nonpregnant women after trauma. During pregnancy, there is an increase in plasma volume and red blood cell mass, and cardiac output increases by 50% during the first trimester. These factors may confer better organ perfusion, improved maternal tolerance to hemorrhage, and increased resistance to the shock state in pregnant women. Perhaps there is something innately protective of higher levels of estrogen and progesterone that we don't currently know about.

Certainly this study creates more questions than it does answers, but hopefully, it will stimulate further large prospective studies to see if there really is a survival benefit with pregnancy. If one exists, researchers then need to determine what part of pregnancy is protective. I do know that researchers in multiple centers across the United States are investigating the effects of progesterone and estrogen in patients with traumatic brain injury to see if there is an effect on improving mortality and morbidity.

D. K. Mullin, MD

Damage Control Resuscitation Is Associated With a Reduction in Resuscitation Volumes and Improvement in Survival in 390 Damage Control Laparotomy Patients
Cotton BA, Reddy N, Hatch QM, et al (The Univ of Texas Health Science Ctr, Houston)
Ann Surg 254:598-605, 2011

Objective.—To determine whether implementation of damage control resuscitation (DCR) in patients undergoing damage control laparotomy (DCL) translates into improved survival.

Background.—DCR aims at preventing coagulopathy through permissive hypotension, limiting crystalloids and delivering higher ratios of plasma and platelets. Previous work has focused only on the impact of delivering higher ratios (1:1:1).

Methods.—A retrospective cohort study was performed on all DCL patients admitted between January 2004 and August 2010. Patients were divided into pre-DCR implementation and DCR groups and were excluded if they died before completion of the initial laparotomy. The *lethal triad* was defined as immediate postoperative temperature less than 95°F, international normalized ratio more than 1.5, or a pH less than 7.30.

Results.—A total of 390 patients underwent DCL. Of these, 282 were pre-DCR and 108 were DCR. Groups were similar in demographics, injury severity, admission vitals, and laboratory values. DCR patients received less crystalloids (median: 14 L vs 5 L), red blood cells (13 U vs 7 U), plasma (11 U vs 8 U), and platelets (6 U vs 0 U) in 24 hours, all $P < 0.05$. DCR patients had less evidence of the lethal triad upon intensive care unit arrival (80% vs 46%, $P < 0.001$). 24-hour and 30-day survival was higher with DCR (88% vs 97%, $P = 0.006$ and 76% vs 86%, $P = 0.03$). Multivariate analysis controlling for age, injury severity, and emergency department variables, demonstrated DCR was associated with a significant increase in 30-day survival (OR: 2.5, 95% CI: 1.10–5.58, $P = 0.028$).

Conclusion.—In patients undergoing DCL, implementation of DCR reduces crystalloid and blood product administration. More importantly, DCR is associated with an improvement in 30-day survival.

▶ Damage control laparotomy is an abbreviated surgical procedure aimed at the rapid control of abdominal hemorrhage and contamination; it is focused on restoring normal physiology at the expense of normal anatomy. Patients often undergo temporary closure of the abdominal wall and are then placed in the intensive care unit for further resuscitation, including correction of coagulopathy, hypothermia, and acidosis. Beginning in 2003, damage control resuscitation (DCR) was developed by military clinicians in Iraq; it strives to prevent or reverse coagulopathy through permissive hypotension, limitation of crystalloids, and delivery of higher ratios of plasma and platelets. DCR is gaining popularity in civilian trauma centers, because patients resuscitated with this approach are less edematous and less coagulopathic after surgery.

This before-and-after study from the University of Texas in Houston demonstrates that when the techniques of DCR are applied to civilian trauma victims, physiologic variables (such as temperature, pH, and international normalized ratio) are improved and survival is increased. Obviously, this process is not something that can be instituted solely by emergency physicians without the agreement of the trauma service; however, all emergency physicians should be aware of these changing methods of resuscitation and be ready to implement them. It might even be advantageous to initiate this conversation with your trauma team.

E. A. Ramoska, MD, MPHE

Definition of mortality for trauma center performance evaluation: A comparative study

Moore L, Turgeon AF, Émond M, et al (Université Laval, Québec, Canada)
Crit Care Med 39:2246-2252, 2011

Objective.—Mortality is widely used as a performance indicator to evaluate the quality of trauma care, but there is no consensus on the most appropriate definition. Our objective was to evaluate the influence of the definition of mortality in terms of the place (in-hospital or postdischarge) and time (30 days and 3, 6, and 12 months) of death on the results of trauma center performance evaluations according to the patients' ages.

Design.—Multicenter retrospective cohort study.

Setting.—Inclusive Canadian provincial trauma system.

Patients.—Adults admitted between 1999 and 2006 with a maximum abbreviated injury severity score ≥3 (n = 47,261).

Interventions.—None.

Measurements and Main Results.—Trauma registry data were linked to vital statistics data to obtain mortality up to 12 months postadmission. Observed mortality was compared to that expected according to provincial population mortality rates. Trauma center performance was evaluated with risk-adjusted mortality estimates. Agreement between performance results based on different definitions of mortality was evaluated with correlation coefficients; >.9 was considered acceptable. Analyses were stratified by predefined age categories (16–64, 65–84, and ≥85 yrs). A total of 3,338 patients (7%) died in-hospital, and 1,794 patients (4%) died postdischarge. Among patients 16–64 yrs old, 30-day hospital mortality represented 83% of all deaths and correlation coefficients across all definitions of mortality were >.9. In patients 65–84 yrs old, 30-day hospital mortality represented 52% of all deaths, observed mortality reached expected rates at around 6 months, and agreement across mortality definitions was low.

Conclusions.—We observed an important variation in performance evaluation results across definitions of mortality, specifically in patients aged ≥65 yrs. Half of the deaths among elders occurred later than 30 days following admission, including a significant number postdischarge. Results suggest that if performance evaluations include elderly patients, data on postdischarge mortality up to 6 months following admission are required.

▶ Mortality is a commonly used indicator of trauma center performance because it is easy to assess, is subject to minimal measurement error, and is of primary importance to both physicians and patients. This retrospective cohort study analyzed data over an 8-year period from the Quebec Trauma Registry. The authors found that the definition of mortality could affect the performance evaluation of trauma centers. In particular, they discovered that among patients over 65 years of age, postdischarge mortality represented nearly half of all deaths and that observed mortality rates were greater than expected for up to 6 months after discharge. On the other hand, in patients aged 16 to 64 years, the majority of deaths occurred within 30 days of admission, and performance evaluation results varied little across definitions of mortality. Because this study was conducted in Canada, it is unclear whether these results would translate to the different health care systems in other countries. However, the results make intuitive sense, and it is my opinion that their conclusions would translate to other nations' trauma systems. In summary, then, if you are evaluating trauma center performance involving geriatric patients, you should include information on postdischarge mortality up to 6 months after admission.

E. A. Ramoska, MD, MPHE

Emergency Department Crystalloid Resuscitation of 1.5 L or More is Associated With Increased Mortality in Elderly and Nonelderly Trauma Patients

Ley EJ, Clond MA, Srour MK, et al (Cedars-Sinai Med Ctr, Los Angeles, CA)
J Trauma 70:398-400, 2011

Background.—Recent evidence suggests a survival advantage in trauma patients who receive controlled or hypotensive resuscitation volumes. This study examines the threshold crystalloid volume that is an independent risk factor for mortality after trauma.

Methods.—This study analyzed prospectively collected data from a Level I Trauma Center between January 2000 and December 2008. Demographics and outcomes were compared in elderly ($\geq$70 years) and nonelderly (<70 years) trauma patients who received crystalloid fluid in the emergency department (ED) to determine a threshold volume that was an independent predictor for mortality.

Results.—A total of 3,137 patients who received crystalloid resuscitation in the ED were compared. Overall mortality was 5.2%. Mortality among the elderly population was 17.3% (41 deaths), whereas mortality in the nonelderly population was 4% (116 deaths). After multivariate logistic regression analysis, fluid volumes of 1.5 L or more were significantly associated with mortality in both elderly (odds ratio [OR]: 2.89, confidence interval [CI] [1.13−7.41], $p = 0.027$) and nonelderly patients (OR: 2.09, CI [1.31−3.33], $p = 0.002$). Fluid volumes up to 1 L were not associated with significantly increased mortality. At 3 L, mortality was especially pronounced in the elderly (OR: 8.61, CI [1.55−47.75] $p − 0.014$), when compared with the nonelderly (OR $=$ 2.69, CI [1.53−4.73], $p = 0.0006$).

Conclusion.—ED volume replacement of 1.5 L or more was an independent risk factor for mortality. High-volume resuscitations were associated with high-mortality particularly in the elderly trauma patient. Our finding supports the notion that excessive fluid resuscitation should be avoided in the ED and when required, operative intervention or intensive care admission should be considered.

▶ This is a retrospective study from Cedars-Sinai Medical Center in Los Angeles that looked at all trauma patients who required crystalloid fluid resuscitation and admission over a 9-year period. The authors found an association between larger volumes of fluid administration (greater than 1.5 L) and mortality, regardless of whether the patient was elderly (70 years and older). They conclude, "excessive fluid resuscitation should be avoided in the ED."

This study has several limitations. First, it is retrospective. Second, and probably more important, it is not possible to adjust for all the possible confounders in a study like this. Although it is possible that larger volumes of fluid are detrimental to trauma patients, it is also possible the reason certain patients received larger volumes of crystalloids was that they were sicker, and therefore they would have had an increased mortality rate in any case. This study, and others like it, should be considered hypothesis generating. It does not prove that excessive fluid resuscitation should be avoided; it merely reports an association and suggests that further research, with a randomized trial, is needed.

E. A. Ramoska, MD, MPHE

EMS Provider Assessment of Vehicle Damage Compared with Assessment by a Professional Crash Reconstructionist
Lerner EB, Cushman JT, Blatt A, et al (Med College of Wisconsin, Milwaukee; Univ of Rochester, NY; CUBRC, Buffalo, NY; et al)
Prehosp Emerg Care 15:483-489, 2011

Objective.—To determine the accuracy of emergency medical services (EMS) provider assessments of motor vehicle damage when compared with measurements made by a professional crash reconstructionist.

Methods.—EMS providers caring for adult patients injured during a motor vehicle crash and transported to the regional trauma center in a midsized community were interviewed upon emergency department arrival. The interview collected provider estimates of crash mechanism of injury. For crashes that met a preset severity threshold, the vehicle's owner was asked to consent to having a crash reconstructionist assess the vehicle. The assessment included measuring intrusion and external automobile deformity. Vehicle damage was used to calculate change in velocity. Paired t-test, correlation, and kappa were used to compare EMS estimates and investigator-derived values.

Results.—Ninety-one vehicles were enrolled; of these, 58 were inspected and 33 were excluded because the vehicle was not accessible. Six vehicles had multiple patients. Therefore, a total of 68 EMS estimates were compared with the inspection findings. Patients were 46% male, 28% were admitted to hospital, and 1% died. The mean EMS-estimated deformity was 18 inches and the mean measured deformity was 14 inches. The mean EMS-estimated intrusion was 5 inches and the mean measured intrusion was 4 inches. The EMS providers and the reconstructionist had 68% agreement for determination of external automobile deformity (kappa 0.26) and 88% agreement for determination of intrusion (kappa 0.27) when the 1999 American College of Surgeons Field Triage Decision Scheme criteria were applied. The mean (± standard deviation) EMS-estimated speed prior to the crash was 48 ± 13 mph and the mean reconstructionist-estimated change in velocity was 18 ± 12 mph (correlation −0.45). The EMS providers determined that 19 vehicles had rolled over, whereas the investigator identified 18 (kappa 0.96). In 55 cases, EMS and the investigator agreed on seat belt use; for the remaining 13 cases, there was disagreement (five) or the investigator was unable to make a determination (eight) (kappa 0.40).

Conclusions.—This study found that EMS providers are good at estimating rollover. Vehicle intrusion, deformity, and seat belt use appear to be more difficult for EMS to estimate, with only fair agreement with the crash reconstructionist. As expected, the EMS provider—estimated speed prior to the crash does not appear to be a reasonable proxy for change in velocity.

▶ Although the Field Triage Decision Scheme was updated by the American College of Surgeons, in conjunction with the Centers for Disease Control and National Highway Traffic Safety Administration, in 2009, only a few states have fully adopted the revised guidelines, and many others are still using the older 1999 scheme. This study conducted at the University of Rochester Medical Center/Strong Memorial Hospital shows why the mechanism of injury section was changed. The authors demonstrate that although emergency medical service (EMS) providers were almost perfect at providing information about whether the vehicle has rolled over, their ability to detect seatbelt usage was only moderate. Moreover, their estimates of passenger compartment intrusion and external vehicle deformity revealed only slight agreement with a trained crash reconstructionist, and their estimates of speed before a crash was not shown to be a useful proxy for change in velocity. Although, in general, the information provided by EMS personnel is extremely valuable, their ability to estimate damage in motor vehicle collisions does not appear to be very accurate. All EMS and trauma systems should consider using the updated 2009 Field Triage Decision Scheme.

E. A. Ramoska, MD, MPHE

Snow shovel—related injuries and medical emergencies treated in US EDs, 1990 to 2006

Watson DS, Shields BJ, Smith GA (The Res Inst at Nationwide Children's Hosp, Columbus, OH)
Am J Emerg Med 29:11-17, 2011

Background.—Injuries and medical emergencies associated with snow shovel use are common in the United States.

Methods.—This is a retrospective analysis of data from the National Electronic Injury Surveillance System. This study analyzes the epidemiologic features of snow shovel—related injuries and medical emergencies treated in US emergency departments (EDs) from 1990 to 2006.

Results.—An estimated 195 100 individuals (95% confidence interval, 140 400-249 800) were treated in US EDs for snow shovel—related incidents during the 17-year study period, averaging 11 500 individuals annually (SD, 5300). The average annual rate of snow shovel—related injuries and medical emergencies was 4.15 per 100 000 population. Approximately two thirds (67.5%) of these incidents occurred among males. Children younger than 18 years comprised 15.3% of the cases, whereas older adults (55 years and older) accounted for 21.8%. The most common diagnosis was soft tissue injury (54.7%). Injuries to the lower back accounted for 34.3% of the cases. The most common mechanism of injury/nature of medical emergency was acute musculoskeletal exertion (53.9%) followed by slips and falls (20.0%) and being struck by a snow shovel (15.0%). Cardiac-related ED visits accounted for 6.7% of the cases, including all of the 1647 deaths in the study. Patients required hospitalization in 5.8% of the cases. Most snow shovel–related incidents (95.6%) occurred in and around the home.

Conclusions.—This is the first study to comprehensively examine snow shovel–related injuries and medical emergencies in the United States using a nationally representative sample. There are an estimated 11 500 snow shovel–related injuries and medical emergencies treated annually in US EDs.

▶ Emergency physicians charged with staffing emergency departments in areas that receive substantial snowfall are familiar with the classic snow-related presentation of the "more senior" male who clutches his chest and collapses while shoveling the driveway but are also aware that the cardiac event is not the only snow-shoveling–associated complication. The authors of this retrospective database review present the spectrum of snow-shovel-related injuries. Despite our attachment to the cardiac story, this represents only 6.7% of presentations. Acute musculoskeletal events, such as overexertion, sprains, or strains, actually represent most complaints, as represented in Fig 2 in the original article. This article is unlikely to change the treating EPs' practice pattern, but it does provide a framework for discussing preventative measures. The authors also suggest alternatives to shoveling, including salt applications, deicing formulations, and snowblowers, which each have their own inherent hazards, whether environmental or physical.

E. C. Bruno, MD

The Relationship Between Annual Hospital Volume of Trauma Patients and In-Hospital Mortality in New York State
Marx WH, Simon R, O'Neill P, et al (SUNY Upstate Med Univ, Syracuse, NY; New York Univ School of Medicine; Kings County Hosp Ctr, Brooklyn, NY; et al)
J Trauma 71:339-346, 2011

Background.—Several studies in the literature have examined the volume-outcome relationship for trauma, but the findings have been mixed, and the associated impact of the trauma center level has not been examined to date. The purposes of this study are to (1) determine whether there is a significant relationship between the annual volume of trauma inpatients treated in a trauma center (with "patients" defined in multiple ways) and short-term mortality of those patients, and (2) examine the impact on the volume-mortality relationship of being a Level I versus Level II trauma center.

Methods.—Data from New York's Trauma Registry in 2003 to 2006 were used to examine the impact of total trauma patient volume and volume of patients with Injury Severity Score (ISS) of at least 16 on in-hospital mortality rates after adjusting for numerous risk factors that have been demonstrated to be associated with mortality.

Results.—The adjusted odds of in-hospital mortality patients in centers with a mean annual volume of less than 2,000 patients was significantly higher (adjusted odds ratio = 1.46, 95% confidence interval, 1.25—1.71) than the odds for patients in higher volume centers. The adjusted odds of mortality for patients in centers with an American College of Surgeons-recommended annual volume of less than 240 patients with an ISS of at least 16 was 1.41 times as high (95% confidence interval, 1.17—1.69) as the odds for patients in higher volume centers. However, for both volume cohorts analyzed, the variation in risk-adjusted in-hospital mortality rate was greater among centers within each volume subset than between these volume subsets.

Conclusion.—When considering the trauma system as a whole, higher total annual trauma center volume (2,000 or higher) and higher volume of patients with ISS ≥16 (240 and higher) are significant predictors of lower in-hospital mortality. Although the American College of Surgeons-recommended 1,200 total volume is not a significant predictor, hospitals in New York with ISS ≥16 volumes in excess of 240 also have total volumes in excess of 2,000. However, when considering individual trauma centers, high volume centers do not consistently perform better than low volume centers. Thus, despite the association between volume and mortality, we believe that the most accurate way to assess trauma center performance is through the use of an accurate, complete, comprehensive database for computing center-specific risk-adjusted mortality rates, rather than volume per se.

▶ There are quite a few studies in the literature documenting the inverse relationship between the volume of a particular entity treated, or procedure performed, and morbidity and mortality rates. This study, from the State University of New York at Syracuse, seems to affirm those conclusions in regards to trauma care: the more you see, the better you do. However, there are so many potentially confounding variables in any study of this type that it is always difficult to know whether the results are correct or whether they are due to some unaccounted for factor. Furthermore, the authors note that the variation in risk-adjusted in-hospital mortality rates was greater among centers within each volume subset than between the volume subsets. This piece of information adds to the supposition that, although there may be a correlation between volume and quality, it is not a straightforward cause-and-effect relationship. Low-volume trauma centers can and do offer quality trauma care, and certain high-volume trauma centers may have higher mortality rates. This debate will continue.

E. A. Ramoska, MD, MPHE

Treatment outcomes of injured children at adult level 1 trauma centers: are there benefits from added specialized care?
Oyetunji TA, Haider AH, Downing SR, et al (Howard Univ College of Medicine, Washington, DC; Johns Hopkins Univ School of Medicine, Baltimore, MD; et al)
Am J Surg 201:445-449, 2011

Background.—Accidental traumatic injury is the leading cause of morbidity and mortality in children. The authors hypothesized that no mortality difference should exist between children seen at ATC (adult trauma centers) versus ATC with added qualifications in pediatrics (ATC-AQ).

Methods.—The National Trauma Data Bank, version 7.1, was analyzed for patients aged <18 years seen at level 1 trauma centers. Bivariate analysis compared patients by ATC versus ATC-AQ using demographic and injury characteristics. Multivariate analysis adjusting for injury and demographic factors was then performed.

Results.—A total sample of 53,702 children was analyzed, with an overall mortality of 3.9%. The adjusted odds of mortality was 20% lower for children seen at ATC-AQ (odds ratio, .80; 95% confidence interval, .68–.94). Children aged 3 to 12 years, those with injury severity scores >25, and those with Glasgow Coma Scale scores <8 all had significant reductions in the odds of death at ATC-AQ.

Conclusions.—Improved overall survival is associated with pediatric trauma patients treated at ATC-AQ.

▶ Previous studies have demonstrated improved survival for children treated at pediatric trauma centers when compared with adult trauma centers (ATC) with added qualifications in pediatrics and ATCs. This current retrospective analysis of 53 702 injured children found that the mortality rate was 4.5% for children who were treated in ATC versus a mortality rate of 3.2% for children cared for in ATC-AQ. This yields a number needed to treat (NNT) of 77. After controlling for demographic factors, injury severity characteristics, and mechanism of injury, the authors still found a 20% reduction in mortality risk for children treated at ATC-AQ when compared with ATC.

There are some limitations to this study. Because of its retrospective nature, there is the possibility of selection bias in children who were brought to ATC versus ATC-AQ. Furthermore, the National Trauma Data Bank is a voluntary database and thus may not be representative of the average trauma center. Nonetheless, this analysis certainly suggests that pediatric trauma patients have reduced mortality when treated at level 1 adult centers that have added qualifications in pediatrics. This information may be used to justify transporting pediatric trauma victims to ATC-AQ over ATC.

E. A. Ramoska, MD, MPHE

2 Resuscitation

Cardiac Arrest

A randomised control trial to determine if use of the iResus© application on a smart phone improves the performance of an advanced life support provider in a simulated medical emergency
Low D, Clark N, Soar J, et al (Royal United Hosp, Bath, UK; Southmead Hosp, Bristol, UK; et al)
Anaesthesia 66:255-262, 2011

This study sought to determine whether using the Resuscitation Council UK's iResus© application on a smart phone improves the performance of doctors trained in advanced life support in a simulated emergency. Thirty-one doctors (advanced life support-trained within the previous 48 months) were recruited. All received identical training using the smart phone and the iResus application. The participants were randomly assigned to a control group (no smart phone) and a test group (access to iResus on smart phone). Both groups were tested using a validated extended cardiac arrest simulation test (CASTest) scoring system. The primary outcome measure was the overall cardiac arrest simulation test score; these were significantly higher in the smart phone group (median (IQR [range]) 84.5 (75.5−92.5 [64−96])) compared with the control group (72 (62−87 [52−95]); $p = 0.02$). Use of the iResus application significantly improves the performance of an advanced life support-certified doctor during a simulated medical emergency. Further studies are needed to determine if iResus can improve care in the clinical setting.

▶ This open-label, randomized, controlled study from the Royal United Hospital in the United Kingdom found that a cognitive aid in the form of an iPhone application (app) improved junior doctors' scores by 12.5 points, on a scale of 24 to 96, using a validated scoring system during a simulated advanced life support (ALS) scenario. Moreover, the participants felt that the app was easy to use and increased their confidence in making decisions. They did not think, from their own perspective, that using the app would be unprofessional or indicate poor training. They expressed a neutral response about whether the public or other health care professionals would view usage in these negative terms.

Other high-risk industries, such as aviation and nuclear power, find the use of cognitive aids integral to their standard operating procedures. The safety culture of medicine is slowly changing in this regard; however, many physicians still appear to feel that the use of cognitive aids makes them appear forgetful, inadequately trained, or incompetent. Perhaps apps for the iPhone and other similar devices will change that perception.

I downloaded this app for my iPhone and found it a little clunky to navigate and use, especially when I wanted to look up a drug recommendation or dosage. In any case, this study is not a review of that particular app but offers a corroboration that apps such as these can be useful tools during a resuscitation, especially for relatively new practitioners.

E. A. Ramoska, MD, MPHE

Adverse events and their relation to mortality in out-of-hospital cardiac arrest patients treated with therapeutic hypothermia

Nielsen N, the Hypothermia Network (Lund Univ, Sweden; et al)
Crit Care Med 39:57-64, 2011

Objectives.—To investigate the association between adverse events recorded during critical care and mortality in out-of-hospital cardiac arrest patients treated with therapeutic hypothermia.

Design.—Prospective, observational, registry-based study.

Setting.—Twenty-two hospitals in Europe and the United States.

Patients.—Between October 2004 and October 2008, 765 patients were included.

Interventions.—None.

Measurements and Main Results.—Arrhythmias (7%—14%), pneumonia (48%), metabolic and electrolyte disorders (5%—37%), and seizures (24%) were common adverse events in the critical care period in cardiac arrest patients treated with therapeutic hypothermia, whereas sepsis (4%) and bleeding (6%) were less frequent. Sustained hyperglycemia (blood glucose >8 mmol/L for >4 hrs; odds ratio 2.3, 95% confidence interval 1.6–3.6, $p < .001$) and seizures treated with anticonvulsants (odds ratio 4.8, 95% confidence interval 2.9–8.1, $p < .001$) were associated with increased mortality in a multivariate model. An increased frequency of bleeding and sepsis occurred after invasive procedures (coronary angiography, intravascular devices for cooling, intra-aortic balloon pump), but bleeding and sepsis were not associated with increased mortality (odds ratio 1.0, 95% confidence interval 0.46–2.2, $p = .91$, and odds ratio 0.30, 95% confidence interval 0.12–0.79, $p = .01$, respectively).

Conclusions.—Adverse events were common after out-of-hospital cardiac arrest. Sustained hyperglycemia and seizures treated with anticonvulsants were associated with increased mortality. Bleeding and infection were more common after invasive procedures, but these adverse events were not associated with increased mortality in our study.

▶ Therapeutic hypothermia (TH) use in patients with return of spontaneous circulation (ROSC) after out-of-hospital cardiac arrest (OHCA) is becoming the standard of care. TH is used for the potential improvement in neurological outcomes and does not address the other organ systems. The authors of this prospective observational international study accumulated data regarding the adverse events—specifically bleeding, infection, and electrolyte abnormalities—that were present in patients receiving TH. In their results, the authors found that arrhythmias, pneumonia, metabolic and electrolyte disorders, and seizures were common events in the critical care phase of the patients' hospital stays. Intuitively, they also found that the use of intravascular devices (intra-aortic balloon pumps, central lines, dialysis catheters, etc) were associated with increased bleeding and infection. Seizure occurred in nearly 25% of patients and was strongly associated with mortality, as was persistent hyperglycemia.

More than half of the enrolled patients were deceased at the predetermined 6-month follow-up point, but most of the remaining patients had a cerebral performance category (CPC) of 1 (74%) or 2 (18%), intensifying previous evidence of improved neurological function with the use of TH. Could one extrapolate that the expired patients were more likely to endure a CPC of 3 or 4 prior to their death within the 6-month follow-up period?

As emergency physicians, when faced with a patient with ROSC after OHCA, the use of TH remains the standard of care in the capable facility. Complications that arise during TH phase may occur and require intervention, but the use of TH should not be avoided because of fear of these adverse events. The potential benefit in neurological outcome and improved quality of life appears to outweigh the risks.

E. C. Bruno, MD

Comparison of first-attempt success between tibial and humeral intraosseous insertions during out-of-hospital cardiac arrest
Reades R, Studnek JR, Garrett JS, et al (Carolinas Med Ctr, Charlotte, NC; et al)
Prehosp Emerg Care 15:278-281, 2011

Background.—Intraosseous (IO) needle insertion is often utilized in the adult population for critical resuscitation purposes. Standard insertion sites include the proximal humerus and proximal tibia, for which limited comparison data are available.

Objective.—This study compared the frequencies of IO first-attempt success between humeral and tibial sites in out-of-hospital cardiac arrest.

Methods.—This observational study was conducted in an urban setting between August 28, 2009, and October 31, 2009, and included all medical cardiac arrest patients for whom resuscitative efforts were performed. Cardiac arrest protocols stipulate that paramedics insert an IO line for initial vascular access. During the first month of the study, the proximal humerus was the preferred primary insertion site, whereas the tibia was preferred throughout the second month. The primary outcome was first-attempt success, defined as secure IO needle position in the marrow cavity and normal fluid flow. Any needle dislodgment during resuscitation was also recorded. The association between first-attempt IO success and initial IO insertion location was analyzed using a test of independent proportions and 95% confidence intervals (CIs) for the difference in proportions.

Results.—There were 88 cardiac arrest patients receiving IO placement, with 58 (65.9%) patients receiving their initial IO attempt in the tibia. The rate of first-time IO success at the tibia was significantly higher than that observed at the humerus (89.7% vs. 60.0%; $p < 0.01$). There were 18 initial successes at the humerus; for six (33.3%) of these, the needle became dislodged during resuscitation, compared with 52 initial successes at the tibia, with three (5.8%) dislodgments. The rate of total success for initial IO placements was significantly lower for the humerus (40.0%) compared with that for the tibia (84.5%; $p < 0.01$) during resuscitation efforts.

Conclusions.—In this subset of patients, tibial IO needle placement appeared to be a more effective insertion site than the proximal humerus. Success rates were higher with a lower incidence of needle dislodgments. Further randomized studies are required in order to validate these results.

▶ This observational study from Mecklenburg County EMS and Carolinas Medical Center (North Carolina) was conducted over the 2 months right after a patient care protocol update specified that every patient in cardiac arrest receive an intraosseous (IO) line for initial vascular access. The paramedics were supposed to use the humerus as the preferred IO site during the first month and the tibia as the preferred site for the second month. There were 92 cardiac arrest patients, 46 patients, in each month. Four patients had no IO line attempted, and therefore the final analysis includes 88 patients.

The first-time success rate for the tibial site was greater than for the humerus. Moreover, the dislodgement rate for the humeral site was greater compared with the tibia. This led the authors to conclude, "tibial IO needle placement appeared to be a more effective insertion site than the proximal humerus." This deduction should be tempered by the following: Although the authors note that there were 46 cardiac arrest patients during each month, the tibia was used as the initial site for 58 patients (66%) and the humerus for only 30 patients. It seems that the paramedics had a preference for the tibial site that may have biased the results. In addition, the humeral site was the preferred site for the first month of the study, and the tibia the preferred site for the second month. It is possible that the increased familiarity with the concept of IO vascular access and the greater experience in placing and securing them may have led to an improved success rate and reduced dislodgment rate for tibial IO lines during the second month of the study.

The IO line is a resurgent technique that warrants attention. Which site will be considered optimal for emergency medical services or for the emergency department remains an open question.

E. A. Ramoska, MD, MPHE

Emergent precordial percussion revisited – pacing the heart in asystole
Monteleone PP, Alibertis K, Brady WJ (Univ of Virginia Health System, Charlottesville)
Am J Emerg Med 29:563-565, 2011

Precordial percussion is a technique by which a manual force is applied repeatedly to the chest of a patient experiencing an unstable bradycardic or asystolic rhythm. The force is used not to defibrillate the myocardium as is the case with the "precordial thump" in pulseless ventricular tachycardia/ventricular fibrillation but rather to initiate a current through the myocardium in the form of an essentially mechanically paced beat. In this review, we discuss the physiology and utility of precordial percussion, or precordial thump, in the emergency setting as a very temporary bridge to more effective and permanent pacing techniques.

▶ Every now and again, someone reminds us of the past in a way that may help imagine the future. The authors of this brief review bring our attention to precordial percussion (a cousin to the precordial thump). The suggestion of these authors is that there may be a way to deliver just the right amount of pacing activity to the heart when standard pacing or other advance cardiac resuscitation techniques might not be available.

However, for a "possible new technique" to be useful, we need to recognize when it would be appropriate to use and when it might be dangerous. The authors suggest that prior to availability of advanced resuscitation tools, precordial percussion, distinct from precordial thumps because of lower applied force, might be used to pace bradyarrhythmias. How would a practitioner know how much force to apply and how frequently to apply the force? Too much force or percussion at the wrong time might initiate an "R on T phenomenon" and lead to ventricular fibrillation.

Can percussions be delivered in a way to provide a perfusing rhythm without already having a monitor on the patient? In a setting where there is a lot of guessing, this may not be that effective; however, for specific cardiac settings, it might be possible to deliver a chance for perfusion before the high-tech equipment arrives.

N. B. Handly, MD, MSc, MS

Self-directed Versus Traditional Classroom Training for Neonatal Resuscitation
Weiner GM, Menghini K, Zaichkin J, et al (St. Joseph Mercy Hosp, Ann Arbor, MI; Seattle Children's Hosp, WA; et al)
Pediatrics 127:713-719, 2011

Objective.—Neonatal Resuscitation Program instructors spend most of their classroom time giving lectures and demonstrating basic skills. We hypothesized that a self-directed education program could shift acquisition of these skills outside the classroom, shorten the duration of the class, and allow instructors to use their time to facilitate low-fidelity simulation and debriefing.

Methods.—Novice providers were randomly allocated to self-directed education or a traditional class. Self-directed participants received a textbook, instructional video, and portable equipment kit and attended a 90-minute simulation session with an instructor. The traditional class included 6 hours of lectures and instructor-directed skill stations. Outcome measures included resuscitation skill (megacode assessment score), content knowledge, participant satisfaction, and self-confidence.

Results.—Forty-six subjects completed the study. There was no significant difference between the study groups in either the megacode assessment score (23.8 [traditional] vs 24.5 [self-directed]; $P = .46$) or fraction that passed the "megacode" (final skills assessment) (56% [traditional] vs 65% [self-directed]; $P = .76$). There were no significant differences in content knowledge, course satisfaction, or postcourse self-confidence. Content knowledge, years of experience, and self-confidence did not predict resuscitation skill.

Conclusions.—Self-directed education improves the educational efficiency of the neonatal resuscitation course by shifting the acquisition of cognitive and basic procedural skills outside of the classroom, which allows the instructor to add low-fidelity simulation and debriefing while significantly decreasing the duration of the course.

▶ This randomized, controlled, single-blinded (the investigator judging the megacode was blinded to group assignment) study evaluated postpartum nurses from St Joseph's Mercy Hospital (Ann Arbor, Michigan) using a previously validated megacode assessment score. The authors found that self-directed learning, beginning 2 weeks before the simulation session, and a 90-minute instructor-led skill session was not inferior to a traditional 6-hour course for a neonatal resuscitation program. The students involved in either type of training were satisfied with the program.

There are a few obvious limitations to this study. It involves a small sample size and a homogeneous population of nurses. Whether these results will translate to the training of physicians, residents, medical students, and the lay public is unclear. Those who are involved in teaching and directing "merit-badge" courses may be able to alter the way courses are presented in the future if further studies validate the findings of this study.

E. A. Ramoska, MD, MPHE

Teamwork and Leadership in Cardiopulmonary Resuscitation
Hunziker S, Johansson AC, Tschan F, et al (Univ Hosp Basel, Switzerland; Univ of Neuchâtel, Switzerland; Beth Israel Deaconess Med Ctr, Boston, MA; et al)
J Am Coll Cardiol 57:2381-2388, 2011

Despite substantial efforts to make cardiopulmonary resuscitation (CPR) algorithms known to healthcare workers, the outcome of CPR has remained poor during the past decades. Resuscitation teams often deviate from algorithms of CPR. Emerging evidence suggests that in addition to technical skills of individual rescuers, human factors such as teamwork and leadership affect adherence to algorithms and hence the outcome of CPR. This review describes the state of the science linking team interactions to the performance of CPR. Because logistical barriers make controlled measurement of team interaction in the earliest moments of real-life resuscitations challenging, our review focuses mainly on high-fidelity human simulator studies. This technique allows in-depth investigation of complex human interactions using precise and reproducible methods. It also removes variability in the clinical parameters of resuscitation, thus letting researchers study human factors and team interactions without confounding by clinical variability from resuscitation to resuscitation. Research has shown that a prolonged process of team building and poor leadership behavior are associated with significant shortcomings in CPR. Teamwork and leadership training have been shown to improve subsequent team performance during resuscitation and have recently been included in guidelines for advanced life support courses. We propose that further studies on the effects of team interactions on performance of complex medical emergency interventions such as resuscitation are needed. Future efforts to better understand the influence of team factors (e.g., team member status, team hierarchy, handling of human errors), individual factors (e.g., sex differences, perceived stress), and external factors (e.g., equipment, algorithms, institutional characteristics) on team performance in resuscitation situations are critical to improve CPR performance and medical outcomes of patients.

▶ This interesting article addresses the "human factors" side of cardiopulmonary resuscitation (CPR). It summarizes the literature in this area and offers suggestions for further research. There are some nuggets to be gleaned from this article that may help when you lead a resuscitation or train others in resuscitation.

There is an association between leadership behavior and performance. Studies have shown that lack of leadership and poor teamwork can result in poor clinical outcomes for groups performing CPR and other emergency tasks. On the other hand, clearer leadership was associated with more efficient cooperation in the team and also with better task performance. Notably, leaders who participated hands-on in the emergency, as opposed to adopting a coordinating role, were less likely to be efficient leaders, and team performance tended to suffer.

The interactions among nurses, residents, and senior physicians during a resuscitation is also worthy of note. First-responding nurses tend to hand over leadership to incoming residents as soon as they arrive. However, not all residents demonstrate rapid acceptance of the leadership role. Given the status differences between experienced nurses and young physicians in training, hesitations and insecurities about adopting a leadership role during CPR are not entirely surprising. Junior doctors need instruction not only in the mechanics of CPR but in the behaviors associated with successfully leading a resuscitation team. Incoming professionals of higher status should not, by default, take over leadership of the resuscitation. Research has found that senior physicians who entered the room later in the crisis supported group performance best by asking questions that brought potential problems to the attention of the leading junior doctors rather than by making directive statements. When high-status team members pose questions, rather than stating directives or giving commands, they create more open interaction, information exchange, and collaboration among the team members.

In high time-pressure situations, individuals and groups may rely on automatic and implicit decision making. However, more explicit communication ("talking to the room") has been related to higher decision making performance in ad hoc medical teams. This behavior ensures that the entire team has a common level of knowledge and reinforces a team structure that promotes the exchange of critical information.

E. A. Ramoska, MD, MPHE

Shock

Association between timing of antibiotic administration and mortality from septic shock in patients treated with a quantitative resuscitation protocol

Puskarich MA, on behalf of the Emergency Medicine Shock Research Network (EMSHOCKNET) (Carolinas Med Ctr, Charlotte, NC; et al)
Crit Care Med 39:2066-2071, 2011

Objective.—We sought to determine the association between time to initial antibiotics and mortality of patients with septic shock treated with an emergency department-based early resuscitation protocol.

Design.—Preplanned analysis of a multicenter randomized controlled trial of early sepsis resuscitation.

Setting.—Three urban U.S. emergency departments.

Patients.—Adult patients with septic shock.

Interventions.—A quantitative resuscitation protocol in the emergency department targeting three physiological variables: central venous pressure, mean arterial pressure, and either central venous oxygen saturation or lactate clearance. The study protocol was continued until all end points were achieved or a maximum of 6 hrs.

Measurements and Main Results.—Data on patients who received an initial dose of antibiotics after presentation to the emergency department were categorized based on both time from triage and time from shock recognition to initiation of antibiotics. The primary outcome was inhospital mortality. Of 291 included patients, mortality did not change with hourly delays in antibiotic administration up to 6 hrs after triage: 1 hr (odds ratio [OR], 1.2; 0.6–2.5), 2 hrs (OR, 0.71; 0.4–1.3), 3 hrs (OR, 0.59; 0.3–1.3). Mortality was significantly increased in patients who received initial antibiotics after shock recognition (n = 172 [59%]) compared with before shock recognition (OR, 2.4; 1.1–4.5); however, among patients who received antibiotics after shock recognition, mortality did not change with hourly delays in antibiotic administration.

Conclusion.—In this large, prospective study of emergency department patients with septic shock, we found no increase in mortality with each hour delay to administration of antibiotics after triage. However, delay in antibiotics until after shock recognition was associated with increased mortality.

▶ The Surviving Sepsis Campaign international consensus guidelines recommend initiating broad-spectrum antibiotic coverage within the first hour of recognizing severe sepsis and septic shock. This study suggests that hourly delays in antibiotic administration either before or after the recognition of septic shock does not affect mortality. The breakpoint is the onset of shock. In this study, patients receiving antibiotics after the recognition of shock had a significant increase in the odds of death.

It should be noted that these results are at odds with the 2006 report by Kumar et al.[1] In that prior study, administration of antimicrobials within the first hour of documented hypotension was associated with a survival rate of 79.9% (somewhat comparable to the 23.8% mortality rate in this current study). However, Kumar found that each hour of delay in antimicrobial administration over the ensuing 6 hours was associated with an average decrease in survival of 7.6%. This time-to-antibiotics mortality relationship was not found in the current study. There could be several explanations for this dichotomy. First, the cohort of subjects in the Kumar study included all intensive care unit patients, rather than emergency department patients as in this study. Second, the Kumar cohort may have had a different baseline severity of illness than the current study. Finally, the institutions in this study all have experience with early sepsis resuscitation protocols and, the vast majority of patients received antibiotics within 3 hours of triage. This means that there were relatively small numbers of patients in the later time points, which led to wide confidence intervals, making it more difficult to draw definitive conclusions regarding associations as time points become progressively longer.

The take-home point should be this: start antibiotics as soon as possible in patients with possible sepsis. There probably is some time relationship regarding antibiotics and mortality, although it is unclear exactly what that relationship is.

E. A. Ramoska, MD, MPHE

Reference

1. Kumar A, Roberts D, Wood KE, et al. Duration of hypotension before initiation of effective antimicrobial therapy is the critical determinant of survival in human septic shock. *Crit Care Med.* 2006;34:1589-1596.

Cardiac Output Determination From Endotracheally Measured Impedance Cardiography: Clinical Evaluation of Endotracheal Cardiac Output Monitor

Maus TM, Reber B, Banks DA, et al (Univ of California San Diego, La Jolla)
J Cardiothorac Vasc Anesth 25:770-775, 2011

Objectives.—To evaluate the accuracy, precision, and trending of a new endotracheally sourced impedance cardiography-based cardiac output (CO) monitor (ECOM; ConMed Corp, Irvine, CA).

Setting.—Two university hospitals.

Participants.—Thirty patients scheduled for elective coronary artery bypass graft (CABG) surgery.

Interventions.—All patients received a pulmonary artery catheter (PAC), arterial catheter, endotracheal CO monitor (ECOM), endotracheal intubation, and transesophageal echocardiographic monitoring. ECOM CO was compared with CO measured with pulmonary artery thermodilution, and left ventricular CO measured with transesophageal echocardiography.

Measurements.—One hundred forty-five pairs of triplicate CO measurements using intermittent bolus pulmonary artery thermodilution (TD) and ECOM were compared at 5 distinct time points: postinduction, postinduction passive leg raise, poststernotomy, post-CABG completion, and post–chest closure. Eighty-seven pairs of triplicate CO measurements using transesophageal echocardiography were obtained at 3 time points: postinduction, post-CABG completion, and post–chest closure and compared with ECOM- and PA-derived CO measurements. The measurements at each time point were compared by using Bland-Altman and polar plot analyses.

Results.—The mean CO ranged from 2.16 to 9.41 L/min. ECOM CO, compared with TD CO, revealed a bias of 0.02 L/min, 95% limits of agreement of −2.26 to 2.30 L/min, and a percent error of 50%. ECOM CO showed trending with TD CO with 91% and 99% of values within 0.5 L/min and 1 L/min limits of agreement, respectively. ECOM CO, compared with TEE CO, revealed a bias of −0.25 L/min, 95% limits of agreement of −2.41 to 1.92 L/min, and a percent error of 48%. ECOM CO showed trending with TEE CO with 83% and 95% of values within 0.5 L/min and 1 L/min limits of agreement, respectively.

Conclusion.—ECOM CO shows an acceptable bias with wide limits of agreement and a large percent error when compared with TD CO or TEE CO; however, it shows acceptable trending of CO to both modalities in patients undergoing cardiac surgery. Further studies are required to evaluate ECOM in other patient populations and clinical situations.

▶ Impedance measurement of cardiac output through the chest wall is noninvasive. However, the technique is subject to errors because the measured changes in thoracic volume with the cardiac cycle are assumed to be due only to stroke volume. Assuming that variations in impedance are a result of cardiac output may not be acceptable, however, if there is pulmonary fluid as in congestive heart failure.

Cardiac output measurement for this new impedance measurement method involves using electrodes placed closer to the aorta on an endotracheal tube. Although the results of comparisons to output measured by pulmonary catheter and transesophageal were less satisfactory than hoped, it does seem that there is a potential for this type of measurement. How well this new tool has to match a pulmonary artery with thermodilution needs to be determined. In some cases, trending with good precision may be enough.

Note that this method should be used only for those patients who are already ill enough to need intubation. Additional work to study how to place cutaneous electrodes to measure the blood outflow more effectively may be the next practical step.

N. B. Handly, MD, MSc, MS

Initial fluid resuscitation of patients with septic shock in the intensive care unit

Carlsen S, for the East Danish Septic Shock Cohort Investigators (Copenhagen Univ Hosp, Rigshospitalet, Denmark)
Acta Anaesthesiol Scand 55:394-400, 2011

Background.—Fluid is the mainstay of resuscitation of patients with septic shock, but the optimal composition and volume are unknown. Our aim was to evaluate the current initial fluid resuscitation practice in patients with septic shock in the intensive care unit (ICU) and patient characteristics and outcome associated with fluid volume.

Methods.—This was a prospective, cohort study of all patients with septic shock ($n = 132$) admitted in six ICUs during a 3-month period. Patients were divided into two groups according to the overall median volume of resuscitation fluid administered during the first 24 h after the diagnosis. Baseline characteristics, other treatments, monitoring and outcome were compared between the groups.

Results.—The mean volume of resuscitation fluid was 4.9 l (median 4.0 l and SD 3.5). Patients in the higher volume group received more crystalloids (3.7 vs. 1.2 l, $P < 0.0001$), colloids (1.8 vs. 0.9 l, $P < 0.0001$), blood products (1.8 vs. 0.6 l, $P = 0.0004$), a higher maximum vasopressor dose (0.37 vs. 0.21 µg/kg/min, $P < 0.0001$) and had a higher initial plasma concentration of lactate (4.0 vs. 3.0 mM, $P = 0.009$) compared with the lower volume group. Simplified acute physiology score II in the lower and higher dose group were 52 and 58 ($P = 0.07$). There were no differences in 30-, 90- or 365-day mortality between the two fluid volume groups.

Conclusion.—In the ICU, patients with septic shock were resuscitated with a combination of crystalloids, colloids and blood products. Although the more severely shocked patients received higher volumes of crystalloids, colloids and blood products, mortality did not differ between the groups.

▶ This observational study from Denmark was conducted during the end of 2007 and describes the current state of fluid resuscitation in patients with septic shock who were admitted to the intensive care unit. Three hospitals were university hospitals, and the other 3 were regional hospitals. Most patients (42%) were admitted from the general wards, 23% were admitted from surgery, 19% from the emergency department, and 14% were transfers from another institution.

The vast majority of the patients (74%) received a combination of crystalloids and colloids, whereas 53% received crystalloids, colloids, and blood products. Virtually all patients (98%) had their fluid treatment supplemented by inotropes or vasopressors; moreover, 35% were given 2 or more of these types of drugs. All patients received broad-spectrum antibiotics, 64% received steroids, and 54% were treated with insulin.

The authors note that the 30-day, 90-day, and 1-year mortality rates were not statistically different between the lower volume fluid group and the higher volume fluid group; however, the number of patients enrolled is small. This study cannot tell us what is the optimal amount of fluid to give to patients in septic shock, nor can it advise us as to which types of fluid are best. What it does do is describe the current state of practice (at least in 2007) in Denmark.

E. A. Ramoska, MD, MPHE

Resuscitation in massive obstetric haemorrhage using an intraosseous needle
Chatterjee DJ, Bukunola B, Samuels TL, et al (Worthing Hosp, UK)
Anaesthesia 66:306-310, 2011

A 38-year-old woman experienced a massive postpartum haemorrhage 30 minutes after emergency caesarean delivery. The patient became severely haemodynamically compromised with an unrecordable blood pressure. Rapid fluid resuscitation was limited by the capacity of the intravenous cannula in place at the time and inability to establish additional vascular access using conventional routes in a timely manner. An intraosseous needle was inserted in the proximal humerus at the first attempt and administration of resuscitation fluid by this route subsequently enabled successful placement of further intravenous lines. Blood and blood products were deployed in conjunction with intra-operative cell salvage and transoesophageal Doppler cardiac output monitoring was used to assess adequacy of volume replacement. Haemorrhage control was finally achieved with the use of recombinant factor VIIa and hysterectomy.

▶ This is yet another case report demonstrating the apparent safety and efficacy of the intraosseous (IO) method of obtaining vascular access. It should be evident to all emergency physicians at this point that they should be familiar with the IO technique. The use of a battery-operated needle driver, such as the EZ-IO driver used in this study, makes the placement of IO needles easy compared with the older style of hand placement with an Osgood needle.

The intraosseous route can be used to administer fluids, resuscitation drugs, blood and blood products, and antibiotics. Moreover, mixed-venous samples may be obtained for blood chemistry, blood gas, and type and cross-match studies.

E. A. Ramoska, MD, MPHE

The role of albumin as a resuscitation fluid for patients with sepsis: A systematic review and meta-analysis
Delaney AP, Dan A, McCaffrey J, et al (Univ of Sydney, Australia; Royal North Shore Hosp, St Leonards, Australia; Belfast City Hosp, UK)
Crit Care Med 39:386-391, 2011

Objective.—To assess whether resuscitation with albumin-containing solutions, compared with other fluids, is associated with lower mortality in patients with sepsis.

Data Sources.—MEDLINE, Embase, and Cochrane Central Register of Controlled Trials databases, the metaRegister of Controlled Trials, and the Medical Editors Trial Amnesty Register.

Study Selection.—Prospective randomized clinical trials of fluid resuscitation with albumin-containing solutions compared with other fluid resuscitation regimens, which included a population or subgroup of participants with sepsis, were included.

Data Extraction.—Assessment of the validity of included studies and data extraction were conducted independently by two authors.

Data Synthesis.—For the primary analysis, the effect of albumin-containing solutions on all-cause mortality was assessed by using a fixed-effect meta-analysis.

Results.—Seventeen studies that randomized 1977 participants were included in the meta-analysis. There were eight studies that included only patients with sepsis and nine where patients with sepsis were a subgroup of the study population. There was no evidence of heterogeneity, $I^2 = 0\%$. The use of albumin for resuscitation of patients with sepsis was associated with a reduction in mortality with the pooled estimate of the odds ratio of 0.82 (95% confidence limits 0.67−1.0, $p = .047$).

Conclusions.—In this meta-analysis, the use of albumin-containing solutions for the resuscitation of patients with sepsis was associated with lower mortality compared with other fluid resuscitation regimens. Until the results of ongoing randomized controlled trials are known, clinicians should consider the use of albumin-containing solutions for the resuscitation of patients with sepsis.

▶ Previous meta-analyses of the use of albumin in critically ill patients have not shown that it is beneficial over crystalloid. This meta-analysis included 17 studies that randomized 1977 participants who were septic and received either albumin or control fluid resuscitation. Its outcome measure was all-cause mortality. A fixed-effect method (which assumes that all studies are estimating the same effect size) was used to poll the data and found that there was a positive effect of albumin on mortality. However, when a random effects model (which assumes that the true effect might vary from study to study) was used to pool the data, the result was not statistically significant. This alternate analytic technique casts doubt on the robustness of their initial finding.

Although this article suggests that albumin may have a beneficial effect on all-cause mortality in septic patients, a definitive answer awaits the completion and publication of additional randomized controlled trials.

E. A. Ramoska, MD, MPHE

Miscellaneous

A fresh take on whole blood
Kaufman R (Brigham and Women's Hosp, Boston, MA)
Transfusion 51:230-233, 2011

Background.—Storing blood as components permits optimal biologic preservation ex vivo, facilitates stringent quality control and targeted replacement therapy, and helps preserve resources. However, fresh whole blood (FWB) is still used by the US military, especially in remote locations where apheresis platelet (aPLT) collections are impractical. However, some surgeons believe that FWB is the best therapy for severely bleeding patients. In addition, stored red blood cells (RBCs) have been found to potentially cause harm to patients, supporting the use of FWB. Whether FWB is clinically superior to RBCs, aPLTs, and fresh-frozen plasma (FFP) and should be used even when component therapy is available was investigated.

Method.—Published comparisons of FWB and component therapy were reviewed. The outcome criteria of the various studies included survival, platelet aggregation, 24-hour postoperative blood loss, postoperative mediastinal or chest tube drainage, and survival plus length of stay in the intensive care unit (ICU). No randomized, controlled trials comparing the two transfusion approaches were available. Also evaluated was whether old blood, having been stored for a considerable period, is safe for patients.

Results.—Outcomes varied widely. Some studies in cardiac surgery suggested that FWB may provide better hemostatic activity than component therapy. Data are limited and conflicting, and survivorship bias may have confounded many studies. It takes longer to issue FWB than aPLTs, and many trauma patients die within the first hour after admission. Therefore severely injured patients may live long enough to receive aPLTs but not long enough to receive FWB, which artificially inflates the survival among those receiving FWB. Adjustments are needed to address this bias.

The term "RBC storage lesion" refers to the in vitro changes that accumulate during RBC storage. It is possible that RBCs grow progressively less healthy and more toxic with longer storage. However, most of the variables in the RBC storage lesion are reversed once the RBCs are transfused into a physiologic environment. A retrospective 2008 study of 6002 cardiac surgery patients by Koch et al showed patients receiving older units of RBCs had significantly higher in-hospital mortality. However, more patients in the "old blood" group received 10 or more RBC units than in the "fresh blood" group, and receiving a high number of transfusions tends to indicate a more severe illness and lower survival. More recent studies show no relationship between age of the blood and survival.

Conclusions.—Ongoing randomized controlled trials are being closely watched to see if they will provide answers regarding the use of FWB versus component therapy and the safety of stored RBCs. Currently FWB should be viewed as a product most useful in extreme environments that is the equivalent of–not better than–its components.

▶ Dr Kaufman reviews some of the work comparing fractionated blood products and whole blood transfusion in this editorial and raises some very interesting questions about the choices we make when giving our patients blood transfusions. The remainder of the volume in which this editorial appears presents some of the more recent primary studies of effects of these types of transfusions.

The history of transfusion with fractionated products is interesting in that there are no outcomes studies on the oxygen-carrying capacity of fractionated red cells versus whole blood. Sure, fractionated red cells may be easier to store, but do they work as well?

Several other of the studies discussed in this editorial also raise some important concerns about study designs. One of the key concepts to understand is that of patient-oriented versus disease-oriented outcomes. In several studies, the fact that outcomes considered mediastinal drainage as a proxy for a measure of hemostasis was mentioned. But this is a disease-oriented measure. Sure, we might suspect that problems with hemostasis are a bad thing, but without relating that drainage to pain or survival or hospital charges (all very much important to the patient), we are likely studying factors that make us feel better.

Another study design discussion was that of survival bias. This was mentioned in the setting of use of whole blood versus fractionated blood because of work that suggested that there was a survival benefit to the use of whole blood in combat injuries. However, the amount of time to intervention is systematically different (whole blood transfusion is not available as rapidly as fractionated blood), so it might be the increased survival among those receiving whole blood that reflected the improved likelihood of survival by the time whole blood was given. A better approach would have been an intention-to-treat design (so subjects who died before receiving whole blood would be grouped with those who did get whole blood) or, as mentioned in Dr Kaufman's editorial, to only consider subjects who have survived in each arm to the time of the latest intervention (in this case, whole blood transfusion).

Composite outcomes are also troublesome; in 1 study discussed, there was an outcome based on survival and number of intensive care unit (ICU) days of stay. Besides the fact that this is a combination of disease- and patient-oriented outcomes, it is actually hard to apply complex outcomes to other settings. What if your hospital has different practices for transitioning patients from ICU to stepdown or floor beds? How would a patient or patient's family understand a decision based on a "possibility of death or number of days in the ICU"?

N. B. Handly, MD, MSc, MS

Efficacy of Field Treatments to Reduce Body Core Temperature in Hyperthermic Subjects

Sinclair WH, Rudzki SJ, Leicht AS, et al (James Cook Univ, Townsville, Queensland, Australia; Australian Army, Canberra, Australian Capital Territory, Australia; et al)
Med Sci Sports Exerc 41:1984-1990, 2009

Purpose.—To contrast the effects of three postcooling techniques in reducing body core temperature (T_c) in exercise-induced hyperthermic participants on the cessation of exercise.

Methods.—Eleven healthy active male volunteers were cooled during a 40-min period using three different methods: ice packs to the neck, axillae, and groin (ICE); water spray and fan (FAN); and 2 L of chilled (20°C) intravenous saline administered during a 20-min period (IV). Rate of decrease in T_c, cardiovascular responses, and any incidence of reported adverse effects were investigated. Trials were presented in a counterbalanced order with the volunteers' body core temperature being elevated to 40.0°C on three occasions via an intermittent walk-run (2 min at 6 km·h^{-1} and 4 min at 10 km·h^{-1}) protocol conducted within a climate-controlled chamber (34.2 ± 0.5°C and 62.3 ± 3.1% relative humidity).

Results.—Rate of Tc reduction during the first 20 min of cooling was greater for FAN compared with ICE (0.09 ± 0.02°C·min^{-1} vs 0.07 ± 0.02°C·min^{-1}, $P < 0.05$), whereas IV did not differ with the other trials (0.08 ± 0.01°C·min^{-1}, $P > 0.05$). Three participants complained of numbness or paresthesia in their arm or hand during administration of the chilled saline, although these symptoms resolved within 5 min of ceasing the infusion.

Conclusions.—All three cooling techniques reduced T_c and would be suitable for first aid application in a field setting during transportation to adequate medical facilities. Chilled IV saline did not produce any contraindications, providing a suitable alternative for T_c cooling.

▶ This study from James Cook University and the Australian Army found that the 3 cooling techniques studied produced a similar reduction in core temperature after 40 minutes of treatment, although the water spray and fan technique was more effective in lowering temperature during the first 20 minutes. Because lowering the temperature rapidly in a hyperthermic patient is desirable, this technique may be the best method; however, there is no reason that all 3 methods could not be used simultaneously. They work through different mechanisms—namely, dilution, conduction, and evaporation—and their cooling effects may be additive.

It should be noted that no abnormal cardiac rhythms were observed during administration of the chilled intravenous saline, despite having an attending physician actively monitor each patient for arrhythmias. There is a theoretical concern that directly cooling the myocardium will induce arrhythmias.

One of the limitations of this study is that it was conducted in young (mean age = 23.5 years), healthy, fit men. Although there is no reason to suspect that women would react differently to the 3 modes of cooling used, the use and effectiveness of the 3 methods in older patients who are have an acute concomitant illness or chronic underlying disease is unknown.

In addition, the authors did not perform a power analysis. With only 11 subjects and no power analysis, we do not know whether there were an insufficient number of participants to detect any difference among the 3 therapies or whether there was actually no difference.

E. A. Ramoska, MD, MPHE

3 Cardiovascular

Acute Myocardial Infarction

A new hydrodynamic approach by infusion of drag-reducing polymers to improve left ventricular function in rats with myocardial infarction
Chen X, Zha D, Xiu J, et al (Southern Med Univ, Guangzhou, Chinau)
Int J Cardiol 147:112-117, 2011

Background.—Recent studies have shown that drag-reducing polymers (DRPs) prolonged survival time in rats with acute myocardial infarction (MI), but their effect on cardiac function post MI remains unknown. This study sought to test the hypothesis that intravenous infusion of DRPs may improve left ventricular (LV) function in rats following surgically induced MI.

Methods.—MI was induced by ligation of the left anterior descending coronary artery in 36 Sprague-Dawley rats, and sham operations were performed in 12 animals. DRPs were then administered to 18 of the MI rats. Echocardiograpy was used to evaluate the changes of impaired LV function and global wall motion. Besides, the hydrodynamic effect of DRPs on microcirculation was also assessed.

Results.—The survival rate at 24 h following MI was significantly different among the sham, MI and DRP groups ($p=0.023$). DRP-treated animals had marked smaller left ventricular end-systolic diameter and better anterior systolic wall thickness comparison with untreated rats. Significant improvement of fractional shortening and ejection fraction were detected in MI rats with DRP. Wall motion score index and contrast score index were both significantly reduced by DRP treatment. DRPs were shown to have beneficial effects on microvascular variables including red blood cell velocity, diameter, blood flow and calculated wall shear stress in third-order arteriole.

Conclusions.—Acute administration of DRPs improved LV function in a rat model of MI possibly by improving microvascular blood flow due to their unique hydrodynamic properties. DRPs may offer a new approach to the treatment of coronary artery ischemic diseases.

▶ Think of the things we do to mitigate the problems of myocardial infarction (MI). We open vessels mechanically (angioplasty) or enzymatically (tissue plasminogen activator); nitroglycerin is used to dilate blood vessels. Aspirin is used to prevent further platelet aggregation and thus further vessel occlusion.

What about optimizing the flow of blood? The use of this technique would complement the techniques we already are using.

The authors call to our attention the beneficial effects of the use of drag-reducing compounds in the setting of MI. In this study, they evaluated performance of the heart with echocardiography for the first 24 hours after experimental MI in rats to show enhanced left ventricular function when drag-reducing polyethylene glycol was administered. Microvascular studies performed in parallel showed that these drag-reducing treatments also improved red blood cell flow in small vessels.

This is an interesting avenue to explore. We have nearly mastered the art of opening blocked vessels, and now this work suggests that we can enhance blood flow through compromised vessels. It seems that all that is left to explore are ways to make "super" blood that can better deliver nutrients and remove metabolites.

N. B. Handly, MD, MSc, MS

Circadian variations of infarct size in acute myocardial infarction

Suárez-Barrientos A, López-Romero P, Vivas D, et al (Hosp Clínico San Carlos, Madrid, Spain; Carlos III (CNIC), Madrid, Spain)
Heart 97:970-976, 2011

Background.—The circadian clock influences a number of cardiovascular (patho)physiological processes including the incidence of acute myocardial infarction. A circadian variation in infarct size has recently been shown in rodents, but there is no clinical evidence of this finding.

Objective.—To determine the impact of time-of-day onset of ST segment elevation myocardial infarction (STEMI) on infarct size.

Methods.—A retrospective single-centre analysis of 811 patients with STEMI admitted between 2003 and 2009 was performed. Infarct size was estimated by peak enzyme release. The relationship between peak enzyme concentrations and time-of-day were characterised using multivariate regression splines. Time of STEMI onset was divided into four 6-hour periods in phase with circadian rhythms.

Results.—Model comparisons based on likelihood ratio tests showed a circadian variation in infarct size across time-of-day as evaluated by peak creatine kinase (CK) and troponin-I (TnI) concentrations (p=0.015 and p=0.012, respectively). CK and TnI curves described similar patterns across time, with a global maximum in the 6:00—noon period and a local minimum in the noon—18:00 period. Infarct size was largest in patients with STEMI onset in the dark-to-light transition period (6:00—noon), with an increase in peak CK and TnI concentrations of 18.3% (p=0.031) and 24.6% (p=0.033), respectively, compared with onset of STEMI in the 18:00—midnight period. Patients with anterior wall STEMI also had significantly larger infarcts than those with STEMI in other locations.

Conclusions.—Significant circadian oscillations in infarct size were found in patients according to time-of-day of STEMI onset. The infarct size was found to be significantly larger with STEMI onset in the dark-to-light transition period (6:00—noon). If confirmed, these results may have a significant impact on the interpretation of clinical trials of cardioprotective strategies in STEMI.

▶ How does time of the day affect your clinical practice? Surely the end of a shift has some effect on how you feel, but the time of day referred to in this article appears to have as important of an effect on the course of your patients' outcomes. You might be aware of the variation in frequency of cardiac presentations and that there is an underlying circadian pattern of cardiovascular physiology.

This is a study of the relationship between circadian rhythm and size of infarcts for those patients receiving percutaneous cardiac intervention. Following on the work done previously in mice, this is the first study looking at this pattern in humans. In this study, the day was broken up into four 6-hour periods, and patients were assigned to these time periods based on the time of onset of symptoms (this might be problematic to determine this time among patients who are not able to establish the onset of symptoms or have atypical anginal symptoms). As for measuring infarct size, the authors chose a proxy measure: the peak amount of cardiac enzymes.

The study was performed by retrospectively analyzing a prospectively collected data set. As such, no number needed to reach statistical significance was provided. Instead, the idea of this study was to explore the hypothesis that there is a pattern. It would be understood that further testing would be necessary to prove the relationship that is suggested by this effort.

An interesting method is used in this study—multivariate regression splines. This is method of model building (data fitting) that allows both nonlinear effects and the potential to break up the domain of possible variables into pieces to best minimize error, at the same time building that model using the least number of variables. For large data sets, this is an appropriate use of computing tools (the software to do this study is available in the open source R statistical language). The learning curve is steep, but perhaps once the kinks have been worked out, it will be useful.

N. B. Handly, MD, MSc, MS

Electrocardiogram Findings in Emergency Department Patients With Syncope

Quinn J, McDermott D (Stanford Univ, Palo Alto, CA; Univ of California San Francisco)
Acad Emerg Med 18:714-718, 2011

Objectives.—To determine the sensitivity and specificity of the San Francisco Syncope Rule (SFSR) electrocardiogram (ECG) criteria for determining cardiac outcomes and to define the specific ECG findings that are the most important in patients with syncope.

Methods.—A consecutive cohort of emergency department (ED) patients with syncope or near syncope was considered. The treating emergency physicians assessed 50 predictor variables, including an ECG and rhythm assessment. For the ECG assessment, the physicians were asked to categorize the ECG as normal or abnormal based on any changes that were old or new. They also did a separate rhythm assessment and could use any of the ECGs or available monitoring strips, including prehospital strips, when making this assessment. All patients were followed up to determine a broad composite study outcome. The final ECG criterion for the SFSR was any nonsinus rhythm or new ECG changes. In this specific study, the initial assessments in the database were used to determine only cardiac-related outcomes (arrhythmia, myocardial infarction, structural, sudden death) based on set criteria, and the authors determined the sensitivity and specificity of the ECG criteria for cardiac outcomes only. All ECGs classified as "abnormal" by the study criteria were compared to the official cardiology reading to determine specific findings on the ECG. Univariate and multivariate analysis were used to determine important specific ECG and rhythm findings.

Results.—A total of 684 consecutive patients were considered, with 218 having positive ECG criteria and 42 (6%) having important cardiac outcomes. ECG criteria predicted 36 of 42 patients with cardiac outcomes, with a sensitivity of 86% (95% confidence interval [CI] = 71% to 94%), a specificity of 70% (95% CI = 66% to 74%), and a negative predictive value of 99% (95% CI = 97% to 99%). Regarding specific ECG findings, any nonsinus rhythm from any source and any left bundle conduction problem (i.e., any left bundle branch block, left anterior fascicular block, left posterior fascicular block, or QRS widening) were 2.5 and 3.5 times more likely associated with significant cardiac outcomes.

Conclusions.—The ECG criteria from the SFSR are relatively simple, and if used correctly can help predict which patients are at risk of cardiac outcomes. Furthermore, any left bundle branch block conduction problems or any nonsinus rhythms found during the ED stay should be especially concerning for physicians caring for patients presenting with syncope.

▶ An electrocardiogram (ECG) is generally a fundamental portion of the workup for a patient presenting after a syncopal event, with the intention of identifying a cardiological etiology. The authors of this study assessed whether the ECG would identify the potential etiology and predict a serious event. As a foundation, the researchers used the San Francisco Syncope Rules ECG criteria: rhythm abnormalities on the ECG (ventricular tachycardia, heart block, paced, supraventricular tachycardia), presence of right branch bundle block, left branch bundle block, ST-segment changes, nonspecific ST-T wave changes, interval variants (PR, QT), presence of ectopy, and presence of Q waves. The authors report a sensitivity of 86%, missing 6 patients whose ECGs were nondiagnostic. The ECG is not to be the only yardstick by which the treating physician measures the merit of the admission; further diagnostic criteria must be used when making this decision. Interestingly, the authors reference significant variations in admission rates among the United States and Canada and Australia, raising the question of defensive medical practices pushing admissions.

E. C. Bruno, MD

Impact of missing data on standardised mortality ratios for acute myocardial infarction: evidence from the Myocardial Ischaemia National Audit Project (MINAP) 2004–7
Gale CP, Cattle BA, Moore J, et al (Univ of Leeds, UK)
Heart 97:1926-1931, 2011

Background.—Standardised mortality ratios (SMR) are often used to depict cardiovascular care. Data missingness, data quality, temporal variation and case-mix can, however, complicate the assessment of clinical performance.

Objectives.—To study Primary Care Trust (PCT) 30-day SMRs for STEMI and NSTEMI whilst considering the impact of missing data for age, sex and IMD score.

Design.—Observational study using data from the Myocardial Ischaemia National Audit Project (MINAP) database to generate PCT SMR maps and funnel plots for England, 2004–2007.

Patients.—217,157 patients: 40.4% STEMI and 59.6% NSTEMI.

Results.—95% CI 30-day unadjusted mortality: STEMI 5.8% to 6.2%; NSTEMI 6.6% to 6.9%; relative risk, 95% CI 1.14, 1.10 to 1.19. Median (IQR) data missingness by PCT for composite of age, sex and IMD score was 1.4% (0.7% to 2.2%). For STEMI and NSTEMI statistically significant predictors of mortality were mean age (STEMI: P<0.001; NSTEMI: P<0.001), proportion of females (STEMI: P<0.001; NSTEMI: P<0.001) and proportion of missing ages (STEMI: P=0.02; NSTEMI: P<0.001). Proportion of missing sex also predicted 30-day mortality for NSTEMI (P=0.01). Maps of SMRs demonstrated substantial mortality variation, but no evidence of North / South divide. There were significant correlations between STEMI and NSTEMI observed (R^2 0.72) and standardised mortality (R^2 0.49) rates. PCT data aggregation gave an acceptable model fit in terms of deviance explained. For STEMI there were 33 (21.7%) regions below the 99.8% lower limit of the associated performance funnel plot, and 28 (18.4%) for NSTEMI; the inclusion of missing data did not affect the distribution of SMRs.

Conclusions.—The proportion of missing data was associated with 30-day mortality for STEMI and NSTEMI, however it did not influence the distribution of PCTs within the funnel plots. There was considerable variation in mortality not attributable to key patient-specific factors, supporting the notion of regional-dependent variation in STEMI and NSTEMI care.

▶ Let's think a moment about things that influence your ability to manage acute coronary syndrome patients: you have to know they are in the emergency department (ED), screening processes start (usually data provided by others to you but you may drop by the bedside, too), and you make some stratification plans that others in the ED will carry out.

The outcomes of this patient depend on patient-oriented data and provider-oriented processes and are even data oriented. In this study, the provider-oriented data are actually regionalized hospital information (so it is not possible to identify particular physicians or nurses whose behaviors are contributing to good or bad outcome), and the data-oriented information is missing data.

The surprising result in this study is that missing data are associated with worsening outcomes. Association is not cause but is a relationship worth exploring. Perhaps among very ill patients, there is not enough time to gather all the data, or the missing data values are conveniently lost to reduce recall to cases.

N. B. Handly, MD, MSc, MS

Myocardial infarction vaccine? Evidence supporting the influenza vaccine for secondary prevention
Natarajan P, Cannon CP (Brigham & Women's Hosp, Boston, MA)
Eur Heart J 32:1701-1703, 2011

Background.—The complex interplay between infection and atherosclerosis has been studied extensively. Among the organisms implicated are herpesviruses, *Chlamydia pneumoniae*, *Mycoplasma pneumoniae*, and periodontal pathogens. The influenza virus is one of the most severe respiratory viral pathogens and the only one for which there is effective prophylaxis and treatment. The effect of influenza vaccination on secondary prevention of coronary heart disease (CHD) was investigated by Phrommintikul et al, who found an absolute risk reduction of nearly 10% for major cardiovascular events over 12 months of follow-up. The evidence supporting the influenza vaccine to provide secondary prevention of CHD was assessed.

Methods.—The most recent study was evaluated along with other investigations into the role of the influenza vaccine for secondary coronary syndrome prevention.

Results.—The FLUVACS randomized controlled trial included patients with recent myocardial infarctions, those having elective percutaneous coronary intervention with no recent or previous acute coronary syndromes, and those with previous revascularization. Patients receiving elective revascularization had no observed benefit from vaccination. Two hundred vaccinated patients with myocardial infarction were less likely to suffer cardiovascular death or recurrent ischemic events over the following year. A cohort study of almost 40,000 patients found no increased short-term risk of acute myocardial infarction or stroke after immunization for influenza, pneumococcus, or tetanus. Preceding systemic respiratory illness did correlate with an increased risk of cardiovascular events in this cohort. The Polish FLUCAD study of 658 patients with stable CHD found that those who received the influenza vaccine had a slightly lower rate of coronary ischemic events than those not vaccinated. Together with the Phrommintikul et al study, these investigations indicate that persons with recent cardiovascular events may derive the greatest benefit from immunization.

An autopsy study of nearly 35,000 patients who died of respiratory illnesses showed that coronary death rate was higher during influenza epidemics. Combining this observation with other findings suggests that current clinical management protocols for non-ST-elevation myocardial infarction and unstable angina may need to be refined for patients with severe systemic illness.

Influenza was persistently related to acute coronary syndromes in these studies. A causative role may exist, with some evidence provided in the setting of atherosclerotic mice inoculated with influenza. These mice had significant infiltration of inflammatory and smooth muscle cells, evidence of platelet aggregation, and thrombus formation in areas of atherosclerotic plaque with no sign of panarteritis. Wild-type mice did not show these findings. In addition, atherosclerotic mice who were inoculated with influenza but showed no viremia also had more viral antigens in coronary atheroma, also not seen in inoculated wild-type mice. Vascular tropism was not present with respiratory syncytial virus (RSV) infection. The high-density lipoprotein cholesterol of mice with influenza infection was less able to protect against oxidation of low-density lipoprotein cholesterol.

Conclusions.—Larger studies are needed before conclusions can be drawn, but the results of mouse models, observational studies, and randomized trials are promising concerning the efficacy of influenza vaccine against CHD. Other acute respiratory pathogens that may be associated with cardiovascular events, such as *Streptococcus pneumoniae*, should also be studied.

▶ These authors summarize the relationship between influenza vaccine and reduced nonlethal cardiac events after a first acute coronary syndrome event. Much of this work follows from the thinking that plaque development and rupture have inflammatory-mediated processes, and most of the damage from influenza infections results from inflammation. So if influenza is particularly good at activating inflammatory pathways, then steps that could reduce influenza infection may offer a way to reduce subsequent myocardial injury.

At the same time vaccination has been found to help reduce injury, some studies of patients with undefined respiratory illness just before a primary cardiac event were found to have worse outcomes. It was not shown that influenza was present, so further steps would need to be taken, perhaps even more precisely to measure the level of inflammation in patients as well as the infectious agent.

This does not mean there is no place for genetic factors in cardiac injury. The sensitivity to inflammatory causes such as influenza infection are likely affected by a patient's underlying genetics.

The authors start us thinking about disease processes in a new light. This could be useful to understand and control disease better.

N. B. Handly, MD, MSc, MS

Oxygen Therapy for Acute Myocardial Infarction—Then and Now. A Century of Uncertainty
Kones R (Cardiometabolic Res Inst, Houston, TX)
Am J Med 124:1000-1005, 2011

For about 100 years, inhaled oxygen has been administered to all patients suspected of having an acute myocardial infarction. The basis for this practice was the belief that oxygen supplementation raised often-deficient arterial oxygen content to improve myocardial oxygenation, thereby reducing infarct size. This assumption is conditional and not evidence-based. While such physiological changes may pertain in some patients who are hypoxemic, considerable data suggest that oxygen therapy may be detrimental in others. Acute oxygen therapy may raise blood pressure and lower cardiac index, heart rate, cardiac oxygen consumption, and blood flow in the cerebral and renal beds. Oxygen also may lower capillary density and redistribute blood in the microcirculation. Several reports now confirm that these changes occur in humans. In patients with both acute coronary syndromes and stable coronary disease, oxygen administration may constrict the coronary vessels, lower myocardial oxygen delivery, and may actually worsen ischemia. There are no large, contemporary, randomized studies that examine clinical outcomes after this intervention. Hence, this long-accepted but potentially harmful tradition urgently needs reevaluation. Clinical guidelines appear to be changing, favoring use of oxygen only in hypoxemic patients, and then cautiously titrating to individual oxygen tensions.

▶ This is a great little review on oxygen therapy for the treatment of acute myocardial infarction (AMI). Still considered by many a mainstay of the treatment of AMI even in the presence of normoxia, the actual practice started around 1900 and should in no way be considered an evidence-based practice. Over the past decade, there have been several systemic reviews done on this topic, including a Cochrane study in 2010, and all came to the same conclusion: there is certainly no benefit accrued from oxygen therapy in uncomplicated AMI patients, but the analyses could not find definitive harm. That said, of the only 3 studies that qualified as appropriate for the analysis, there were 14 deaths out of 387 patients. Of these, 3 times as many patients randomized to oxygen treatment died. This was not statistically significant given the small numbers but should raise some eyebrows. So too should a recent study based on the Project IMPACT database involving 6326 adults with nontraumatic cardiac arrest admitted to 120 US intensive care units after resuscitation. Hyperoxia was present in 18% of patients, and it conferred an odds ratio for death of 1.8, indicating that arterial hyperoxia was independently associated with increased in-hospital mortality compared with either normoxia or hypoxia.

Until a definitive randomized controlled trial is performed, the doctrine of primum non nocere should be followed, and patients with AMI with hypoxia should be treated with inhaled oxygen. Otherwise, physicians cannot be faulted for either using or not using oxygen, but the latter may eventually be proven to be the treatment of choice. The Air Versus Oxygen in myocardial Infarction Study (AVOID) is in progress and will hopefully give us some more definitive answers.

D. K. Mullin, MD

Emergency physician—initiated cath lab activation reduces door to balloon times in ST-segment elevation myocardial infarction patients
Kontos MC, Kurz MC, Roberts CS, et al (Virginia Commonwealth Univ, Richmond)
Am J Emerg Med 29:868-874, 2011

Objectives.—We evaluated the impact of emergency physician (EP)—initiated primary percutaneous coronary intervention (PCI) via a single-group page on door to balloon (D2B) interval times in patients with ST-segment elevation myocardial infarction.

Methods.—Consecutive ST-segment elevation myocardial infarction patients presenting to the emergency department between February 2004 and September 2008 were divided into 4 groups: group 1, PCI performed on an ad hoc basis after cardiology consultation; group 2, primary PCI activated via a single-group page only on-call cardiology consultation; group 3, primary PCI with EP cardiac catheterization laboratory (CCL) activation via the same page strategy; group 4, prehospital CCL activation based on prehospital diagnostic electrocardiogram. Composite D2B and relevant time intervals were measured for each time group.

Results.—A total of 295 consecutive patients undergoing emergent angiography were included. Times decreased for most time intervals from groups 1 to 4. Although there was no significant change in composite D2B or any measured interval time with the introduction of PCI after emergent cardiology consultation, each decreased significantly after implementing an EP-initiated PCI strategy except CCL2B (D2B 95 to 77 minutes, D2E 14 to 10 minutes, D2CCL 71 to 50 minutes). Further significant reductions in D2B time were achieved among all patients after the institution of emergency medicine services activation of the CCL (D2B 77 to 64 minutes, D2CCL 50 to 38 minutes, CCL2B 28 to 22 minutes).

Conclusions.—A systematic process of initiating D2B recommendations, including EP-initiated CCL activation via a single-group page, significantly reduces D2CCL and D2B times (Figs 1 and 2).

▶ For patients presenting with ST-segment elevation myocardial infarction (STEMI) on the initial electrocardiogram (ECG), prompt reperfusion is critical for improving outcomes, reducing myocardial infarct size, and preventing subsequent adverse cardiac events including heart failure, arrhythmia, and death. Primary percutaneous intervention (PCI) appears to be the reperfusion treatment of choice, because previous data show that it is associated with significantly better outcomes than treatment with fibrinolytics. The American College of Cardiology/American Heart Association recommend that patients with STEMI

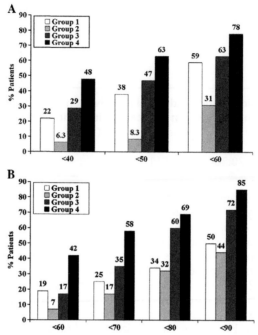

FIGURE 1.—Proportion of patients having door to CCL less than 40, 50, and 60 minutes (A) and door to PCI less than 60, 70, 80, and 90 minutes (B). (Reprinted from the American Journal of Emergency Medicine, Kontos MC, Kurz MC, Roberts CS, et al. Emergency physician—initiated cath lab activation reduces door to balloon times in ST-segment elevation myocardial infarction patients. *Am J Emerg Med.* 2011;29:868-874. Copyright 2011, with permission from Elsevier.)

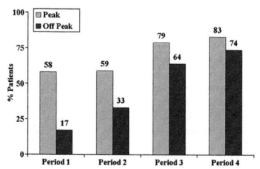

FIGURE 2.—Time in minutes for door to CCL and door to PCI for patients presenting during peak and off-peak hours. (Reprinted from the American Journal of Emergency Medicine, Kontos MC, Kurz MC, Roberts CS, et al. Emergency physician—initiated cath lab activation reduces door to balloon times in ST-segment elevation myocardial infarction patients. *Am J Emerg Med.* 2011;29:868-874. Copyright 2011, with permission from Elsevier.)

have reperfusion therapy with PCI as quickly as possible, with a goal door-to-balloon (D2B) time of less than 90 minutes.

The purpose of this study was to determine the effectiveness of one of the recommended interventions from the American College of Cardiology D2B

Program—namely, emergency physician cardiac catheterization laboratory activation (CCL). Group 1 consisted of the first historical group when fibrinolytic therapy was the primary reperfusion therapy and PCI was performed only on an ad hoc basis after cardiology consultation. Group 2 was this hospital's next attempt of D2B in less than 90 minutes and CCU fellow activation. After the CCU fellow was called and the patient was evaluated, the fellow would activate the "STEMI page," thus activating the CCL. Group 3 was CCL activation by the emergency physician actually seeing the patient. Group 4 included cases in which the CCL was activated by the emergency physician based on the emergency medical services ECG, thus the patient was not in the emergency department when the STEMI page was called. As you can see from Fig 1, Groups 3 and 4 were far superior in terms of D2B times; Fig 2 shows this improvement in D2B times was even more impressive during off-peak hours.

This is the way to go at all hospitals with PCI capabilities. If you're an emergency physician and you aren't the person activating the CCL for STEMIs, you need to bring the change. Take this article and the American College of Cardiology D2B program guidelines to a meeting with hospital administrators and the hospital cardiologists, and no doubt you will change some minds. This is soon to become standard of care at all hospitals with PCI capabilities.

D. K. Mullin, MD

Atrial Fibrillation

A Clinical Prediction Model to Estimate Risk for 30-Day Adverse Events in Emergency Department Patients With Symptomatic Atrial Fibrillation

Barrett TW, Martin AR, Storrow AB, et al (Vanderbilt Univ School of Medicine, Nashville, TN)
Ann Emerg Med 57:1-12, 2011

Study Objective.—Atrial fibrillation affects more than 2 million people in the United States and accounts for nearly 1% of emergency department (ED) visits. Physicians have little information to guide risk stratification of patients with symptomatic atrial fibrillation and admit more than 65%. Our aim is to assess whether data available in the ED management of symptomatic atrial fibrillation can estimate a patient's risk of experiencing a 30-day adverse event.

Methods.—We systematically reviewed the electronic medical records of all ED patients presenting with symptomatic atrial fibrillation between August 2005 and July 2008. Predefined adverse outcomes included 30-day ED return visit, unscheduled hospitalization, cardiovascular complication, or death. We performed multivariable logistic regression to identify predictors of 30-day adverse events. The model was validated with 300 bootstrap replications.

Results.—During the 3-year study period, 914 patients accounted for 1,228 ED visits. Eighty patients were excluded for non—atrial-fibrillation-related complaints and 2 patients had no follow-up recorded. Of 832 eligible patients, 216 (25.9%) experienced at least 1 of the 30-day adverse events. Increasing age (odds ratio [OR] 1.20 per decade; 95% confidence interval [CI] 1.06 to 1.36 per decade), complaint of dyspnea (OR 1.57; 95% CI 1.12 to 2.20), smokers (OR 2.35; 95% CI 1.47 to 3.76), inadequate ventricular rate control (OR 1.58; 95% CI 1.13 to 2.21), and patients receiving β-blockers (OR 1.44; 95% CI 1.02 to 2.04) were independently associated with higher risk for adverse events. C-index was 0.67.

Conclusion.—In ED patients with symptomatic atrial fibrillation, increased age, inadequate ED ventricular rate control, dyspnea, smoking, and β-blocker treatment were associated with an increased risk of a 30-day adverse event.

▶ In this retrospective chart review, the authors determined which risk factors were associated with adverse events within a 30-day follow-up period. By determining the important risk factors, the authors could then create a prediction rule to prospectively identify which patients presenting with symptomatic atrial fibrillation are in jeopardy of a poor outcome, defined as a 30-day emergency department return visit for an atrial fibrillation—related complaint, unscheduled hospital admission for an atrial fibrillation—related complaint, 30-day cardiovascular complication, and patient death as a result of an atrial fibrillation—related problem. According to the risk analysis, the authors found 5 clinical situations that predicted a worse outcome: increased age, smoking, dyspnea, inadequate ventricular rate control in the emergency department, and home beta-blocker use. Knowledge of these conditions may guide the treating emergency physician in determining whether to admit or discharge the patient. Interestingly, the researchers found that 18.2% of discharged patients had a 30-day adverse event, compared with 28.4% of the admitted patients. Although the authors' complication definition is conservative, this complication rate raises the question of whether most patients presenting with atrial fibrillation should, at minimum, be admitted for observation.

E. C. Bruno, MD

Low-dose diltiazem in atrial fibrillation with rapid ventricular response
Lee J, Kim K, Lee CC, et al (Seoul Natl Univ, Sungnam-si, Gyeonggi-do, Republic of Korea; Stony Brook Univ Hosp, NY; et al)
Am J Emerg Med 29:849-854, 2011

Objectives.—Diltiazem is one of the most commonly used medications to control the rapid ventricular response in atrial fibrillation (AF). The recommended starting dose is an intravenous bolus of 0.25 mg/kg over 2 minutes. To avoid hypotension, we have empirically used a lower dose of diltiazem. We compared the efficacy and safety of different doses of diltiazem in rapid AF.

Methods.—A retrospective chart review was undertaken in patients who presented to the emergency department with rapid AF. Patients were divided into 3 groups according to diltiazem dosage: low dose ($\leq$0.2 mg/kg), standard dose (>0.2 and $\leq$0.3 mg/kg), and high dose (>0.3 mg/kg). We compared the rates of therapeutic response (adequate rate control) and complications (such as hypotension). Multivariate regression analysis was used to determine the effect of diltiazem dose on the occurrence of complications.

Results.—A total of 180 patients were included in the analysis. There were no significant differences in the rates of therapeutic response for the low-, standard-, and high-dose groups (70.5%, 77.1%, and 77.8%; $P = .605$). The rates of hypotension in the low-, standard-, and high-dose groups were 18%, 34.9%, and 41.7%, respectively. After adjusting confounding variables, the rate of hypotension was significantly lower in the low-dose group in comparison with the standard-dose group (adjusted odds ratio, 0.39; 95% confidence interval, 0.16-0.94).

Conclusions.—Low-dose diltiazem might be as effective as the standard dose in controlling rapid AF and reduce the risk of hypotension.

▶ Diltiazem is commonly used to initiate rate control in patients presenting with atrial fibrillation with rapid ventricular response. Unfortunately, patients may experience complications, specifically hypotension, with the administration of diltiazem. With the goal of minimizing complications while maintaining effectiveness, the authors of this study evaluated patient response to low, standard, and high diltiazem dosing. The authors concluded that the low-dose (0.20 mg/kg) bolus of diltiazem was equally effective at rate control, without the complication of hypotension. Increasing doses, increases in rate control, and complications suggested a dose response phenomenon. When cardioversion with rhythm conversion is unattainable, rate control becomes the target. Anecdotal experience suggests that preloading the patient with intravenous calcium may attenuate the hypotension. When this is not an option, low-dose diltiazem seems like a reasonable technique and affords the physician the ability to repeat the dose. If a patient becomes unstable from the diltiazem bolus, cardioversion may become a necessity.

E. C. Bruno, MD

Congestive Heart Failure

Beyond dyspnoea as an endpoint in acute heart failure trials
Gheorghiade M, Ruschitzka F (Northwestern Univ, Chicago, IL; Univ of Zurich, Switzerland)
Eur Heart J 32:1442-1445, 2011

Background.—Acute heart failure syndrome (AHFS) is new-onset or recurrent signs and symptoms of heart failure (HF) that gradually or rapidly grow worse and need emergency treatment. Dyspnea is the most common presenting symptom in patients hospitalized for AHFS, which suggests it is a clinically relevant therapeutic target and endpoint for clinical trials and regulatory approval efforts. Often standard therapy alone can improve dyspnea and other HF signs and symptoms, but many patients show persistent evidence of HF even when they are sent home. The post-discharge mortality and HF rehospitalization rates within 60 to 90 days are also high, up to 15% and 30%, respectively. New agents are needed that can safely improve HF during hospitalization and reduce early post-discharge events. Metra and associates studied whether early relief of dyspnea, defined as moderate to marked improvement after 24 and 48 hours, is related to changes in body weight and mortality 14 and 30 days after receiving rolofylline or placebo. Rolofylline did not improve a composite primary endpoint of death or HF rehospitalization, signs and symptoms of HF, or worsening renal function. A retrospective analysis of this study revealed that early dyspnea relief was associated with lower post-discharge mortality even after adjustments for some known prognostic factors. It was hypothesized that dyspnea would be a suitable surrogate for safety and/or an endpoint for mortality in AHFS trials. This offers several attractive features, but the data indicate that patients experiencing early relief of dyspnea had less severe HF at baseline. Current evidence suggests that improved clinical predictors of prognosis such as body weight, serum sodium levels, renal function, neurohormone levels, and central hemodynamics do not translate clinically into a direct mortality benefit.

Analysis.—Prognostic indicators are not necessarily causative mediators. Also, the mediator for one therapeutic intervention may not be a mediator for others, with known or unknown side effects sometimes obscuring benefits. Dyspnea is not a substitute for clinical outcomes such as rehospitalization for HF and mortality as endpoints in AHFS clinical trials. It is an important measure of symptomatic improvement and serves as an approval endpoint for Food and Drug Administration (FDA) and European Medicines Agency (EMA) trials. It indicates efficacy for short-term symptomatic relief.

Role as Primary Endpoint.—Standard therapy is the most effective and safest approach for improving symptoms such as dyspnea. However, some patients are discharged after inadequate treatment of dyspnea. Most patients are not severely dyspneic after 6 hours of standard therapy alone unless there is a contributing factor. However, many trials enroll patients up to 48 hours after admission for HF, thereby selecting patients who are the most refractory to standard therapy and the most likely to have lower blood pressure and baseline renal dysfunction, which may influence a treatment's efficacy. Few current studies use a standardized method to measure dyspnea and ensure data collection reproducibility, although a standard method has now been developed and should be useful in future attempts. Patients with very high pulmonary capillary wedge pressure (PCWP) may have minimal dyspnea, whereas patients with relatively lower PCWP can have severe dyspnea. HF rarely occurs in isolation; often there are medical co-morbid conditions that contribute to the dyspnea. Therefore dyspnea severity often does not correlate with other HF signs and symptoms. Finally, dyspnea is self-reported and can be perceived differently by different patient populations across the world.

Conclusions.—The high prevalence of dyspnea in patients with AHFS shows it is an important primary efficacy endpoint for short-term symptom improvement in clinical trials and regulatory approval processes. For it to continue as an important endpoint, it must be measured early, determined using uniform methods, and correlated with other relevant clinical signs and symptoms and biomarkers. Endpoints that focus on a single symptom ignore other symptoms and/or biomarkers of congestion and/or myocardial injury that may be highly relevant. A clinical composite endpoint requires moderate or marked improvement early in treatment. Conventional approaches permit patients who deteriorate and improve just because of more intense background therapy to be considered clinically improved. Clinical composite endpoints minimize the "noise" of background therapy intensification. Conventional approaches also eliminate patients who deteriorate and drop out of a study. Clinical composite approaches minimize bias inherent in considering just "completers" by including all patients, especially those whose clinical course worsened to the point that they dropped out of the study. Composite endpoints also consider not just signs and symptoms but also improved or preserved organ function that occurs as long as it is not at the expense of longer-term safety. The degree of "acceptable risk" is related to the degree and type of benefit produced.

▶ How do you reassure yourself that your interventions have improved the status of a patient who comes to the emergency department with heart failure? I think we are likely to use some easily observed characteristic such as dyspnea; however, would we judge it the same way? Is "the patient looks a lot better now" useful? Of course it is, but how would we apply the "better" in a standardized way?

The authors of this editorial considered that outcomes in heart failure research such as dyspnea may not be appropriate for every test. They mentioned one trial medication that improved dyspnea but increased dysrhythmias so that the long-term outcome of death was actually not better.

They also discussed the analysis of another study that suggested that as many as 50% of patients admitted did not have any improvement in their dyspnea. Was this because many patients were not ill enough to demonstrate significant respiratory distress? Or maybe there are some differences in what judgments are made when discharging patients who have been admitted in acute heart failure.

It is probably the case that better descriptions of subjects upon entry to a study need to be made—whether that is based on a physiologic status or comorbidities. For dyspnea, measurements must be standardized and then reliably used.

N. B. Handly, MD, MSc, MS

Hypertensive heart failure: patient characteristics, treatment, and outcomes
Peacock F, For the Stat Investigators (The Cleveland Clinic, OH; et al)
Am J Emerg Med 29:855-862, 2011

Background.—Acute heart failure (AHF) is a common, poorly characterized manifestation of hypertensive emergency. We sought to describe characteristics, treatment, and outcomes of patients with severe hypertension complicated by AHF.

Methods and Results.—The observational retrospective Studying the Treatment of Acute hypertension (STAT) registry records data on emergency department and hospitalized patients receiving intravenous therapy for blood pressure (BP) greater than 180/110 mm Hg in 25 US hospitals. A subset of patients with HF was defined as pulmonary edema on chest x-ray (CXR) or an elevated B-type natriuretic peptide level (BNP > 500 or NTproBNP > 900 pg/mL) in patients with creatinine level 2.5 mg/dL or less. Remaining STAT patients, after excluding those with a primary neurologic diagnosis, constitute the non-HF cohort. An adverse composite outcome was defined as mechanical ventilation, intensive care unit (ICU) admission, hospital length of stay more than 1 week, or death within 30 days. Of 1199 patients, 302 (25.2%) had AHF. Acute HF patients and non-AHF patients were similar in age, sex, and overall mortality, but AHF patients were more commonly African American, with a history of HF, diabetes or chronic obstructive pulmonary disease, and prior hypertension admissions. Heart failure patients had higher creatinine and natriuretic peptide levels but lower ejection fraction. They were more likely admitted to the ICU; receive electrocardiograms, bilevel positive airway pressure ventilation, and CXRs; and be readmitted within 90 days. Finally, BP decreases lower than 120 mm Hg within 12 hours were associated with an increased rate of the composite adverse outcome.

Conclusions.—Acute HF as a manifestation of hypertensive emergency is common, more likely in African Americans, and requires more clinical resources than patients with non–HF-related severe hypertension. Accurate BP control is critical, as declines less than 120 mm Hg were associated with increased adverse event rates (Table 6).

▶ Hypertensive crises, consisting of urgencies (without end-organ damage) and emergencies (with end-organ damage) are common and may result in 3% of all emergency department visits and up to 25% of all true medical emergencies. Hypertensive emergency end organ damage includes cerebral infarction, intracranial hemorrhage, pulmonary edema, hypertensive encephalopathy, aortic dissection, myocardial infarction, unstable angina with dynamic ST changes, acute renal failure, microangiopathic hemolytic anemia, and retinopathy. This

TABLE 6.—Blood Pressure Control Over Time Among HF Patients

	Composite Outcome (Mechanical Ventilation, ICU Admission, Hospital Length of Stay ≥7 d, Death at 30 d)		
	Yes (n = 195), n (%)	No (n = 107), n (%)	P
Systolic BP has been <120 within 1 h	9 (4.6)	2 (1.9)	.34[a]
Systolic BP has been <120 within 2 h	18 (9.2)	4 (3.7)	.08
Systolic BP has been <120 within 3 h	22 (11)	6 (5.6)	.10
Systolic BP has been <120 within 6 h	32 (16)	8 (7.5)	.029
Systolic BP has been <120 within 12 h	45 (23)	10 (9.4)	.003

Only outcomes associated with a BP less than 120 mm Hg are shown, as lowering the BP to levels greater than 120 mm Hg were not associated with any statistical improvements in adverse clinical outcome rates.
[a]Fisher exact test used due to the small cell values.

study paid most attention to the relationship between severe hypertension and heart failure.

The most critical finding in this study was that lowering blood pressure too aggressively, that is, systolic blood pressure less than 120, resulted in an increased risk of adverse events (see Table 6). Although this study was retrospective and in no way conclusive, emergency physicians should pay very close attention to its results. Physicians should treat patient symptoms and not numbers. Future prospective studies are needed to determine the best therapy, timing, and blood pressure targets for patients presenting with hypertension and heart failure/pulmonary edema, but I believe the majority of data supports high-dose nitroglycerin along with intravenous Lasix as first-line therapy. Care should be taken not to be too aggressive with blood pressure control. In my experience, the risk of dropping a patient's blood pressure too low is greatest in the period just after intubation when most of the patient's sympathetic drive is attenuated.

D. K. Mullin, MD

Natriuretic peptide testing in EDs for managing acute dyspnea: a meta-analysis
Trinquart L, Ray P, Riou B, et al (Evidence-based Medicine Ctr, Paris, France; UPMC Univ Paris 06, France)
Am J Emerg Med 29:757-767, 2011

Purposes.—The aim of the study was to assess the usefulness of systematic natriuretic peptide testing in the management of patients presenting with acute dyspnea to emergency departments (EDs).

Methods.—We performed a systematic review and meta-analysis of randomized controlled trials assessing the usefulness of B-type natriuretic peptide (BNP) or its N-terminal fragment (NT-proBNP) in the management of patients presenting with dyspnea into ED. We searched Medline, Embase, and conference proceedings without restriction on neither language nor publication year. Selection of studies, data collection, and assessment of risk of bias were performed by 2 reviewers independently and in duplicate. Outcomes included hospital admission rate, time to discharge, and length of hospital stay, mortality and rehospitalization rates, and total direct medical costs. Combined risk ratios were estimated using fixed or random effects model. Duration and cost data were not combined.

Findings.—Four randomized controlled trials, representing 2041 patients, were selected. In 4 trials, there was a tendency for hospital admission to be reduced in the intervention group (combined risk ratio, 0.95; 95% confidence interval, 0.89-1.01). Time to discharge was significantly reduced in 2 trials, whereas there was no significant reduction in hospital length of stay in 3 trials. There was no significant effect on in-hospital and 30-day mortality rates or rehospitalization rates (3 trials reporting each outcome). Two trials found significant reduction in direct costs.

Conclusions.—The current evidence remains inconclusive on whether systematic natriuretic peptide testing is useful for the management of patients presenting to ED with acute dyspnea.

▶ B-type natriuretic peptide (BNP) testing is commonplace in many emergency departments (ED) in the United States to assist the emergency physician when evaluating the dyspneic patient. Researchers in the attached meta-analysis ventured to determine whether the BNP diagnostic test results were actually useful in the evaluation and management of ED patients presenting with acute dyspnea. The data points were not only related to ED parameters. Paring down to the most relevant randomized clinical trials, the authors convey that the routine use of BNP testing is meager. Although length of stay and direct hospital costs were decreased, the rates of admission and/or readmission were unaffected. These conclusions may be related to the primary complaint. Patients presenting with undifferentiated dyspnea, where congestive heart failure is well within the differential, may be admitted regardless of the results of a BNP test. Once the diagnosis is made during the admission, BNP may provide guidance about overall clinical improvement for the ward-based physicians.

E. C. Bruno, MD

Short-term Mortality Risk in Emergency Department Acute Heart Failure
Peacock WF, Nowak R, Christenson R, et al (Cleveland Clinic Foundation, OH; Henry Ford Health System, Detroit, MI; Univ of Maryland School of Medicine, Baltimore; et al)
Acad Emerg Med 18:947-958, 2011

Objectives.—Few tools exist that provide objective accurate prediction of short-term mortality risk in patients presenting with acute heart failure (AHF). The purpose was to describe the accuracy of several biomarkers for predicting short-term death rates in patients diagnosed with AHF in the emergency department (ED).

Methods.—The Biomarkers in ACute Heart failure (BACH) trial was a prospective, 15-center, international study of patients presenting to the ED with nontraumatic dyspnea. Clinicians were blinded to all investigational markers, except troponin and natriuretic peptides, which used the local hospital reference range. For this secondary analysis, a core lab was used for all markers except troponin. This study evaluated patients diagnosed with AHF by the on-site emergency physician (EP).

Results.—In the 1,641 BACH patients, 466 (28.4%) had an ED diagnosis of AHF, of whom 411 (88.2%) had a final diagnosis of AHF. In the ED-diagnosed HF patients, 59% were male, 69% had a HF history, and 19 (4.1%) died within 14 days of their ED visit. The area under the curve (AUC) for the 14-day mortality receiver operating characteristic (ROC) curve was 0.484 for brain natriuretic peptide (BNP), 0.586 for N-terminal pro-B-type natriuretic peptide (NT-proBNP), 0.755 for troponin (I or T),

0.742 for adrenomedullin (MR-proADM), and 0.803 for copeptin. In combination, MR-proADM and copeptin had the best 14-day mortality prediction (AUC = 0.818), versus all other markers.

Conclusions.—MR-proADM and copeptin, alone or in combination, may provide superior short-term mortality prediction compared to natriuretic peptides and troponin. Presented results are explorative due to the limited number of events, but validation in larger trials seems promising.

▶ Acute congestive heart failure (aCHF) patients carry a significant mortality risk. Patients discharged from the emergency department have a 4% risk of death, whereas those patients warranting admission have a 5.7% risk.[1] The ability to identify which patients presenting with aCHF are more likely to have a catastrophic event would be ideal, and the authors of this project evaluated which, if any, clinically relevant biomarkers could predict an adverse event. Rather than using previously determined time endpoints of 30 or 90 days, the methods used more emergency medicine applicable outlooks of 7 and 14 days. The biomarkers assayed included B-type natriuretic peptide (BNP), midregion pro-atrial natriuretic peptide (MR-proANP), midregion pro-adrenomedullin (MR-proADM), copeptin, and troponin. Whereas MR-proADM, copeptin, and troponin all predicted short-term mortality (14-day), the combination of MR-proADM and copeptin was superior to each individual biomarker, with statistical significance, to predict both short- and long-term mortality. The growing availability of laboratory testing may soon lead to point-of-care testing of these biomarkers in patients presenting with acute dyspnea that is believed to be aCHF. In this study, the treating emergency physician determined the diagnosis of aCHF, based on the complete clinical assessment. Regrettably, codiagnoses were present in more than 33% of patients, which included pneumonia, acute coronary syndrome, arrhythmia, pulmonary embolism, and the dreaded catch-all "other." The EP, even in the presence of aCHF, must consider alternative etiologies for the patient's dyspnea. One confounding variable to this study's results is the extensive list of financially relevant relationships disclosed by the authors, which could allow for external influence and bias.

E. C. Bruno, MD

Reference

1. Lee DS, Schull MJ, Alter DA, et al. Early deaths in patients with heart failure discharged from the emergency department: a population-based analysis. *Circ Heart Fail.* 2010;3:228-235.

Miscellaneous

Acute myocarditis presenting as acute coronary syndrome: role of early cardiac magnetic resonance in its diagnosis

Monney PA, Sekhri N, Burchell T, et al (Barts and The London NHS Trust, UK)
Heart 97:1312-1318, 2011

Background.—In patients presenting with acute cardiac symptoms, abnormal ECG and raised troponin, myocarditis may be suspected after normal angiography.

Aims.—To analyse cardiac magnetic resonance (CMR) findings in patients with a provisional diagnosis of acute coronary syndrome (ACS) in whom acute myocarditis was subsequently considered more likely.

Methods and Results.—79 patients referred for CMR following an admission with presumed ACS and raised serum troponin in whom no culprit lesion was detected were studied. 13% had unrecognised myocardial infarction and 6% takotsubo cardiomyopathy. The remainder (81%) were diagnosed with myocarditis. Mean age was 45 ± 15 years and 70% were male. Left ventricular ejection fraction (EF) was $58 \pm 10\%$; myocardial oedema was detected in 58%. A myocarditic pattern of late gadolinium enhancement (LGE) was detected in 92%. Abnormalities were detected more frequently in scans performed within 2 weeks of symptom onset: oedema in 81% vs 11% (p<0.0005), and LGE in 100% vs 76% (p<0.005). In 20 patients with both an acute (<2 weeks) and convalescent scan (>3 weeks), oedema decreased from 84% to 39% (p<0.01) and LGE from 5.6 to 3.0 segments (p=0.005). Three patients presented with sustained ventricular tachycardia, another died suddenly 4 days after admission and one resuscitated 7 weeks following presentation. All 5 patients had preserved EF.

Conclusions.—Our study emphasises the importance of access to CMR for heart attack centres. If myocarditis is suspected, CMR scanning should be performed within 14 days. Myocarditis should not be regarded as benign, even when EF is preserved.

▶ Presentation concerning acute coronary syndrome, based on history, physical examination, and abnormal electrocardiogram findings, generally receive emergent cardiology evaluation and intervention. Cardiac catheterization is the intervention of choice but is nondiagnostic in approximately 10% of the cases. One alternate diagnosis is acute myocarditis. The authors of this observational cohort study suggest that cardiac magnetic resonance (CMR) imaging is the follow-up diagnostic tool to further evaluate for myocarditis. They present the CMR imaging protocol used at their facility. Patients were subsequently diagnosed with acute myocarditis in 81% of cases. Interestingly, CRM also found a missed myocardial infarction (MI) in 13% of the cases. Although emergency physicians are likely not responsible for the ordering of the CRM diagnostic test, knowledge of the missed MI rate is paramount, especially when consulting cardiologists about patients returning with chest pain postcardiac catheterization. In smaller hospitals with the requisite equipment, 24-hour availability of CRM is likely a battleground between radiologists and cardiologists.

E. C. Bruno, MD

Autologous Cardiomyotissue Implantation Promotes Myocardial Regeneration, Decreases Infarct Size, and Improves Left Ventricular Function
Wykrzykowska JJ, Rosinberg A, Lee SU, et al (Harvard Med School, Boston MA; Lenox Hill Hosp, NY; Kwangju Christian Hosp, Gwangju, Korea; et al)
Circulation 123:62-69, 2011

Background.—Cell therapy for myocardial infarction (MI) may be limited by poor cell survival and lack of transdifferentiation. We report a novel technique of implanting whole autologous myocardial tissue from preserved myocardial regions into infarcted regions.

Methods and Results.—Fourteen rats were used to optimize cardiomyotissue size with peritoneal wall implantation (300 μm identified as optimal size). Thirty-nine pigs were used to investigate cardiomyotissue implantation in MI induced by left anterior descending balloon occlusion (10 animals died; male-to-female transplantation for tracking with in situ hybridization for Y chromosome, n=4 [2 donors and 2 MI animals]; acute MI implantation cohort at 1 hour, n=13; and healed MI implantation at 2 weeks, n=12). Assessment included echocardiography, magnetic resonance imaging, hemodynamics, triphenyltetrazolium chloride staining, and histological and molecular analyses. Tracking studies demonstrated viable implants with donor cells interspersed in the adjacent myocardium with gap junctions and desmosomes. In the acute MI cohort, treated animals compared with controls had improved perfusion by magnetic resonance imaging (1.2 ± 0.01 versus 0.86 ± 0.05; $P<0.01$), decreased MI size (magnetic resonance imaging: left ventricle, $2.2 \pm 0.5\%$ versus $5.4 \pm 1.5\%$, $P=0.04$; triphenyltetrazolium chloride: anterior wall, $10.3 \pm 4.6\%$ versus $28.9 \pm 5.8\%$, $P<0.03$), and improved contractility (dP/dt, 1235 ± 215 versus 817 ± 817; $P<0.05$). In the healed MI cohort, treated animals had less decline in ejection fraction between 2 and 4 week assessment ($-3 \pm 4\%$ versus $-13 \pm -4\%$; $P<0.05$), less decline in $\pm$ dP/dt, and smaller MI (triphenyltetrazolium chloride, $21 \pm 11\%$ versus $3 \pm 8\%$; $P=0.006$) than control animals. Infarcts in the treated animals contained more mdr-1[+] cells and fewer c-kit[+] cells with a trend for decreased expression of matrix metalloproteinase-2 and increased expression of tissue inhibitor of metalloproteinase-2.

Conclusion.—Autologous cardiomyotissue implanted in an MI area remains viable, exhibits electromechanical coupling, decreases infarct size, and improves left ventricular function.

▶ Let's remind ourselves about types of prevention of disease by using the example of cardiac disease. Primary prevention would be the efforts to avoid any damage in the first place. Steps would include smoking avoidance and control of blood pressure and diabetes. Secondary prevention would include the steps to minimize the damage occurring at the time of a myocardial infarction, such as with aspirin and tissue plasminogen activator. Tertiary prevention would be applied to restore function after an acute myocardial infraction has already destroyed tissue. This is a report of an interesting approach for tertiary prevention.

The authors demonstrate a technique for injecting healthy septal cells into the central portion of an anterior infarct. These cells were observed to grow, make electrical connections, and preserve cardiac function. Part of their success is a result of enhancements in technique for transplanting myocardial tissue.

This is an interesting approach that needs further study, ultimately in humans. If successful in humans, I can imagine emergency physicians talking to our patients about this type of procedure.

N. B. Handly, MD, MSc, MS

Cardiac bone marrow cell therapy: the proof of the pudding remains in the eating

Janssens SP (Univ of Leuven, Belgium)
Eur Heart J 32:1697-1700, 2011

This editorial refers to 'Intracoronary infusion of mononuclear cells from bone marrow or peripheral blood compared with standard therapy in patients after acute myocardial infarction treated by primary percutaneous coronary intervention: results of the randomized controlled HEBE trial'[†], by A. Hirsch *et al.*, on page 1736, and 'Intracoronary autologous mononucleated bone marrow cell infusion for acute myocardial infarction: results of the randomized multicenter BONAMI trial'[‡], by J. Roncalli *et al.*, on page 1748.

▶ This editorial has a primary value in placing 2 recent studies of the use of adult bone marrow cells in treatment of post—myocardial infarction (MI) patients among prior experiments.

The safety of the cell therapy has not been a problem to date, and the 2 recent studies do not provide any different conclusions.

Study designs previously have not been consistent, some have not been randomized, and others have different inclusion criteria. The 2 discussed in this editorial were randomized and open (not blinded) and had somewhat different outcome measures. Meanwhile, no significant improvements in outcomes over standard therapy were found.

It could be that we have not found the right patients who would benefit from treatment, or perhaps we have not waited long enough to see the improvements. Regardless, the field of post-MI treatment is still waiting for breakthroughs.

N. B. Handly, MD, MSc, MS

CLUE: a randomized comparative effectiveness trial of IV nicardipine versus labetalol use in the emergency department

Peacock WF, Varon J, Baumann BM, et al (The Cleveland Clinic, OH; The Univ of Texas Health Science Ctr at Houston and The Univ of Texas Med Branch at Galveston; Cooper Univ Hosp, Camden, NJ; et al)
Critical Care 15:R157, 2011

Introduction.—Our purpose was to compare the safety and efficacy of food and drug administration (FDA) recommended dosing of IV nicardipine versus IV labetalol for the management of acute hypertension.

Methods.—Multicenter randomized clinical trial. Eligible patients had 2 systolic blood pressure (SBP) measures ≥180 mmHg and no contraindications to nicardipine or labetalol. Before randomization, the physician specified a target SBP ± 20 mmHg (the target range: TR). The primary endpoint was the percent of subjects meeting TR during the initial 30 minutes of treatment.

Results.—Of 226 randomized patients, 110 received nicardipine and 116 labetalol. End organ damage preceded treatment in 143 (63.3%); 71 nicardipine and 72 labetalol patients. Median initial SBP was 212.5 (IQR 197, 230) and 212 mmHg (IQR 200,225) for nicardipine and labetalol patients ($P = 0.68$), respectively. Within 30 minutes, nicardipine patients more often reached TR than labetalol (91.7 vs. 82.5%, $P = 0.039$). Of 6 BP measures (taken every 5 minutes) during the study period, nicardipine patients had higher rates of five and six instances within TR than labetalol (47.3% vs. 32.8%, $P = 0.026$). Rescue medication need did not differ between nicardipine and labetalol (15.5 vs. 22.4%, $P = 0.183$). Labetalol patients had slower heart rates at all time points ($P < 0.01$). Multivariable modeling showed nicardipine patients were more likely in TR than labetalol patients at 30 minutes (OR 2.73, $P = 0.028$; C stat for model = 0.72).

Conclusions.—Patients treated with nicardipine are more likely to reach the physician-specified SBP target range within 30 minutes than those treated with labetalol.

▶ In this randomized clinical trial, the researchers present the first emergency department comparison of nicardipine and labetolol for the management of acute hypertensive crisis. The researchers' primary goal was to quickly (within 30 minutes) obtain blood pressure control in the hypertensive patient and were able to demonstrate that patients receiving nicardipine were within predetermined blood pressure range more consistently than labetolol. Interestingly, more than 60% of patients enrolled in the study already had evidence of end-organ damage prior to any intervention. When cessation of further end-organ damage is necessary, nicardipine's increased success rate makes it a more attractive decision. Additionally, patients with established end-organ damage were more likely to respond to the nicardipine. This approached statistical significance.

If the initial medication choice is unsuccessful, rescue medications were selected. Rescue medications essentially translated to a crossover approach, because nicardipine and labetalol were the most commonly selected rescue substances.

E. C. Bruno, MD

Abnormally high prevalence of major components of the metabolic syndrome in subjects with early-onset idiopathic venous thromboembolism
Di Minno MND, Tufano A, Guida A, et al ("Federico II" Univ, Naples, Italy)
Thromb Res 127:193-197, 2011

Background.—Although patients with idiopathic VTE are at higher than normal risk of asymptomatic atherosclerosis and of cardiovascular events, the impact of cardiovascular risk factors on VTE is poorly understood.

Objective.—To assess the prevalence of the metabolic syndrome and of its components in patients with early-onset idiopathic VTE.

Methods.—As many as 323 patients referred to our Thrombosis Ward for a recent (<6-months) early-onset idiopathic venous thromboembolism (VTE), were compared with 868 gender- and age-matched subjects, in whom a history of venous thrombosis had been excluded, referred during the same period time to our Ward. All had undergone a clinical assessment for smoking habits and for the presence of the components of the metabolic syndrome.

Results.—The metabolic syndrome was detected in 76/323 cases (23.5%) and in 81/868 controls (9.3%) (p<0.001; OR:2.990; 95% C.I.:2.119-4.217). Smoking was more common in patients with idiopathic VTE than in controls. In addition to the metabolic syndrome as a whole, its major individual determinants (arterial hypertension, impaired fasting glucose plasma levels, abdominal obesity, hypertriglyceridemia, low HDL-cholesterol) significantly correlated with idiopathic VTE (p always <0.05). The prevalence of thrombotic events was lower in females than in males (p=0.000; OR:2.217), the latter being most often hypertensives, smokers, hypertriglyceridemics, carriers of a metabolic syndrome and of impaired fasting glucose than females. In a multivariate analysis, arterial hypertension, impaired fasting glucose, abdominal obesity, and hypercholesterolemia independently predicted idiopathic venous events.

Conclusions.—Both metabolic syndrome as a whole and its major components individually considered, independently predict early-onset idiopathic VTE (Table 4).

▶ Reviewing recorded data from their thrombosis ward, the authors of this Italian study looked to determine if metabolic syndrome was an independent risk factor for development of venous thromboembolism (VTE). Simply having a separate ward for thrombotic disease may increase the validity of this study. The studied population included patients with idiopathic VTE, defined by the absence of recognized risk factors (pregnancy, active malignancy, recent [< 3 months] surgery or trauma, fracture, immobilization, acute medical illness, use of oral contraceptives, long-distance travel, personal or family history of

TABLE 4.—Predictors of Idiopathic VTE: Linear Regression*

	β	p
Smoking habit	0.121	0.000
Impaired fasting glucose (IFG)	0.061	0.032
Visceral obesity	0.111	0.000
Hypertension	0.129	0.000
Low HDL-cholesterol	0.095	0.001
Inherited thrombophilia	0.062	0.024
Male Sex	0.118	0.000
Hypertriglyceridemia		0.880

*Method: Stepwise. Dependent variable VTE: Variable entered if p<0.05; removed if p>0.05.

arterial and/or venous thrombosis, or repeated spontaneous abortions). Metabolic syndrome markers (abdominal obesity, impaired fasting glucose levels, hypertension, and dyslipidemia [high triglycerides and low HDL-cholesterol]) were assessed in a dichotomous fashion (present or not) to pinpoint independent threats for VTE. Although not applicable in the emergency department, hypercoagulability panels were drawn to look for genetic mutation risks for VTE as well. With statistical significance, patients with metabolic syndrome were more likely to develop idiopathic VTE when compared with controls (23.3% vs 9.3%). Individual metabolic syndrome components also portend negative events, as seen in Table 4. These results should push emergency physicians to consider VTE in the patient who may otherwise be thought to be low risk according to a Wells score or PERC rule.

E. C. Bruno, MD

ED technicians can successfully place ultrasound-guided intravenous catheters in patients with poor vascular access
Schoenfeld E, Boniface K, Shokoohi H (George Washington Univ Med Ctr, DC)
Am J Emerg Med 29:496-501, 2011

Objective.—The objective of the study was to assess the success rate of emergency department (ED) technicians in placing ultrasound (US)-guided peripheral intravenous (IV) catheters.

Methods.—In this prospective, observational trial, 19 ED technicians were taught to use US guidance to obtain IV access. Training sessions consisted of didactic instruction and hands-on practice. The ED technicians were then prospectively followed. The US guidance for IV access was limited to patients with difficult access. The primary outcome was successful peripheral IV placement.

Results.—A total of 219 attempts were recorded, with a success rate of 78.5% (172/219). There was a significant correlation between operator experience and success rate. Complications were reported in 4.1% of patients and included 5 arterial punctures and 1 case of a transient paresthesia.

Conclusions.—Emergency department technicians can be taught to successfully place US-guided IVs in patients with difficult venous access. Teaching this skill to ED technicians increases the pool of providers available in the ED to obtain access in this patient population.

▶ Obtaining intravenous (IV) access in patients for whom that access is difficult is a common problem in the emergency department (ED). Requiring a physician to use alternate, time-consuming vascular access procedures in these patients can degrade physician efficiency and take them away from more urgent duties. As ultrasound becomes more commonplace in emergency medicine, it is only natural that its use will be expanded to other personnel. This study from George Washington University shows that emergency medical technicians (EMTs) can be taught to place ultrasound-guided IV catheters after a brief training session. Although the success rate in this study was slightly lower than in previous studies examining physicians and nurses, the data did demonstrate a learning curve. The greater the previous number of successful ultrasound-guided IVs placed, the higher the success rate. Furthermore, ED technicians with more years of experience in placing nonultrasound-guided IVs also had a higher success rate. Busy EDs, especially those with a sizeable number of difficult IV—access patients, should consider this strategy to decrease physician interruptions and potentially increase efficiency.

E. A. Ramoska, MD, MPHE

4 Gastrointestinal

A pilot study on potential new plasma markers for diagnosis of acute appendicitis
Thuijls G, Derikx JPM, Prakken FJ, et al (Maastricht Univ Med Centre, the Netherlands)
Am J Emerg Med 29:256-260, 2011

Background.—Diagnosis of acute appendicitis (AA) remains a surgical dilemma, with negative appendectomy rates of 5% to 40% and perforation suggestive for late operative intervention in 5% to 30%. The aim of this study is to evaluate new plasma markers, representing early neutrophil activation, to improve diagnostic accuracy in patients suspected for AA.

Materials and Methods.—Fifty-one patients who underwent surgery for AA were included (male-female = 28:23), and blood was sampled. Plasma concentrations of 2 neutrophil proteins were measured: lactoferrin (LF) and calprotectin (CP). Controls consisted of 27 healthy volunteers. C-reactive protein (CRP) and white blood cell count (WBC) concentrations were measured for routine patient care.

Results.—Median plasma concentrations for LF and CP were significantly higher in 51 patients with proven AA (665 and 766 ng/mL, respectively) than in 27 healthy volunteers (198 and 239 ng/mL, respectively), $P < .001$).

No clinically relevant correlation exists between the plasma levels of LF and CP and the conventional laboratory tests for CRP and WBC.

Conclusions.—Circulating LF and CP levels are significantly elevated in patients with appendicitis and are detectable in plasma using relatively simple and low-cost enzyme-linked immunosorbent assays. Furthermore, plasma levels of LF and CP give additional information to conventional markers WBC and CRP, making them potential new markers for AA diagnosis.

▶ The authors examined the plasma levels of 2 proteins expected to be elevated in acute appendicitis. These proteins, lactoferrin and calprotectin, had been found to be released by degranulating neutrophils as part of the inflammatory response.

In this study, the levels of these 2 proteins in patients with confirmed appendicitis were compared with those from healthy control subjects. Significant differences in the levels for both proteins were in fact found between the appendicitis sufferers and the healthy control subjects.

However, to really use these markers, 2 things have to happen. One is that a cutoff level of the quantity of these proteins that discriminates appendicitis from no appendicitis needs to be established. Second, values for these 2 proteins need to be collected from a broader variety of patients, not just those with appendicitis and those who are totally healthy (we would be interested in measuring the levels of these proteins in patients suffering from abdominal pain regardless of the underlying disease). Emergency department physicians are rarely going to have difficulties distinguishing between patients suffering from appendicitis and those who are healthy. The authors are correct that we need help in identifying those patients with abdominal pain who have appendicitis.

For the study described in this article, collection of samples had to occur before knowing if the patient actually had appendicitis. Over the course of the study, there must have been many more samples stored than were analyzed—certainly samples from patients who had abdominal pain without appendicitis would have been collected. It would have been easy to do a proper sensitivity and specificity test after matching diagnoses to samples. After all, it could not have been that measuring the level of the proteins was the obstacle for not doing a better study because the authors state that the tests were low costs.

We can think a bit more about the process of identifying cutoff levels to distinguish between those who need operative management and those who do not. There are 2 extremes we can consider here for the cutoff and defining of our patients. Because the authors did provide the scattergrams, we can actually discuss the extremes. One would be to find a group that had members who exclusively had the disease (no healthy patients) and would need to go to the operating room (no false positives). A simple cutoff above the greatest value of protein among the healthy patients would be used. However, about half of the patients with appendicitis had lactoferrin levels lower than the greatest level found in healthy subjects. For calprotectin, a little less than half of the patients with appendicitis had levels lower than the greatest level found in healthy subjects. Essentially half of the patients with appendicitis would not go to the operating room. The other approach would be to use the tests to find a group that contained all the patients with appendicitis (the group would include some healthy patients). Presumably all the patients in this group would need operative management (no false negatives). In this case, a simple cutoff below the lowest value found for patients with appendicitis would be used. For lactoferrin, about 90% of the healthy patients would be included in the appendicitis group. Using calprotectin, about 75% of the healthy patients would be included in the appendicitis group. Some risk of false positives or false negatives may be accepted and a cutoff choice between the 2 values discussed here may be established; however, the overlaps of memberships among those with appendicitis and those without are quite notable.

My analysis is somewhat simplistic because there may be some additional discriminative power of combining the 2 tests together. The information to better apply this combination cutoff is not shown in these results.

It may turn out that the level of these proteins could be helpful in identifying appendicitis from among other causes of abdominal pain. But I wonder whether there will be much discrimination using these protein levels between those with and those without appendicitis when comparing the results of patients who all have abdominal pain.

N. B. Handly, MD, MSc, MS

Acute cholecystitis in the elderly: use of computed tomography and correlation with ultrasonography
McGillicuddy EA, Schuster KM, Brown E, et al (Yale Univ School of Medicine, New Haven, CT)
Am J Surg 202:524-527, 2011

Background.—Elderly patients diagnosed with acute cholecystitis (AC) may undergo both ultrasonography (US) and computed tomography (CT).
Methods.—A total of 475 patients (age, >64 y) with AC were included.
Results.—Groups included US alone (n = 240), CT alone (n = 60), and CT + US (n = 168). Sixty patients (35.7%) in the US + CT group had inflammation in both studies, 34 (20.2%) had inflammation only on US, and 32 (19.0%) had inflammation only on CT. In the US + CT group, detection of cholelithiasis was not different, but mean common bile duct size did not correlate. There was no difference among the groups in age, sex, medical service admission, nonambulatory status, dementia, diabetes, or coronary artery disease. Peritonitis, leukocytosis, and acidosis were more frequent in the 2 groups undergoing CT. The cholecystectomy rate was lowest (and the complication rate was highest) in the CT + US group.
Conclusions.—CT often is used in the diagnosis of AC in the elderly, especially those with more acute presentations. CT and US findings may be complementary in AC.

▶ The evaluation of elderly patients with abdominal pain is certainly among the more difficult procedures that emergency physicians must perform. The elderly patient may complain of vague abdominal pain and present with few or no alarming findings despite the occurrence of a catastrophic process. On average, more than two-thirds of elderly patients presenting to the emergency department with abdominal pain are admitted, and nearly one-fifth go directly to the operating room. The most common surgical emergency is acute cholecystitis (AC).

This study, which was a retrospective review of all patients aged older than 65 admitted to a single hospital over a 10-year period with AC, was done to determine factors associated with using CT in the diagnosis of AC. Although the right upper quadrant ultrasound is considered the diagnostic adjunct of choice in the initial diagnosis of AC, the CT scan is generally used in the investigation of acute abdominal pain when other diagnoses such as diverticulitis, appendicitis, perforation, obstruction, abdominal aortic aneurysm, aortic dissection, mesenteric ischemia, and other diagnoses are more likely than AC. The results of this study should not be terribly surprising for most. Fifty percent of elderly patients with a final diagnosis of AC underwent a CT scan, likely because they showed the classic presentation of AC. Interestingly, in the group that had both a CT scan and right upper quadrant ultrasound, 12 patients without ultrasound findings had CT scan findings consistent with AC, and 23 patients with a negative CT scan had ultrasound findings concerning for AC.

Because this was a retrospective review of patients given a final diagnosis of AC, it was unable to demonstrate the major benefit of CT scan in undifferentiated abdominal pain—that being its ability to assist in ruling out other life-threatening intra-abdominal catastrophes. That said, rather than viewing the ultrasound as the modality of choice in ruling in or ruling out AC, clinicians may view ultrasound and CT scan as complementary.

D. K. Mullin, MD

Amoxicillin plus clavulanic acid versus appendicectomy for treatment of acute uncomplicated appendicitis: an open-label, non-inferiority, randomised controlled trial

Vons C, Barry C, Maitre S, et al (Hôpital Antoine Béclère (Assistance Publique-Hôpitaux de Paris and Université Paris XI), Clamart, France; Université Paris-Sud and Université Paris Descartes, France; et al)
Lancet 377:1573-1579, 2011

Background.—Researchers have suggested that antibiotics could cure acute appendicitis. We assessed the efficacy of amoxicillin plus clavulanic acid by comparison with emergency appendicectomy for treatment of patients with uncomplicated acute appendicitis.

Methods.—In this open-label, non-inferiority, randomised trial, adult patients (aged 18—68 years) with uncomplicated acute appendicitis, as assessed by CT scan, were enrolled at six university hospitals in France. A computer-generated randomisation sequence was used to allocate patients randomly in a 1:1 ratio to receive amoxicillin plus clavulanic acid (3 g per day) for 8—15 days or emergency appendicectomy. The primary endpoint was occurrence of postintervention peritonitis within 30 days of treatment initiation. Non-inferiority was shown if the upper limit of the two-sided 95% CI for the difference in rates was lower than 10 percentage points. Both intention-to-treat and per-protocol analyses were done. This trial is registered with ClinicalTrials.gov, number NCT00135603.

Findings.—Of 243 patients randomised, 123 were allocated to the antibiotic group and 120 to the appendicectomy group. Four were excluded from analysis because of early dropout before receiving the intervention, leaving 239 (antibiotic group, 120; appendicectomy group, 119) patients for intention-to-treat analysis. 30-day postintervention peritonitis was significantly more frequent in the antibiotic group (8%, n=9) than in the appendicectomy group (2%, n=2; treatment difference $5 \cdot 8$; 95% CI $0 \cdot 3—12 \cdot 1$). In the appendicectomy group, despite CT-scan assessment, 21 (18%) of 119 patients were unexpectedly identified at surgery to have complicated appendicitis with peritonitis. In the antibiotic group, 14 (12% [$7 \cdot 1—18 \cdot 6$]) of 120 underwent an appendicectomy during the first 30 days and 30 (29% [$21 \cdot 4—38 \cdot 9$]) of 102 underwent appendicectomy between 1 month and 1 year, 26 of whom had acute appendicitis (recurrence rate 26%; $18 \cdot 0—34 \cdot 7$).

Interpretation.—Amoxicillin plus clavulanic acid was not non-inferior to emergency appendicectomy for treatment of acute appendicitis. Identification of predictive markers on CT scans might enable improved targeting of antibiotic treatment.

▶ Cut the red wire. Cut the blue wire. With a sense of immediacy, throw the object, which explodes just before striking the wall. The object in question is the appendix, and the appendectomy scenario is the picture painted to patients and their families. Although appendicitis remains a surgical condition, recent evidence cited in this article suggest that nonoperative management with antibiotics is a viable option. The authors of this French noninferiority project endeavored to prove that nonoperative management of acute appendicitis is not an acceptable alternative. Referencing a 3% rate of complication, specifically postoperative bowel obstruction, the authors indicated that, if successful, treatment with antibiotics and supportive care would improve the risk-to-benefit ratio. Required patient demographics would include noncomplicated disease, limited comorbidities, no indication of malignancy, and reliable follow-up. The authors found that the risk of peritonitis within 30 days, a practice primary endpoint, was significantly higher in the antibiotics-only group, refuting previous evidence. If the antibiotics-only group was shown to be noninferior, a change in dogma would be possible. Not knowing the malpractice climate in France or the expectations of the French people when diagnosed with appendicitis, would this practice take hold in the United States? Also, would physicians be encouraged to prescribe amoxicillin plus clavulanic acid for all patients with gastrointestinal symptoms and nonspecific abdominal pain?

E. C. Bruno, MD

Effect of delay in presentation on rate of perforation in children with appendicitis
Narsule CK, Kahle EJ, Kim DS, et al (Hasbro Children's Hosp and Warren Alpert Med School of Brown Univ, Providence, RI)
Am J Emerg Med 29:890-893, 2011

Introduction.—Appendicitis is the most common emergency operation in children. The rate of perforation may be related to duration from symptom onset to treatment. A recent adult study suggests that the perforation risk is minimal in the first 36 hours and remains at 5% thereafter. We studied a pediatric population to assess symptom duration as a risk factor for perforation.

Methods.—We prospectively studied all children older than 3 years who underwent an appendectomy over a 22-month period.

Results.—Of 202 patients undergoing appendectomies, 197 had appendicitis. Median age was significantly lower in the perforated group, but temperature and leukocytosis were not. As expected, length of hospital stay was longer in the perforated group (4-13 vs 2-6 days). The incidence of perforation was 10% if symptoms were present for less than 18 hours. This incidence rose in a linear fashion to 44% by 36 hours. Prehospital delays were greater in patients with perforated appendicitis. However, in-hospital delay (from presentation to surgery) was less than 5 hours in the perforated group and 9 hours in the nonperforated group.

Discussion.—Appendiceal perforation in children is more common than in adults and correlates directly with duration of symptoms before surgery. Perforation is more common in younger children. Unlike in adults, the risk of perforation within 24 hours of onset is substantial (7.7%), and it increases in a linear fashion with duration of symptoms. In our experience, however, perforation correlates more with prehospital delay than with in-hospital delay.

▶ A perforated appendix, when discovered preoperatively, can increase the urgency of further interventions. Considering all patients diagnosed with appendicitis and taken for operative intervention, the authors compared the differences between patients identified with perforations to those without perforation. Patients who tended to have perforations were generally younger and presented later in the course of the illness. These results emphasized both the challenges of evaluating young patients with fever and/or gastrointestinal illnesses and the importance of early assessment and rapid intervention. Contrary to perpetuated dogma, the authors found no statistically significant difference in white blood cell count or temperature when comparing the perforated group to the nonperforated group. Excluded from the study population were 6 cases of pathologically normal appendices, but no mention was made how the diagnosis of appendicitis was made to prompt the negative appendix laparotomy. This would calculate to an acceptable negative laparotomy rate of approximately 3%.

E. C. Bruno, MD

Is nasogastric tube lavage in patients with acute upper GI bleeding indicated or antiquated?

Pallin DJ, Saltzman JR (Brigham and Women's Hosp, Boston, MA)
Gastrointest Endosc 74:981-984, 2011

Background.—Nasogastric (NG) lavage is commonly performed for patients suspected of having acute upper gastrointestinal (GI) bleeding. A bloody NG aspirate is a good predictor of discovering a high-risk lesion on upper endoscopy, but NC lavage is also one of the most painful procedures commonly performed in the emergency department (ED). Evidence-based medicine indicates that the correlation between a positive NG aspirate and finding a high-risk lesion represents a surrogate endpoint and does not confirm patient benefit. With no prospective randomized trial results available the value of NG lavage and urgency of endoscopy has rested on clinical criteria alone or the use of validated GI bleeding risk prognostic scores. However, a trial using an observational design was conducted to approximate a randomized trial.

Methods.—Of the 632 patients admitted with upper GI bleeding, 386 patients were divided into 193 closely matched pairs using propensity matching. One patient in each pair had NG lavage and one did not. The relevant outcomes assessed included 30-day mortality, length of hospital stay, transfusion requirement, and need for emergency surgery. The process of care, performance, and timing of endoscopy were also evaluated.

Results.—Mortality at 30 days and hospital length of stay were similar for those who had NG lavage and those who did not. Slightly more blood was used for the NG lavage patients, and they were also slightly more likely to need emergency surgery compared to those who did not have this procedure. The latter differences were not significant. Patients who had NG lavage were more like to undergo endoscopy than those who did not and to have the imaging done earlier. NG lavage did not, however, help patients in terms of outcome.

Conclusions.—NG lavage does not improve the care of patients in the ED who have acute upper GI bleeding. Although a positive NG lavage finding correlates with high-risk lesions, performing this procedure does not predict clinical outcome. Thus for patients with acute upper GI bleeding NG lavage should not be considered necessary.

▶ This is a great editorial done by an emergency physician and a gastroenterologist from Brigham and Women's Hospital. It comes to the same conclusion that I have had for several years about the use of nasogastric (NG) lavage in the management of upper gastrointestinal (GI) bleeding—that the practice of NG lavage is antiquated and does not help patients in the emergency department with acute upper GI bleeding.

The authors mention that NG lavage is an intuitively logical procedure for the evaluation of the patient suspected of having acute upper GI bleeding. Additionally, a grossly bloody aspirate appears to be a good predictor of finding a high-risk lesion. Previous studies have found that 45% of patients with a blood aspirate had high-risk lesions on endoscopy versus 15% of those with only a clear or bilious aspirate. Unfortunately, NG lavage is one of the most painful procedures an emergency physician can perform on a patient. A previous study of the 15 most common procedures performed in the emergency department found that NG lavage was the most painful, more so than abscess incision and drainage, fracture reduction, urethral catheterization, lumbar puncture, and arterial blood gas collection.

Just because a positive NG lavage correlates to a high-risk lesion does not imply patient benefit. The important, precise evidentiary question is whether a negative finding on NG lavage can accurately identify patients in whom endoscopy can be safely delayed. As per these authors, when using the most conservative approach to current data, the positive predictive value was 32%, and the negative predictive value 85%. When using the most liberal approach, the positive and negative predictive values were 45% and 80%, respectively. Is a negative predictive value of 80% to 85% sufficient to reassure gastroenterologists that endoscopy can wait? These authors think not!

Current recommendations state that most patients with acute upper GI bleeding should undergo an early endoscopy within 24 hours of presentation. Emergency physicians, in consultation with gastroenterologists, must decide which patients need even more emergent endoscopy. Unfortunately for physicians, and fortunately for patients, NG lavage should not factor in that decision.

D. K. Mullin, MD

Peritoneal fluid cultures rarely alter management in patients with ascites
Chinnock B, Gomez R, Hendey GW (Univ of California San Francisco-Fresno)
J Emerg Med 40:21-24, 2011

Study Objective.—The objective of this study is to determine if the peritoneal fluid culture results in the ascites patient being evaluated for spontaneous bacterial peritonitis (SBP) in the Emergency Department (ED) are used by the inpatient physician to appropriately alter empiric antibiotic treatment.

Methods.—We performed a retrospective study of all ascitic fluid samples sent from the ED between January 1, 2002 and December 31, 2004. Exclusion criteria included peritoneal fluid samples sent from peritoneal dialysis patients and those undergoing diagnostic peritoneal lavage for trauma. Medical records were examined to determine culture results, initial antibiotic choices, and subsequent changes in antibiotics by the inpatient physician in response to the culture results. The primary outcome measure was the percentage of cases in which ED peritoneal fluid culture results caused inpatient physicians to appropriately change antibiotic coverage.

Results.—There were 201 ascitic fluid samples, of which 7 (3.5%; 95% confidence interval [CI] 1.4%−7.0%) had a pathogen identified. Of these, only 1 (0.5%; 95% CI .01%−2.4%) resulted in an appropriate change in empiric antibiotic therapy. Although there were additional opportunities for appropriately using the culture results to change the antibiotic coverage in 2 (1%; 95% CI 0.1%−3.6%) patients, coverage was not changed. In fact, it was changed inappropriately in these 2 patients, and in an additional patient on appropriate empiric therapy.

Conclusions.—The yield from ascitic fluid cultures was low, and when positive, did not appropriately change management according to microbiologic criteria.

▶ The cirrhotic patient presenting with abdominal pain remains a diagnostic dilemma because spontaneous bacterial peritonitis (SBP) is well within the differential, along with other intra-abdominal processes. Reluctantly, emergency physicians can be finessed by the admitting team, citing diagnostic and therapeutic reasons, into performing a paracentesis. With concerns of complications related to coagulopathy, one questions whether the paracentesis is actually necessary—that is, do the results of the paracentesis, particularly fluid culture, direct care decisions? The researchers of this retrospective review scrutinized charts of cirrhotic patients who received paracentesis for presumed SBP to determine whether culture results influenced antibiotic selection. Although the authors concluded that the culture results did not alter management, the results raise a separate question. Should paracentesis be performed at all?

Of 201 procedures, only 7 (3.5%) had positive culture results. In this study, a patient was more likely (4.5%) to have a contaminated culture, and the overwhelming majority of the microbial tests were negative (92%). An emergency physician treating a cirrhotic patient presenting with abdominal pain should consider SBP, even starting empiric antibiotics, but should also rule out other intra-abdominal pathology concurrently.

E. C. Bruno, MD

Randomized Clinical Trial of Rapid Versus 24-Hour Rehydration for Children With Acute Gastroenteritis
Powell CVE, Priestley SJ, Young S, et al (Royal Children's Hosp, Melbourne, Australia; Sunshine Hosp, Melbourne, Australia; et al)
Pediatrics 128:e771-e778, 2011

Objective.—To compare the efficacy of 2 nasogastric rehydration regimens for children with acute viral gastroenteritis.

Methods.—Children 6 to 72 months of age with acute viral gastroenteritis and moderate dehydration were recruited from emergency departments (EDs) at 2 metropolitan, pediatric, teaching hospitals. After clinical assessment of the degree of dehydration, patients were assigned randomly to receive either standard nasogastric rehydration (SNR) over 24 hours in the hospital ward or rapid nasogastric rehydration (RNR) over 4 hours in the ED. Primary (>2% weight loss, compared with the admission weight) and secondary treatment failures were assessed.

Results.—Of 9331 children with acute gastroenteritis who were screened, 254 children were assigned randomly to receive either RNR ($n = 132$ [52.0%]) or SNR ($n = 122$ [48.0%]). Baseline characteristics for the 2 groups were similar. All patients made a full recovery without severe adverse events. The primary failure rates were similar for RNR (11.8% [95% confidence interval [CI]: 6.0%—17.6%]) and SNR (9.2% [95% CI: 3.7%—14.7%]; $P = .52$). Secondary treatment failure was more common in the SNR group (44% [95% CI: 34.6%—53.4%]) than in the RNR group (30.3% [95% CI: 22.5%—38.8%]; $P = .03$). Discharge from the ED after RNR failed for 27 patients (22.7%), and another 9 (7.6%) were readmitted to the hospital within 24 hours.

Conclusions.—Primary treatment failure and clinical outcomes were similar for RNR and SNR. Although RNR generally reduced the need for hospitalization, discharge home from the ED failed for approximately one-fourth of the patients.

▶ Children presenting with signs and symptoms of acute gastroenteritis and related dehydration require fluid resuscitation. The administration of oral rehydration therapy is a viable alternative to standard intravenous therapy. The authors of this attached study advocate the use of oral rehydration therapy, administered through a nasogastric tube, citing lower risk of complications, including electrolyte imbalances, cerebral edema, and/or phlebitis. The speed of rehydration has been called into question. In this prospective, randomized, clinical trial, researchers compared rapid rehydration (over 4 hours) with standard rehydration (over 24 hours). They demonstrated similar outcomes in each group. Although rapid rehydration resulted in less need for hospital admission, approximately 25% of patients in this group returned within 24 hours for readmission to the hospital.

All patients received the most noxious emergency medicine procedure, the nasogastric tube, yet the authors provided antiemetic medications to none of them. A more suitable approach to these stable patients is to encourage them to drink the required trial of oral rehydration therapy after receiving an antiemetic.

E. C. Bruno, MD

The Treatment of Pediatric Gastroenteritis: A Comparative Analysis of Pediatric Emergency Physicians' Practice Patterns

Freedman SB, Sivabalasundaram V, Bohn V, et al (Univ of Toronto, Ontario, Canada; et al)
Acad Emerg Med 18:38-45, 2011

Objectives.—Acute gastroenteritis is a very common emergency department (ED) diagnosis accounting for greater than 1.5 million outpatient visits and 200,000 hospitalizations annually among children in the United States. Although guidelines exist to assist clinicians, they do not clearly address topics for which evidence is new or limited, including the use of antiemetic agents, probiotics, and intravenous (IV) fluid rehydration regimens. This study sought to describe the ED treatments administered to children with acute gastroenteritis and to compare management between Canadian and U.S. physicians practicing pediatric emergency medicine (PEM).

Methods.—Members of PEM research networks located in Canada and the United States were invited to participate in a cross-sectional, Internet-based survey. Participants were included if they are attending physicians and provide care to patients <18 years of age in an ED.

Results.—In total, 235 of 339 (73%) eligible individuals responded. A total of 103 of 136 Canadian physicians (76%) report initiating oral rehydration therapy (ORT) in children with moderate dehydration, compared with 44 of 94 (47%) of their U.S. colleagues ($p < 0.001$). The latter more often administer antiemetic agents to children with vomiting (67% vs. 45%; $p = 0.001$). American physicians administer larger IV fluid bolus volumes ($p < 0.001$) and over shorter time periods ($p = 0.001$) and repeat the fluid boluses more frequently ($p < 0.001$). Probiotics are routinely recommended by only 35 of 230 respondents (15%).

Conclusions.—The treatment of pediatric gastroenteritis varies by geographic location and differs significantly between Canadian and American PEM physicians. Oral rehydration continues to be underused, particularly in the United States. Probiotic use remains uncommon, while ondansetron administration has become routine. Children frequently receive IV rehy-dration, with the rate and volume administered being greater in the United States.

▶ Emergency physicians strive to meet or exceed the standard of care, and when a subspecialty within emergency medicine exists, the members of these subspecialties strongly influence the definition of the standard. This cross-sectional survey of pediatric emergency medicine (PEM) physicians assessed practice patterns in the management and disposition of children with presumed acute gastroenteritis (AGE), indirectly defining the standard of care. The article did not seek to define AGE, nor did it suggest compliance with a specific guide-line. The survey simply asked PEM physicians about their general approach to AGE. The surveyors found that PEM physicians generally use oral rehydration therapy (ORT), with oral rehydration solution as the fluid of choice, and pair ORT with the antiemetic ondansetron. However, PEM physicians are not rec-ommending the use of probiotics, antidiarrheal agents, antisecretory agents, or supplemental zinc with any frequency.

The survey disclosures divulge the general practice pattern of PEM physi-cians in the management of pediatric patients with AGE and provides EPs with guidance for treatment and documented support when discussing the management options with patients, parents, and families.

E. C. Bruno, MD

Clinical triage decision vs risk scores in predicting the need for endotherapy in upper gastrointestinal bleeding
Farooq FT, Lee MH, Das A, et al (Gastro One, Memphis, TN; Univ Hosps Case Med Ctr, Cleveland, OH; Mayo Clinic, Scottsdale, AZ)
Am J Emerg Med 30:129-134, 2012

Background.—Acute upper gastrointestinal hemorrhage (UGIH) is a common reason for hospitalization with substantial associated morbidity, mortality, and cost. Differentiation of high- and low-risk patients using established risk scoring systems has been advocated.

The aim of this study was to determine whether these scoring systems are more accurate than an emergency physician's clinical decision making in predicting the need for endoscopic intervention in acute UGIH.

Methods.—Patients presenting to a tertiary care medical center with acute UGIH from 2003 to 2006 were identified from the hospital database, and their clinical data were abstracted. One hundred ninety-five patients met the inclusion criteria and were included in the analysis. The clinical Rockall score and Blatchford score (BS) were calculated and compared with the clinical triage decision (intensive care unit vs non-intensive care unit admission) in predicting the need for endoscopic therapy.

Results.—Clinical Rockall score greater than 0 and BS greater than 0 were sensitive predictors of the need for endoscopic therapy (95% and 100%) but were poorly specific (9% and 4%), with overall accuracies of 41% and 39%. At higher score cutoffs, clinical Rockall score greater than 2 and BS greater than 5 remained sensitive (84% and 87%) and were more specific (29% and 33%), with overall accuracies of 48% and 52%. Clinical triage decision, as a surrogate for predicting the need for endoscopic therapy, was moderately sensitive (67%) and specific (75%), with an overall accuracy (73%) that exceeded both risk scores.

Conclusions.—The clinical use of risk scoring systems in acute UGIH may not be as good as clinical decision making by emergency physicians.

▶ This retrospective study from the Division of Gastroenterology and Liver Disease at University Hospitals Case Medical Center in Cleveland looked at patients admitted through the emergency department with upper gastrointestinal hemorrhage (UGIH) and whether they required endoscopic therapy. The need for endoscopic therapy was defined as injection of saline, epinephrine, or sclerosants and application of clips, bands, or thermal therapy (heat probe, bipolar electrocoagulation, and argon plasma coagulation) as well as bleeding that resulted in death or required emergency surgery, transjugular intrahepatic portosystemic shunt, or balloon tamponade. It purports to show that clinical decision making by emergency physicians is at least as good as, and more likely better than, using a risk scoring system in predicting the need for endoscopic therapy in UGIH. That inference is certainly consistent with the conclusions of other efforts that have sought to develop clinical prediction rules for complex medical problems. In general, it appears that the decision-making acumen of experienced clinicians seems to outperform clinical decision rules for complicated medical issues.

However, there is a major limitation to this study. The clinical triage decision of admission to the intensive care unit (ICU) versus admission to a non-ICU setting was used as a surrogate marker for predicting the need for endoscopic therapy. Just because an emergency physician thinks a patient belongs in the ICU does not equate with the need for endoscopic therapy. Moreover, the decision to admit to an ICU may also be affected by various other factors, such as bed availability and recommendations from consulting physicians.

E. A. Ramoska, MD, MPHE

5   Neurology

An analysis of admissions from 155 United States hospitals to determine the influence of weather on stroke incidence
Cowperthwaite MC, Burnett MG (NeuroTexas Inst at St. David's HealthCare, Austin)
J Clin Neurosci 18:618-623, 2011

Weather is the most frequently proposed factor driving apparent seasonal trends in stroke admissions. Here, we present the largest study of the association between weather and ischemic stroke in the USA to date. We consider admissions to 155 United States hospitals in 20 states during the five-year period from 2004 to 2008. The data set included 196,439 stroke admissions, which were classified as ischemic ($n = 98,930$), hemorrhagic ($n = 18,960$), or transient ischemic attack ($n = 78,549$). Variations in stroke admissions were tested to determine if they tracked seasonal and transient weather patterns over the same time period. Using autocorrelation analyses, no significant seasonal changes in stroke admissions were observed over the study period. Using time-series analyses, no significant association was observed between any weather variable and any stroke subtype over the five-year study. This study suggests that seasonal associations between weather and stroke are highly confounded, and an association between weather and stroke is virtually non-existent. Therefore, previous studies reporting an association between specific weather patterns and stroke should be interpreted with caution.

▶ The human cognitive process likes to look for patterns. In the emergency or obstetrics worlds, you may hear someone talk about increased patient arrival based on the phase of the moon. There are likely patterns in the circadian cycle that influence cardiac events and probably other physiological responses. In this study, the authors examine relationships between weather and the incidence of stroke.

There has been some work in the past that suggested that stroke incidence and weather are related in some way, but the results of the studies are inconsistent. In this study, the authors have access to a large database of stroke admissions and local weather.

They made the decision to look for relations between stroke incidence and acute weather changes occurring over 24 to 72 hours (they found no such pattern). However, there may not be a reason to filter out absolute values of weather: could strokes be more likely when the weather is hot? The authors were in a good position to test weather patterns other than just acute changes over days.

There may be another design flaw because the authors chose to group ischemic and hemorrhagic strokes with transient ischemic attacks. Ischemic and transient ischemic events may be closely enough related to be considered together, but hemorrhagic strokes may well represent enough difference in immediate triggers that all 3 of these strokes should not be grouped as a single dependent variable.

N. B. Handly, MD, MSc, MS

Biomarkers for Stroke: In Search of Fingerprints
Bettermann K (Penn State College of Medicine, Hershey, PA)
J Stroke Cerebrovasc Dis 20:173-176, 2011

Background.—Cardiac enzymes are widely used to diagnose acute myocardial infarction but comparable biomarkers for acute brain injury, such as stroke, remain elusive. The complexity of the ischemic cascade makes it difficult to isolate brain-specific biomarkers. Any marker of brain tissue injury must also be able to cross the blood-brain barrier and be released into the bloodstream in quantities sufficient to be detected on a blood test.

Ideal Characteristics.—Stoke biomarkers must be brain-specific, sufficiently sensitive and specific, detectable in blood within minutes of symptom onset, and inexpensively and readily measurable. The biomarker's concentration should reflect lesion size, location, and functional outcome. Predictive value must be comparable to the sensitivity and specificity of brain magnetic resonance imaging (MRI), which is the gold standard for stroke diagnosis. Stroke biomarkers would be reliable and cost-effective clinically only if they help diagnose and classify stroke, anticipate outcome, and assess complication risks. They should also help diagnose acute stroke in patients who lack access to advanced neuroimaging and provide timely identification and triage of patients to thrombolysis or interventional therapy. Stroke biomarkers would also ideally differentiate ischemic from hemorrhagic stroke and stroke from other conditions. If sufficiently sensitive and specific for diagnosing transient ischemic attack and evolving infarction, biomarkers could be used to trigger hospital admission for acute management for at-risk patients, thus avoiding misdiagnosis and discharge without the right treatment. Currently no single or panel of biomarkers has proved sufficiently specific and sensitive and been validated by large clinical trials.

Current Candidates.—A panel of 26 biomarkers permitted the diagnosis of ischemic stroke within 24 hours of symptom onset (sensitivity 90%, specificity 90%). This panel included protein S100B, matrix metallopeptidase 9 (MMP-9), vascular cell adhesion molecule, and von Willebrand factor. Brain natriuretic peptide, C-reactive protein, D-dimer, MMP-9, and protein S100B were able to diagnose ischemic stroke (sensitivity 81%, specificity 70%). N-methyl diaspartate receptor peptide, an indicator of glutamate excitotoxicity associated with acute stroke pathophysiology, has diagnosed acute ischemic stroke within 3 hours of symptom onset (sensitivity 97%, specificity 98%). Combined with biomarkers for intracranial hemorrhage, N-methyl diaspartate receptor peptide differentiated hemorrhagic from ischemic stroke (sensitivity 79%, specificity 98%). Midregional proatrial natriuretic peptide (MR-proANP) levels were elevated in patients with more severe stroke, history of heart failure, atrial fibrillation, and increased mortality, with the risk of poor outcome at 3 months four times higher than for patients without elevated levels. MR-proANP levels are higher in patients with cardioembolic stroke than in those with noncardioembolic stroke, making this biomarker potentially useful in etiologic distinctions, which can guide stroke prevention strategies. Copeptin has also been related to poor outcome and increased mortality after ischemic stroke.

Biomarkers studied for the ability to predict hemorrhagic transformation after thrombolytic therapy include apolipoproteins CI and CIII. These proteins were expressed at different levels after stroke within 6 hours of symptom onset. CIII could differentiate ischemic from hemorrhagic stroke (sensitivity 94%, specificity 87%).

Advances in proteomics offer promise for identifying multiple potential stroke biomarkers. Similar strides in genomics target millions of genes and their protein products over a short period, showing patterns in gene up-regulation and down-regulation related to brain injury and cell repair. Although messenger RNA expression studies are highly promising, few results are available. Gene array analysis identified virsinin-like protein 1 as a potential acute blood-borne marker of ischemic stroke. Spinal fluid studies have identified PARK7 protein and nucleoside diphosphate kinase A as possible candidates. Ischemic stroke was diagnosed by PARK7 (sensitivity 58%, specificity 90%) and by nucleoside diphosphate kinase A (sensitivity 67%, specificity 90%).

Participants in coagulation and platelet activation are also being studied. Human studies of stroke with oligonucleotide microarrays show reproducible gene expression patterns within 4 hours after ischemic stroke. Genes expressing amphiphysin and interleukin-1 receptor 2 can help identify ischemic stroke subtypes. Real-time polymerase chain reaction studies reflect and predict tissue and related clinical outcomes.

Stroke prediction biomarkers should be able to identify persons at risk for an initial or recurrent stroke and guide therapeutic decisions by analyzing the effectiveness of interventions. Both genetic and genomic factors related to vascular disease reflect a predisposition to stroke. Only 60% of all strokes are related to modifiable factors; the other 40% are likely related to genetic, environmental, or unknown mechanisms. Stroke risk in general and high-risk populations can be assessed using genome-wide relationships, gene expression profiling, proteomics, and metabolomics. Gene expression profiling allows assessment of the entire transcriptome from RNA expression to protein and metabolite production, capturing genetic variations that change functional status as well as environmentally induced alterations in gene expression. The effectiveness of therapy can also be monitored over time. Variants of gene expression that increase the risk of stroke are already used in assessing young stroke patients, who often have nontraditional causes of stroke.

Conclusions.—The studies that have been done or are underway show multiple potential applications of stroke biomarkers. Much must still be learned before stroke biomarkers can be used routinely to improve diagnosis and patient management. Clinical usefulness and cost-effectiveness also must be established before biomarkers can be reliably employed in clinical practice.

▶ This editorial and short review of the state of research in stroke biomarkers is instructive for both the goals and strategies in this endeavor. Of course, we want timeliness, accuracy of results to avoid errors, broad applicability for managing all types of stroke occurrence, and even the ability to predict outcomes.

This is a big order to fill, not surprisingly. Markers from brain tissue ordinarily are unlikely to cross the blood-brain barrier (perhaps those that appear after stroke do indicate the disruption of this barrier), and those that diffuse into the cerebrospinal fluid are not as easily accessible as would be markers in peripheral blood.

Imagine a substance A is found after a stroke with relative good accuracy and specificity. An attempt may be made to neutralize the now identified Marker A to somehow reduce the consequences of stroke, but without success. This kind of result is not that surprising; markers are not necessarily the same as mediators of disease.

We would benefit not only from markers but also from methods to test for those markers that are less invasive and simple to use. Biosensors that could detect such markers through intact skin would likely improve the application of the measures.

N. B. Handly, MD, MSc, MS

TWO ACES: Transient Ischemic Attack Work-Up as Outpatient Assessment of Clinical Evaluation and Safety
Olivot J-M, Wolford C, Castle J, et al (Stanford Univ Med Ctr, CA; Pritzker School of Medicine, Evanston, IL)
Stroke 42:1839-1843, 2011

Background and Purpose.—To evaluate a novel emergency department-based TIA triage system.

Methods.—We developed an approach to TIA triage and management based on risk assessment using the $ABCD^2$ score in combination with early cervical and intracranial vessel imaging. It was anticipated that this triage system would avoid hospitalization for the majority of TIA patients and result in a low rate of recurrent stroke. We hypothesized that the subsequent stroke rate among consecutively encountered patients managed with this approach would be lower than predicted based on their ABCD^2 scores.

Results.—From June 2007 to December 2009, 224 consecutive patients evaluated in the Stanford emergency department for a possible TIA were enrolled in the study. One hundred fifty-seven were discharged to complete their evaluation at the outpatient TIA clinic; 67 patients were hospitalized. One hundred sixteen patients had a final diagnosis of TIA/minor stroke or possible TIA. The stroke rates at 7, 30, and 90 days were 0.6% (0.1%−3.5%) for patients referred to the TIA clinic and 1.5% (0.3%−8.0%) for the hospitalized patients. Combining both groups, the overall stroke rate was 0.9% (0.3%−3.2%), which is significantly less than expected based on ABCD^2 scores (P=0.034 at 7 days and P=0.001 at 90 days).

Conclusions.—This emergency department-based inpatient versus outpatient TIA triage system led to a low rate of hospitalization (30%). Recurrent stroke rates were low for both the hospitalized and outpatient subgroups.

▶ This paper from the Stanford Stroke Center assesses their experience with an emergency department (ED)-based transient ischemic attack (TIA) triage system using the ABCD^2 score and cervical and intracranial vascular imaging. They discharged 157 of 224 consecutive patients (70%) who were evaluated in the ED for suspicion of TIA over a 2-year and 4-month period. The median time between ED encounter and TIA clinic follow-up was 3 days (interquartile range = 2-5). Only 30% of the patients were seen within the first 3 days, whereas two-thirds were seen more than 3 days after the ED visit. Four patients declined to attend the TIA clinic, and 1 patient (0.6%, 95% confidence interval = 0.01%-3.04%) had a stroke and was hospitalized before the expected clinic visit. Many of the patients (92%) had vascular imaging before the clinic visit; however, nearly two-thirds of these studies were performed in the ED before the patient was discharged. Even with this, however, the authors note that the median delay to MRI/MRA was longer than that currently recommended by the American Heart Association (recommendation = 24 hours). One serious limitation to generalizing these results is that the population studied may have a higher socioeconomic status than other populations and for this reason might be more likely to follow up and/or adhere to secondary stroke prevention recommendations.

It must have taken a fair amount of ED resources to get vascular imaging in the 91 patients who had it before they were discharged. The authors do not mention the length of stay for any of the study patients, whether admitted or discharged. Did the extra time in the ED needed to complete this workup contribute to crowding? Finally, we are still left with the fact that one patient had a stroke before being able to follow up in the TIA clinic (the upper limit of the 95% confidence interval is 3%). Would this 1 adverse event have led to legal action? Would the expense of addressing this adverse event have surpassed the cost savings of the entire strategy? These questions remain unanswered. At this point in time, whether this approach can be effective and efficient in a community hospital ED serving a different patient population is anyone's guess.

E. A. Ramoska, MD, MPHE

Use of biomarkers in triage of patients with suspected stroke

Vanni S, Polidori G, Pepe G, et al (Azienda Ospedaliero-Universitaria Careggi, Florence, Italy; et al)
J Emerg Med 40:499-505, 2011

Background.—The absence of a rapidly available and sensitive diagnostic test represents an important limitation in the triage of patients with suspected stroke.

Objectives.—The aim of the present study was to investigate the triage accuracy of a novel test that measures blood-borne biomarkers (triage stroke panel, TSP) and to compare its accuracy with that of the Cincinnati Prehospital Stroke Scale (CPSS).

Methods.—Consecutive patients with suspected stroke presenting to the Emergency Departments of three Italian hospitals underwent triage by a trained nurse according to the CPSS and had blood drawn for TSP testing. The TSP simultaneously measures four markers (B-type natriuretic peptide, D-dimer, matrix metalloproteinase-9, and $S100\beta$) presenting a single composite result, the Multimarker Index (MMX). Stroke diagnosis was established by an expert committee blinded to MMX and CPSS results.

Results.—There were 155 patients enrolled, 87 (56%) of whom had a final diagnosis of stroke. The area under the receiver operating characteristic (ROC) curve for CPSS was 0.77 (95% confidence interval [CI] 0.70–0.84) and that of MMX was 0.74 (95% CI 0.66–0.82) ($p = 0.285$). Thus, both tests, when used alone, failed to recognize approximately 25% of strokes. The area under the ROC curve of the combination of the two tests (0.86, 95% CI 0.79–0.91) was significantly greater than that of either single test ($p = 0.01$ vs. CPSS and $p < 0.001$ vs. TSP).

Conclusions.—In an emergency care setting, a panel test using multiple biochemical markers showed triage accuracy similar to that of CPSS. Further studies are needed before biomarkers can be introduced in the clinical work-up of patients with suspected stroke.

▶ Great! Just what we need—another biomarker controversy. The use of cardiac biomarkers in the emergency department is fraught with hazard and misunderstanding. Into the fray comes this study conducted in 3 emergency departments from 3 regions of Italy. It investigates the use of a point-of-care fluorescence immunoassay for diagnosing stroke.

Although the authors state, "The area under the ROC curve of the combination of the two tests was significantly greater than that of either single test," there was still considerable overlap of the confidence intervals. Whether this represents a real increase in diagnostic accuracy is unclear. Moreover, remember that this is a derivation study attempting to define the point at which the Multimarker Index value might be useful and how it should be combined with the Cincinnati Prehospital Stroke Scale. All of this will need to be validated in an independent study. Needless to say, this is an interesting concept that is "not yet ready for prime time."

E. A. Ramoska, MD, MPHE

Steroids for migraine headaches: a randomized double-blind, two-armed, placebo-controlled trial

Fiesseler FW, Shih R, Szucs P, et al (Morristown Memorial Hosp, NJ; et al)
J Emerg Med 40:463-468, 2011

Background.—Recurrence of migraine headache after treatment in the emergency department (ED) is common. Conflicting evidence exists regarding the utility of steroids in preventing migraine headache recurrence at 24—48 h.

Objective.—To determine if steroids decrease the headache recurrence in patients treated for migraine headaches in the ED.

Methods.—Double-blind placebo-controlled, two-tailed randomized trial. Patients aged >17 years with a moderately severe migraine headache diagnosed by treating Emergency Physician were approached for participation. Enrollees received either dexamethasone (10 mg i.v.) if intravenous access was utilized or prednisone (40 mg by mouth × 2 days) if no intravenous access was obtained. Each medication was matched with an identical-appearing placebo. Patients were contacted 24—72 h after the ED visit to assess headache recurrence.

Results.—A total of 181 patients were enrolled. Eight were lost to follow-up, 6 in the dexamethasone group and 2 in the prednisone arm. Participants had a mean age of 37 years ($\pm$ 10 years), with 86% female. Eighty-six percent met the International Headache Society Criteria for migraine headache. Of the 173 patients with completed follow-up, 20/91 (22%) (95% confidence interval [CI] 13.5—30.5) in the steroid arm and 26/82 (32%) (95% CI 21.9—42.1) in the placebo arm had recurrent headaches ($p = 0.21$).

Conclusion.—We did not find a statistically significant decrease in headache recurrence in patients treated with steroids for migraine headaches.

▶ A previous meta-analysis suggests that the use of steroids, specifically dexamethasone, is effective in decreasing these rebound headaches.[1] The authors of this randomized double-blind project sought to determine whether steroids prevented the recurrence of migraines in their study population. Patients were randomized to receive intravenous dexamethasone, oral prednisone, or placebo. No statistically significant difference between the steroid group and placebo group could be demonstrated, suggesting that steroid administration is unnecessary. The sample size may compromise the results in this case (n = 173) when compared with the pooled data of the meta-analysis (n = 742). A larger multi-center trial modeled after the included one may produce a more reliable answer to the clinical question. One caveat would be to eliminate narcotics as a rescue medication. The authors added that 57% of the study's population received narcotics. With the narcotic receivers more likely to return to the emergency department for narcotics and their migraines, these patients may be skewing the data.

E. C. Bruno, MD

Reference

1. Singh A, Alter HJ, Zaia B. Does the addition of dexamethasone to standard therapy for acute migraine headache decrease the incidence of recurrent headache for patients treated in the emergency department? A meta-analysis and systematic review of the literature. *Acad Emerg Med.* 2008;15:1223-1233.

Sensitivity of computed tomography performed within six hours of onset of headache for diagnosis of subarachnoid haemorrhage: prospective cohort study

Perry JJ, Stiell IG, Sivilotti MLA, et al (Univ of Ottawa, Ontario, Canada; Queen's Univ, Kingston, Ontario, Canada; et al)
BMJ 343:d4277, 2011

Objective.—To measure the sensitivity of modern third generation computed tomography in emergency patients being evaluated for possible subarachnoid haemorrhage, especially when carried out within six hours of headache onset.

Design.—Prospective cohort study.

Setting.—11 tertiary care emergency departments across Canada, 2000-9.

Participants.—Neurologically intact adults with a new acute headache peaking in intensity within one hour of onset in whom a computed tomography was ordered by the treating physician to rule out subarachnoid haemorrhage.

Main Outcome Measures.—Subarachnoid haemorrhage was defined by any of subarachnoid blood on computed tomography, xanthochromia in cerebrospinal fluid, or any red blood cells in final tube of cerebrospinal fluid collected with positive results on cerebral angiography.

Results.—Of the 3132 patients enrolled (mean age 45.1, 2571 (82.1%) with worst headache ever), 240 had subarachnoid haemorrhage (7.7%). The sensitivity of computed tomography overall for subarachnoid haemorrhage was 92.9% (95% confidence interval 89.0% to 95.5%), the specificity was 100% (99.9% to 100%), the negative predictive value was 99.4% (99.1% to 99.6%), and the positive predictive value was 100% (98.3% to 100%). For the 953 patients scanned within six hours of headache onset, all 121 patients with subarachnoid haemorrhage were identified by computed tomography, yielding a sensitivity of 100% (97.0% to 100.0%), specificity of 100% (99.5% to 100%), negative predictive value of 100% (99.5% to 100%), and positive predictive value of 100% (96.9% to 100%).

Conclusion.—Modern third generation computed tomography is extremely sensitive in identifying subarachnoid haemorrhage when it is carried out within six hours of headache onset and interpreted by a qualified radiologist.

▶ Acute headache is a common complaint seen in the emergency department, and emergency physicians are compelled to address the potential for subarachnoid hemorrhage (SAH) as the etiology for the headache. The current standard workup is computed tomography (CT) of the head, followed by lumbar puncture (LP), if the CT is nondiagnostic. After the arduous task of obtaining written consent, performance of the LP can be technically challenging, especially in certain patient populations (obese, previous spinal surgery, etc). The need for the LP after CT is based on previously reported CT sensitivity of approximately 90% to identify SAH. The authors of this prospective study suggest that newer CT technology (third-generation scanners) are more sensitive and could obviate the need for the dreaded LP. Although performed at multiple tertiary care centers, the reading radiologists only needed familiarity with CT head imaging and did not need to be a dedicated neuroradiologist. This makes the approach more generalizable to the community facility. If the images are obtained within 6 hours of the onset of the headache, the sensitivity approaches 100%. With the increased ability to identify bleeding, a negative CT head scan appears to be an adequate evaluation in the patient who is low risk for SAH.

E. C. Bruno, MD

Low-Dose Recombinant Tissue-Type Plasminogen Activator Enhances Clot Resolution in Brain Hemorrhage: The Intraventricular Hemorrhage Thrombolysis Trial
Naff N, Williams MA, Keyl PM, et al (Sinai Hosp of Baltimore, MD; Johns Hopkins Univ School of Medicine, Baltimore, MD; et al)
Stroke 42:3009-3016, 2011

Background and Purpose.—Patients with intracerebral hemorrhage and intraventricular hemorrhage have a reported mortality of 50% to 80%. We evaluated a clot lytic treatment strategy for these patients in terms of mortality, ventricular infection, and bleeding safety events, and for its effect on the rate of intraventricular clot lysis.

Methods.—Forty-eight patients were enrolled at 14 centers and randomized to treatment with 3 mg recombinant tissue-type plasminogen activator (rtPA) or placebo. Demographic characteristics, severity factors, safety outcomes (mortality, infection, bleeding), and clot resolution rates were compared in the 2 groups.

Results.—Severity factors, including admission Glasgow Coma Scale, intracerebral hemorrhage volume, intraventricular hemorrhage volume, and blood pressure were evenly distributed, as were adverse events, except for an increased frequency of respiratory system events in the placebo-treated group. Neither intracranial pressure nor cerebral perfusion pressure differed substantially between treatment groups on presentation, with external ventricular device closure, or during the active treatment phase. Frequency of death and ventriculitis was substantially lower than expected and bleeding events remained below the prespecified threshold for mortality (18% rtPA; 23% placebo), ventriculitis (8% rtPA; 9% placebo), symptomatic bleeding (23% rtPA; 5% placebo, which approached statistical significance; $P=0.1$). The median duration of dosing was 7.5 days for rtPA and

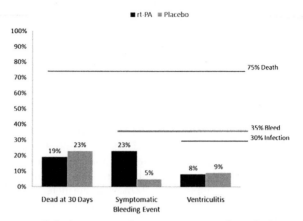

FIGURE 1.—Prespecified safety triggers and events. None was significant (death at 30 days, $P=1.00$; symptomatic bleeding event, $P=0.106$; ventriculitis, $P=1.00$). (Reprinted from Naff N, Williams MA, Keyl PM, et al. Low-dose recombinant tissue-type plasminogen activator enhances clot resolution in brain hemorrhage: the intraventricular hemorrhage thrombolysis trial. *Stroke.* 2011;42:3009-3016, with permission from American Heart Association, Inc.)

12 days for placebo. There was a significant beneficial effect of rtPA on rate of clot resolution.

Conclusions.—Low-dose rtPA for the treatment of intracerebral hemorrhage with intraventricular hemorrhage has an acceptable safety profile compared to placebo and historical controls. Data from a well-designed phase III clinical trial, such as CLEAR III, will be needed to fully evaluate this treatment (Fig 1).

▶ This is a treatment I never thought I'd see attempted—recombinant tissue-type plasminogen activator (rtPA) for the treatment of intracerebral hemorrhage associated with intraventricular hemorrhage. Emergency physicians are all accustomed to hearing about how intravenous rtPA causes intracerebral hemorrhage, but this treatment entails using low-dose rtPA given via an external ventricular device (into the lateral ventricles) to increase intraventricular clot lysis. These external ventricular devices must have already been placed to treat obstructive hydrocephalus. Patients were randomized to receive either low-dose rtPA or normal saline through the ventriculostomy every 12 hours until computed tomographic evidence of clot resolution was sufficient to remove the catheter or until a safety end point (symptomatic bleeding, infection, or death) occurred.

Interestingly, the total death rate in this trial was only 21%, compared with the predicted mortality of approximately 75% (calculated from a previously well-validated severity algorithm). The mortality rate was slightly lower in the rtPA group, but given the small sample size, this only meant that 1 additional person died in the placebo group. Not surprisingly, the rate of symptomatic bleeding and asymptomatic bleeding increased in the group receiving the rtPA (see Fig 1). The rate of blood clot resolution was significantly greater in the rtPA group, and this was associated with a higher rate of successful removal of the catheter at the end of administration.

This study was neither designed nor powered to assess functional outcome but rather to test safety. It did, however, have some interesting trends. Probably the most interesting finding was that the overall mortality rate was so much lower than predicted for both rtPA and placebo (21% vs 75%). Perhaps this was due to good intensive care unit care and regular patient monitoring (the Hawthorne effect), or perhaps it was because all patients had to have had a ventriculostomy catheter placed to relieve acute obstructive hydrocephalus. There is a much larger ongoing phase III clinical trial, CLEAR III that will hopefully give us more conclusive data. That said, this treatment is promising, and we may hear more about it in the future.

D. K. Mullin, MD

D. K. Mullin, MD

6 Infections and Immunologic Disorders

Blood Cultures at Central Line Insertion in the Intensive Care Unit: Comparison with Peripheral Venipuncture
Stohl S, Benenson S, Sviri S, et al (Hadassah Hebrew Univ Med Centre, Jerusalem, Israel)
J Clin Microbiol 49:2398-2403, 2011

Blood cultures are a key diagnostic test for intensive care unit (ICU) patients; however, contaminants complicate interpretations and lead to unnecessary antibiotic administration and costs. Indications for blood cultures and central venous catheter (CVC) insertions often overlap for ICU patients. Obtaining blood cultures under the strict sterile precautions utilized for CVC insertion might be expected to decrease culture contamination. This retrospective study compared the results of blood cultures taken at CVC insertion, at arterial line insertion, and from peripheral venipuncture in order to validate the advantage of CVC insertion cultures. Cultures from indwelling lines were excluded. Results of 14,589 blood cultures, including 2,736 (19%) CVC, 1,513 (10%) arterial line, and 10,340 (71%) peripheral cultures taken over 5.5 years in two ICUs (general and medical) were analyzed. CVC cultures were contaminated more frequently than arterial line or peripheral cultures (225/2,736 [8%] CVC, 48/1,513 [3%] arterial line, and 378/10,340 (4%) peripheral cultures [$P < 0.001$ for CVC versus peripheral and CVC versus arterial line cultures]). True pathogens were found more frequently in CVC insertion cultures (334/2,736 [12%] CVC, 155/1,513 [10%] arterial line, and 795/10,340 [8%] peripheral cultures [$P < 0.001$ for CVC versus peripheral cultures; $P = 0.055$ for CVC versus arterial line cultures; $P < 0.001$ for peripheral versus arterial line cultures]). Contamination and true-positive rates were similar for culture sets from the two ICUs for each given culture source. Despite superior sterile precautions, cultures taken at the time of central line insertion had a higher contamination rate than did either peripheral or arterial line blood cultures. This may be related to the increased manipulations required for CVC insertion.

▶ Which source of blood cultures would you think had the lower rate of contamination: peripheral vein collection or freshly placed central lines?

The authors reviewed culture results from 2 intensive care units over multiple years to find that contaminants occur more frequently among blood samples taken at the time of central line insertion. At the same time, they found that true infections are more frequent among central line collections than peripheral vein collections in a relatively parallel setting (samples collected within 24 hours of each other). A useful comparison was to look at results from cultures from arterial lines.

So what is different between the 2 methods that might explain these results? The authors suggest we think about the blood culture process as a collection of several subprocesses.

Preparation seems to favor the central line process to have less contaminants—drapes, skin preparation, gloves, and other barrier protection are routine.

Finding the vessel and aspirating blood may favor the peripheral vein process—smaller needles and less subsurface manipulation is done in this setting. There are some bacteria likely to be lingering in the subsurface volumes that cannot be cleaned by surface prep. Longer time to complete placement of the central line might also provide occasion for contaminant bacteria to reach the sterile area or attach to catheters from air, patient, or operators.

Loading the culture bottles might also favor the peripheral vein collection process because, on average, peripheral blood volumes collected are likely to be less than central line volumes. The larger volume of blood added to a culture bottle increases the likelihood of the successful growth of bacteria, whether the bacteria is a contaminant or true pathogen. (The authors found that the success of finding true pathogens was greater with blood from central line insertions compared with a peripheral vein source, which would support the blood volume rationale.)

The actual injection of collected blood into culture bottles may not advantage one method over another.

What are the results from your institution? How can we improve the collection of blood for culture?

N. B. Handly, MD, MSc, MS

Blood Cultures in the Emergency Department Evaluation of Childhood Pneumonia

Shah SS, Dugan MH, Bell LM, et al (The Children's Hosp of Philadelphia, PA; et al)
Pediatr Infect Dis J 30:475-479, 2011

Background.—Blood cultures are frequently obtained in the emergency department (ED) evaluation of children with community-acquired pneumonia (CAP).

Objectives.—To determine the prevalence of bacteremia in children presenting to the ED with CAP, identify subgroups at increased risk for bacteremia, and quantify the effect of positive blood cultures on management.

Methods.—This case—control study was nested within a cohort of children followed up at 35 pediatric practices. Patients from this cohort who were ≤18 years of age, evaluated in the ED in 2006—2007, and diagnosed with CAP were eligible. Cases were those with bacteremia. Controls included those with negative blood cultures and those without blood cultures performed.

Results.—A total of 877 (9.6%) of 9099 children with CAP were evaluated in the ED. The mean age was 3.6 years; 53% were male. Blood cultures were obtained from 291 children (33.2%). Overall, the prevalence of bacteremia was 2.1% (95% confidence interval [CI]: 0.8%—4.4%). Bacteremia occurred in 2.6% (95% CI: 1.0%—5.6%) with an infiltrate on chest radiograph and in 13.0% (95% CI: 2.8%—33.6%) with complicated pneumonia. *Streptococcus pneumoniae* accounted for 4 of the 6 cases of bacteremia. Blood culture results altered management in 5 of the 6 bacteremic patients; 1 had an appropriate broadening and 4 had an appropriate narrowing of coverage. The contamination rate was 1.0% (95% CI: 0.2%—3.0%).

Conclusion.—Children presenting to the ED for evaluation of CAP are at low-risk for bacteremia. Although positive blood cultures frequently altered clinical management, the overall impact was small because of the low prevalence of bacteremia.

▶ I feel better when I see evidence that blood cultures are not needed for emergency department (ED) patients diagnosed with community-acquired pneumonia. In the busy ED, coordinating as well as documenting the draw and then sending the samples to the lab is a challenge. These authors found that among the pediatric patients they surveyed, only 1 needed to change the antibiotic for coverage. The remaining 5 patients were found to have bacteria sensitive to a narrower-spectrum antibiotic. The authors said this latter group also represented a change in clinical management but hardly as important as the discovery of the 1 patient who needed coverage for an infection that was not being treated by the antibiotic initiated in the ED.

However, there are some things about this study that are troubling. The authors used discharge diagnoses of pneumonia by *International Classification of Diseases, Ninth Revision* to identify index cases even if the chest x-ray was negative. This makes it difficult to compare children in this study to others because it is likely that practice patterns (sometimes local and subjective) might affect the application of this diagnosis to the patients.

Additionally, the authors overlooked the possibility that patients who did not receive blood cultures in the ED (most of these were patients who were discharged from the ED) might, if they had been checked, have had positive cultures. In fact, the authors chose to modify their found rate of bacteremia by the 1 positive culture found among the 28 of these initially untested 586 patients who were cultured within 3 days of the ED index visit. Is it possible that among the remaining uncultured children, there was no chance of a positive noncontaminated culture? I am not sure how we can answer these questions unless a study performs the gold standard test (blood cultures) on all patients. Maybe we can find a group of patients who have nonconsequential bacteremia.

N. B. Handly, MD, MSc, MS

Cost-effectiveness of an emergency department-based early sepsis resuscitation protocol

Jones AE, Troyer JL, Kline JA (Carolinas Med Ctr, Charlotte, NC; Univ of North Carolina at Charlotte)
Crit Care Med 39:1306-1312, 2011

Objectives.—Guidelines recommend that sepsis be treated with an early resuscitation protocol such as early goal-directed therapy. Our objective was to assess the cost-effectiveness of implementing early goal-directed therapy as a routine protocol.

Design.—Prospective before and after study.

Setting.—Large urban hospital emergency department with >110,000 visits/yr.

Patients.—The target population was patients with consensus criteria for septic shock. We excluded those with age <18 yrs, no aggressive care desired, or need for immediate surgery.

Interventions.—Clinical and cost data were prospectively collected on two groups: 1) patients from 1 yr before; and 2) 2 yrs after implementing early goal-directed therapy as standard of care. Before phase patients received non-protocolized care at attending discretion. The primary outcomes were 1-yr mortality, discounted life expectancy, and quality-adjusted life-years. Using costs and quality-adjusted life-years, we constructed an incremental cost-effectiveness ratio and performed a net monetary benefit analysis, producing the probability that the intervention was cost-effective given different values for the willingness to pay for a quality-adjusted life-year.

Results.—Two hundred eighty-five subjects, 79 in the before and 206 in the after phases, were enrolled. Treatment with early goal-directed therapy was associated with an increased hospital cost of $7,028 and an increase in both discounted sepsis-adjusted life expectancy and quality-adjusted life years of 1.5 and 1.3 yrs, respectively. Early goal-directed therapy use was associated with a cost of $5,397 per quality-adjusted life-years gained and the net monetary benefit analysis indicates a 98% probability ($p = .038$) that early goal-directed therapy is cost-effective at a willingness to pay of $50,000 per quality-adjusted life-years.

Conclusion.—Implementation of early goal-directed therapy in the emergency department care of patients with severe sepsis is cost-effective.

▶ This before-and-after study from the Carolinas Medical Center uses sophisticated methods to perform a cost-effectiveness analysis of their implementation of an early goal-directed therapy (EGDT)/sepsis protocol in the emergency department (ED). This was not a research protocol to look at sepsis treatment in the ED but rather a change in the ED's standard of care expected of all physicians who encountered patients with sepsis. They found that their change in standard operating procedure resulted in care that was cost-effective from a societal standpoint.

Cost-effectiveness analyses can be confusing to read and interpret, and the results are always contingent on the assumptions made by the authors. A strength of this study is that it used 2 methods to determine cost-effectiveness and performed different sensitivity analyses to see whether their conclusions held up despite varying assumptions. Limitations include that this was a single-site study, a Hawthorne effect (where results are affected just because someone is looking), and the fact that treatment and technology may have changed over the 3 years of the study. All in all, however, these results suggest that mortality is reduced and quality-adjusted life years are increased at an acceptable cost to the health care system by implementing an aggressive protocol when EGDT is used routinely in the ED for the care of sepsis patients.

E. A. Ramoska, MD, MPHE

7 Pediatric Emergency Medicine

Cardiovascular

A pilot study of the feasibility of heart screening for sudden cardiac arrest in healthy children
Vetter VL, Dugan N, Guo R, et al (Univ of Pennsylvania School of Medicine, Philadelphia)
Am Heart J 161:1000-1006.e3, 2011

Background.—In children, sudden cardiac arrest (SCA) is associated with structural and electrical cardiac abnormalities. No studies have systematically screened healthy school children in the United States for conditions leading to SCA to identify those at risk.

Methods.—From June 2006 to June 2007, we screened 400 healthy 5- to 19-year-olds (11.8 ± 3.9 years) in clinical offices at The Children's Hospital of Philadelphia using a medical and family history questionnaire, weight, height, blood pressure, heart rate, cardiac examination, electrocardiogram (ECG), and echocardiogram (ECHO). Our goals were to determine the feasibility of adding an ECG to history and physical examination and to identify a methodology to be used in a larger multicenter study. A secondary objective was to compare identification of cardiovascular abnormalities by history and physical examination, ECG, and ECHO.

Results.—Previously undiagnosed cardiac abnormalities were found in 23 subjects (5.8%); an additional 20 (5%) had hypertension. Potentially serious cardiac conditions were identified in 10 subjects (2.5%); 7 were suspected or identified by ECG and 3 more only by ECHO. Only 1 of the 10 had symptoms (previously dismissed); none had a positive family history.

Conclusions.—It is feasible to screen for conditions associated with SCA in healthy children by adding ECG to history and physical examination. In this nongeneralizable sample, ECG identified more cases compared to history and physical examination alone, with further augmentation from ECHOs. Improvements in ECG and echocardiographic normative standards, representing age, gender, race, and ethnicity, are needed to increase the efficacy of screening in a young population.

▶ Although not incorporated in the everyday practice of general emergency medicine, emergency physicians may volunteer to perform sports medical clearance physical examinations for children in their communities. The rationale for the evaluation is to identify those children at risk for sudden cardiac arrest (SCA). In the attached pilot study, the researchers questioned whether the addition of an electrocardiogram (ECG) to the standard survey (history, physical, and questionnaire) improved the physician's ability to find at-risk children. Pediatric patients (age 5-19) were enrolled, and each received an ECG and an echocardiogram. They were able to diagnose potentially serious conditions in 2.5% patients, in whom the previous standard evaluation would have failed. The use of the ECG was 3 times more effective than the history and physical at identification of concerning abnormalities.

This altruistic act of performing sports physicals is not without risk. Screening surveys and a standard evaluation appear to have gaps, which may be partially closed with the noninterventional ECG analysis. The addition of an ECG may become a necessary step in this process in an attempt to prevent SCA in pediatric patients.

E. C. Bruno, MD

A pilot study of the feasibility of heart screening for sudden cardiac arrest in healthy children
Vetter VL, Dugan N, Guo R, et al (Univ of Pennsylvania School of Medicine, Philadelphia)
Am Heart J 161:1000-1006.e3, 2011

Background.—In children, sudden cardiac arrest (SCA) is associated with structural and electrical cardiac abnormalities. No studies have systematically screened healthy school children in the United States for conditions leading to SCA to identify those at risk.

Methods.—From June 2006 to June 2007, we screened 400 healthy 5- to 19-year-olds (11.8 ± 3.9 years) in clinical offices at The Children's Hospital of Philadelphia using a medical and family history questionnaire, weight, height, blood pressure, heart rate, cardiac examination, electrocardiogram (ECG), and echocardiogram (ECHO). Our goals were to determine the feasibility of adding an ECG to history and physical examination and to identify a methodology to be used in a larger multicenter study. A secondary objective was to compare identification of cardiovascular abnormalities by history and physical examination, ECG, and ECHO.

Results.—Previously undiagnosed cardiac abnormalities were found in 23 subjects (5.8%); an additional 20 (5%) had hypertension. Potentially serious cardiac conditions were identified in 10 subjects (2.5%); 7 were suspected or identified by ECG and 3 more only by ECHO. Only 1 of the 10 had symptoms (previously dismissed); none had a positive family history.

Conclusions.—It is feasible to screen for conditions associated with SCA in healthy children by adding ECG to history and physical examination. In this nongeneralizable sample, ECG identified more cases compared to history and physical examination alone, with further augmentation from ECHOs. Improvements in ECG and echocardiographic normative standards, representing age, gender, race, and ethnicity, are needed to increase the efficacy of screening in a young population.

▶ So how would you screen children for risk of sudden cardiac arrest (SCA)? Screening for risk is not the same as definitively knowing the disease is present, at least not in cases in which the evaluation for risk of disease can be complicated, potentially harmful, or simply expensive. Catheterization of each child before being recruited to play sports? This is just not reasonable.

Cardiac dysrhythmias are important causes of SCA in children, so the authors chose to add electrocardiograms (ECGs) to the screening process of history and exam, as has been done previously outside the United States.

In this study, pediatric cardiologists reviewed all of the ECGs. The use of cardiology consults would be an additional cost or resource needed to complete the ECG screening process. It might be expected that there is not only a personnel cost but a time cost because the ECG is not going to be interpreted at the same time as the office visit. Is this significant?

We do not know just how well this expanded type of screening will perform in identifying children at risk, although this pilot suggests that it may be quite a useful tool. Meanwhile, regardless of screening efforts, we are still going to be seeing youngsters suffering from SCA-like or even some syncopal or near-syncopal events in emergency departments. We know the ECG is a good tool and will be ready to use it.

N. B. Handly, MD, MSc, MS

Beneficial Effects of Terlipressin in Pediatric Cardiac Arrest
Yildizdaş D, Horoz ÖÖ, Erdem S (Çukurova Univ, Adana, Turkey)
Pediatr Emerg Care 27:865-868, 2011

Objective.—Vasopressin and its analog, terlipressin (TP), are potent vasopressors that may be useful therapeutic agents in the treatment of cardiac arrest (CA), septic and catecholamine-resistant shock, and esophageal variceal hemorrhage. The American Heart Association 2000 guidelines recommend its use for adult ventricular fibrillation arrest, and the American Heart Association 2005 guidelines note that it may replace the first or second epinephrine dose. There is little reported experience with TP in cardiopulmonary resuscitation (CPR) of children. The purpose of this retrospective case series was to report successful return of spontaneous circulation after the rescue administration of vasopressin after prolonged CA and failure of conventional CPR, advanced life support, and epinephrine therapy in children.

Methods.—Nine pediatric patients with asystole, aged 11 months to 14 years, who experienced 12 episodes of refractory CA and did not respond to conventional therapy. Terlipressin was administered as intravenous bolus doses of 20 mcg/kg to standard cardiopulmonary resuscitation.

Results.—Return of spontaneous circulation was monitored and achieved in 6 of the 12 episodes. The mean duration of CPR was 24.8 minutes in these 12 episodes of CA with TP administration, with a range of 10 to 50 minutes (median, 23 minutes). Five survivors were discharged home without sequelae and with good neurologic status (score 1 by the pediatric cerebral performance category).

Conclusions.—The combination of TP to epinephrine during CPR may have a beneficial effect in children with CA. However, the recommendations for its use in the pediatric literature are based on limited clinical data.

▶ In pediatrics, the vasoactive pressor recommended for cardiac arrest is epinephrine. In adult resuscitation, vasopressin has been used; however, the use of it in pediatrics is limited. Terlipressin, a synthetic analog of vasopressin, has similar pharmacodynamic profile with a longer half-life. There have been some case reports of some success with pediatric septic shock. This retrospective chart review found that about 56% of patients in arrest survived and were discharged home without neurologic sequelae. This study is greatly limited by the small sample size and the nature of its retrospective methodology. Further studies are warranted before considering terlipressin as an adjunct to our current Pediatric Advanced Life Support protocols.

E. C. Quintana, MD, MPH

Endocrinology

How Well Does Serum Bicarbonate Concentration Predict the Venous pH in Children Being Evaluated for Diabetic Ketoacidosis?

Nadler OA, Finkelstein MJ, Reid SR (Legacy Emanuel Med Ctr, Portland, OR; Children's Hosps and Clinics of Minnesota, Minneapolis; Children's Hosps and Clinics of Minnesota, St Paul)
Pediatr Emerg Care 27:907-910, 2011

Objective.—The objective of the study was to determine whether serum bicarbonate (HCO_3) concentration can accurately predict venous pH in the evaluation of diabetic ketoacidosis (DKA).

Methods.—A retrospective review of patients who presented to a children's hospital emergency department and received an *International Classification of Diseases, Ninth Revision* code related to DKA or diabetes mellitus was performed. To be eligible for inclusion and data abstraction, patients had blood sampled simultaneously for venous blood gas and metabolic panel. A linear regression model was created using pH (dependent variable) and HCO_3 (predictor). The diagnostic performance and accuracy of HCO_3 to discriminate abnormal pH were evaluated using receiver operating characteristic curve analysis.

Results.—Three hundred patients met the inclusion criteria. The linear relationship between pH and HCO_3 using the Pearson correlation coefficient was found to be $R = 0.89$ (confidence interval [CI], 0.83−0.95; $R^2 = 0.79$). Receiver operating characteristic curve analysis that maximized sensitivity and specificity demonstrated that a HCO_3 18.5 or less predicts pH less than 7.3 (area under the curve $= 0.97$; CI, 0.94−0.99; sensitivity, 93%; specificity, 91%), and a HCO_3 10.5 or less predicts pH less than 7.1 (area under the curve $= 0.97$; CI, 0.95−0.99; sensitivity, 97%; specificity, 88%).

Conclusions.—Serum bicarbonate accurately predicts abnormal venous pH in children with DKA. Venous pH determination may not be necessary for all patients being evaluated for DKA.

▶ Determination of whether a child with hyperglycemia and previously diagnosed insulin-dependent diabetes mellitus is in mild diabetic ketoacidosis (DKA) is a particular dilemma for the community physician. Using diagnostic tests such as basic metabolic panel, urinalysis, serum ketone level, and venous blood gas, the emergency physician tries to decide whether the patient is dehydrated with ketosis or is in DKA. The initial management, including intravenous fluids, antiemetics, and identification of the potential etiology (dietary indiscretion, insulin noncompliance, infection, etc) is relatively straightforward. However, if DKA is suspected, the patient will presumably need pediatric intensive care unit admission or transfer to a facility with the requisite resources. The authors of this retrospective review suggest that serum bicarbonate level is adequate to identify acidosis and correlates with the venous blood gas (VBG) measurement. They were able to identify a linear relationship between the serum bicarbonate and VBG analysis. Unfortunately, neither test predicted the presence or absence of ketonemia or ketonuria. This study does provide the emergency physician the option of not ordering the VBG, but this would be more clinically relevant if the physician is still using arterial blood gas.

E. C. Bruno, MD

ENT

A Placebo-Controlled Trial of Antimicrobial Treatment for Acute Otitis Media

Tähtinen PA, Laine MK, Huovinen P, et al (Turku Univ Hosp, Finland; Natl Inst for Health and Welfare, Turku, Finland)
N Engl J Med 364:116-126, 2011

Background.—The efficacy of antimicrobial treatment in children with acute otitis media remains controversial.

Methods.—In this randomized, double-blind trial, children 6 to 35 months of age with acute otitis media, diagnosed with the use of strict criteria, received amoxicillin−clavulanate (161 children) or placebo (158 children) for 7 days. The primary outcome was the time to treatment failure from the first dose until the end-of-treatment visit on day 8. The definition of treatment failure was based on the overall condition of the child (including adverse events) and otoscopic signs of acute otitis media.

Results.—Treatment failure occurred in 18.6% of the children who received amoxicillin—clavulanate, as compared with 44.9% of the children who received placebo (P<0.001). The difference between the groups was already apparent at the first scheduled visit (day 3), at which time 13.7% of the children who received amoxicillin—clavulanate, as compared with 25.3% of those who received placebo, had treatment failure. Overall, amoxicillin—clavulanate reduced the progression to treatment failure by 62% (hazard ratio, 0.38; 95% confidence interval [CI], 0.25 to 0.59; P<0.001) and the need for rescue treatment by 81% (6.8% vs. 33.5%; hazard ratio, 0.19; 95% CI, 0.10 to 0.36; P<0.001). Analgesic or antipyretic agents were given to 84.2% and 85.9% of the children in the amoxicillin—clavulanate and placebo groups, respectively. Adverse events were significantly more common in the amoxicillin—clavulanate group than in the placebo group. A total of 47.8% of the children in the amoxicillin-clavulanate group had diarrhea, as compared with 26.6% in the placebo group (P<0.001); 8.7% and 3.2% of the children in the respective groups had eczema (P=0.04).

Conclusions.—Children with acute otitis media benefit from antimicrobial treatment as compared with placebo, although they have more side effects. Future studies should identify patients who may derive the greatest benefit, in order to minimize unnecessary antimicrobial treatment and the development of bacterial resistance. (Funded by the Foundation for Paediatric Research and others; ClinicalTrials.gov number, NCT00299455.)

▶ Acute otitis media (AOM) is a common infection in pediatrics. Although antibiotics were initially the primary treatment for AOM, several articles have recommended an observation period before treatment. This randomized, double-blind, placebo-controlled study evaluated the efficacy of antibiotics in the resolution of AOM signs and symptoms. Amoxicillin-clavulanate would reduce the risk of treatment failure. It was interesting that they chose 40 mg of amoxicillin per kilogram of body weight per day plus 5.7 mg of clavulanate per kilogram per day, divided into 2 daily doses, instead of the current recommendations of 80 to 90 mg/kg per day of amoxicillin divided into 2 daily doses. Treatment failure occurred in 18.6% with antibiotics with an overall risk reduction of treatment failure of 62% (P < .001). In other words, to avoid treatment failure in 1 child, almost 4 children need to be treated with amoxicillin-clavulanate. Rescue treatment was decreased by 81%. Contralateral AOM developed in almost 8% of children with antibiotics and 18.6% in placebo group. There was no statistically significant difference in the use of analgesic or antipyretic agents. Parents of day care attendees in the antibiotic group missed significantly fewer work days than the placebo group (81 days vs 101 days, respectively, P = .005). The overall condition and otoscopic signs were better in the antibiotic group compared with placebo (P > .001). Treatment with amoxicillin-clavulanate significantly accelerated the resolution of fever, poor appetite, decreased activity, and irritability; however, there was no significant effect on otalgia. An adverse event occurred in more than half of the patients in the amoxicillin-clavulanate group (52.8%, $P = .003$). The most commonly reported adverse events were diarrhea and eczema. No mastoiditis was reported. Although this study is suggestive of early treatment of AOM, it can be also interpreted differently. It showed that half the children in the placebo group did not have treatment failure and two-thirds did not need rescue treatment. Not all patients with acute otitis media need antimicrobial treatment. It will be important in the future to characterize patients who do not need it.

E. C. Quintana, MD, MPH

How Do Parents of Preverbal Children With Acute Otitis Media Determine How Much Ear Pain Their Child Is Having?
Shaikh N, Kearney DH, Colborn DK, et al (Univ of Pittsburgh School of Medicine, PA; et al)
J Pain 11:1291-1294, 2010

The objective of this study was to determine how parents of preverbal children determine whether their child is having otalgia. We constructed 8 cases describing a 1-year-old child with acute otitis media (AOM) using various combinations of the following 6 observable symptoms: fussiness, ear tugging, eating less, fever, sleeping difficulty, and playing less. Parents of children with a history of AOM presenting for well or sick appointments to an ambulatory clinic were asked to assign a pain level to each case on a visual analog scale. Sixty-nine parents participated in the study. Each of the 6 behaviors was associated with increased pain levels ($P < .0001$). Ear tugging and fussiness had the highest impact on the assigned pain levels. Higher level of parental education and private insurance were associated with higher reported pain levels ($P = .007$ and $P = .001$, respectively). Because interpretation of symptoms appears to be influenced by socioeconomic status, we question the utility of using an overall pain score from a 1-item parent scale as an outcome measure in clinical trials that include preverbal children.

Perspective.—Parents of preverbal children with acute otitis media use observable behaviors to determine their child's pain level. Interpretation of symptoms, however, appears to be influenced by socioeconomic status. Thus, we question the utility of using a 1-item parental pain scale in clinical trials that include preverbal children.

▶ It is not uncommon for a parent to bring a child to the emergency department for otalgia, especially in the middle of the night. Their main concern is acute otitis media (AOM). In many trials, the antimicrobial efficacy is based on otalgia resolution. However, in preverbal children, parental pain assessment in AOM is not clear. This study presented a 1-year-old with AOM in different symptom scenarios: ear tugging, fussiness, sleeping difficulty, fever, eating less, and playing less. Parents were enrolled and assigned a pain score to each scenario case. Most parents were African American (71%) with public insurance (77%) and were not college graduates (79%). Univariate analysis showed that each of 6 symptoms were statistically significant for increased levels of pain ($P < .0001$).

This supports that parents use observable behaviors to determine their child's level of pain. Ear tugging and fussiness seem to be the most important symptoms influencing parental pain perception based on multivariate analysis. These findings are also suggestive that there are many factors influencing their pain perception. Maternal education and insurance status greatly influence pain assessment. It shouldn't be surprising that there are plenty of behavioral and nonbehavioral factors that influence parental pain assessment. Based on this study, asking parents about ear tugging and fussiness will most likely address their concerns about otalgia.

This study was limited by its small sample and the homogeneity of parental population, so external validity could be challenged. However, it an interesting starting point on the biopsychosocial model of pain that is well accepted in the adult population with pain.

E. C. Quintana, MD, MPH

Hematology/Oncology

Changes in Platelet Count as a Predictive Tool in Sickle Cell Acute Vaso-Occlusive Crises: A Pediatric Study
Shanley LA, Ebeling M, Titus MO (Univ of Texas—Southwestern, Dallas; Med Univ of South Carolina, Charleston)
Clin Pediatr 50:657-661, 2011

Objective.—Studies have shown that platelets play an important role in the pathophysiology of vaso-occlusive crises (VOC) in sickle cell disease. This study investigates whether changes in platelet indices from baseline can be predictive of complications during acute pain crisis.

Methods.—Data were obtained from pediatric sickle cell patients in the well-clinic setting and compared with data gathered during VOC (n = 67). Primary outcome was complicated (admission, acute chest syndrome, transfusion, etc) versus uncomplicated (discharge from emergency department without subsequent return) course.

Results.—Patients with uncomplicated courses had larger platelet declines (53.7) than those with complicated courses (14.8, $P = .005$).

Conclusions.—The study suggests that patients with uncomplicated VOC are more likely to experience a larger decline in platelets. The predictive value is limited by the need to have preexisting steady-state data and relatively small decline. Ongoing studies are needed to identify useful laboratory data to help predict severity of VOC.

▶ Children with sickle cell disease frequently present to emergency departments (EDs) for management of vaso-occlusive crisis. This retrospective cross-sectional descriptive study of children with sickle cell complaints used platelet count as predictor of clinical severity. The platelet counts were then compared between ED visits to the patient's outpatient or steady-state values. Platelets were compared between the complicated and uncomplicated sickle cell crisis groups at the ED visit, which showed no statistical difference

(*P* = .29). However, when comparing clinic with ED counts, the group without complications did show a statistically significant larger drop in platelet values (53.7, *P* = .005) than their counterparts (14.8, *P* = .41). This study contributes to the small but growing body of literature discussing whether objective findings of a complete blood count can have clinical predictability of sickle cell disease outcomes. The study also suggests that patients in sickle cell crisis may demonstrate a significant drop from their steady state to vaso-occlusive crisis platelet counts, perhaps reflecting a protective mechanism of the spleen in sequestering platelets and preventing peripheral vaso-occlusion. Unfortunately, isolated platelet counts obtained in the ED do not differentiate between patients with complications versus those without. Clinical correlation is needed.

E. C. Quintana, MD, MPH

Pediatric vasooclusive crisis and weather conditions
Rogovik AL, Persaud J, Friedman JN, et al (BC Children's Hosp, Vancouver, Canada; The Hosp for Sick Children, Toronto, Ontario, Canada)
J Emerg Med 41:559-565, 2011

Background.—Previous studies have demonstrated associations of frequency of vasoocclusive crisis with weather conditions in adults, although relationships have been inconsistent.

Objectives.—Our objective was to determine if there is an association between weather conditions and pediatric emergency department (ED) visits, hospital admissions, and day and severity of pain precipitation for vasoocclusive crisis (VOC).

Methods.—A retrospective observational study was performed at a large tertiary care pediatric center. We reviewed health records of all VOC patients under the age of 18 years with a chief complaint of pain and performed correlations between daily and average weekly and monthly weather conditions and frequency of painful crises.

Results.—A total of 430 visits for VOC to the ED were documented from January 2005 to December 2006. Significant correlations were noted between the daily and weekly number of painful crises and colder temperatures ($\rho = -0.11$, $p = 0.004$ for daily data and $r = 0.25$, $p = 0.01$ weekly) and wind speed ($\rho = 0.13$, $p < 0.001$ and $r = 0.25$, $p = 0.01$). The monthly number of painful crises was moderately correlated with temperatures ($r = -0.42$, $p = 0.04$). The average monthly pain score was higher in more humid months ($r = 0.44$, $p = 0.03$).

Conclusion.—We found significant correlations of VOC with weather conditions where colder temperatures and higher wind speed were associated with a higher incidence of VOC in children. Health care providers as well as parents should be aware of these findings and ensure that preventive measures are instituted in patients at risk (Fig 1).

▶ It is sometimes thought that presentations of chronic diseases are related to weather changes. One study demonstrated that increased admissions for sickle

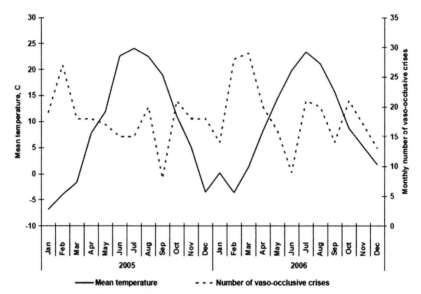

FIGURE 1.—Monthly number of vasoocclusive crises and mean outside temperatures during the 2-year study period. (Reprinted from Journal of Emergency Medicine, Rogovik AL, Persaud J, Friedman JN, et al. Pediatric vasoocclusive crisis and weather conditions. *J Emerg Med.* 2011;41:559-565. © 2011, with permission from Elsevier.)

cell vaso-occlusive crisis (VOC) were significantly associated with increased wind speed and low humidity, and another study found an association between wind speed and the onset of pain. One hundred sixty-nine patients were documented during this study. The mean age of patients was 10.6 ± 4.5 (range, 1−18) years; 241 (56%) were girls. The mean pain score as recorded on arrival at the emergency department (ED) was 8.2 on a 10-point scale, and the median duration of pain before coming to the ED was 24 hours. Eighty percent of patients were admitted. Significant correlation was noted between colder temperatures and the daily and weekly number of painful episodes starting and with the number of daily and weekly visits. Wind speed was significantly positively correlated with the daily and weekly number of starting painful episodes, weekly number of visits, and daily admitted patients; however, the correlations were weak. Although daily pain score did not correlate with weather, the average monthly pain score was higher in humid months. This study found that lower temperatures were significantly correlated with a higher incidence of VOC on a daily, weekly, and monthly basis (Fig 1). In conclusion, there were significant correlations of VOC with weather conditions, in which colder temperatures and higher wind speed were associated with a higher incidence of sickle cell VOC in children. These results lend support to other clinical and physiologic studies suggesting that skin cooling is associated with sickle cell VOC.

E. C. Quintana, MD, MPH

Changes in Platelet Count as a Predictive Tool in Sickle Cell Acute Vaso-Occlusive Crises: A Pediatric Study

Shanley LA, Ebeling M, Titus MO (Univ of Texas—Southwestern, Dallas; Med Univ of South Carolina, Charleston)
Clin Pediatr 50:657-661, 2011

Objective.—Studies have shown that platelets play an important role in the pathophysiology of vaso-occlusive crises (VOC) in sickle cell disease. This study investigates whether changes in platelet indices from baseline can be predictive of complications during acute pain crisis.

Methods.—Data were obtained from pediatric sickle cell patients in the well-clinic setting and compared with data gathered during VOC (n = 67). Primary outcome was complicated (admission, acute chest syndrome, transfusion, etc) versus uncomplicated (discharge from emergency department without subsequent return) course.

Results.—Patients with uncomplicated courses had larger platelet declines (53.7) than those with complicated courses (14.8, $P = .005$).

Conclusions.—The study suggests that patients with uncomplicated VOC are more likely to experience a larger decline in platelets. The predictive value is limited by the need to have preexisting steady-state data and relatively small decline. Ongoing studies are needed to identify useful laboratory data to help predict severity of VOC.

▶ Low platelet counts can certainly be alarming when patients present with sickle cell crises involving aplastic changes. Meanwhile, platelet counts and activity may be useful markers of a number of acute intravascular changes in both children and adults. Whether the changes in platelet count reflect an asplenic crisis or a less serious disease pattern is critical information needed for our decision making.

This article follows the patterns of platelet levels in children with sickle cell disease when making comparisons between levels noted at outpatient clinic levels and vaso-occlusive crisis levels (steady state [SS] and emergency department state [ED-S], respectively).

In the SS setting, platelet levels were higher than normal, which was suggested by the authors to be likely a result of decreased splenic clearance. If this difference in splenic clearance is as the authors describe, more careful comparisons of the very young who still have relatively functional spleens versus older children who are largely functionally asplenic would show the pattern of increased numbers of platelets with age. Furthermore, the levels of platelets were found to drops significantly among the ED-S subjects but more so for those individuals whose ED course was less complex (not needing admission or transfusion).

Of course, comparing levels with "normal" can be problematic. Often times we do not know about possible variations in the levels of anything that is diurnal, associated with activity/exercise or diet, or, in the case of sickle cell disease, possible variations in disease. Still, whether SS levels of platelets are above normal or not, the drop in count associated with crisis is still worth noting.

How well these findings can be applied to adults or even to children with more severe sickle cell crises is not clear. Children have the advantage of more complete primary or outpatient care (to allow for baseline levels of platelets to be known).

Like many other practice rule models, this one will require validation among larger subject numbers. However, it raises some interesting biological questions about other aspects of sickle cell disease.

N. B. Handly, MD, MSc, MS

Infectious Disease

A pilot study of the ability of the forced response test to discriminate between 3-year-old children with chronic otitis media with effusion or with recurrent acute otitis media
Casselbrant ML, Mandel EM, Seroky JT, et al (Children's Hosp of Pittsburgh of UPMC and the Univ of Pittsburgh School of Medicine, PA)
Acta Otolaryngol 131:1150-1154, 2011

Conclusions.—When used to test 3-year-old children within 3 months of tympanostomy tube placement for recurrent acute otitis media (rAOM) or chronic otitis media with effusion (cOME) the forced response test (FRT) showed relatively minor differences in the active and passive functions of the eustachian tube. While the sample size was small, the high variability in all test parameters suggests that the FRT alone is not capable of distinguishing between children with different expressions of otitis media.

Objective.—The FRT was designed to measure the passive and active properties of the eustachian tube. We evaluated the ability of that test to discriminate groups of children with rAOM or cOME.

Methods.—Twenty-two ears (15 children) with a confirmed history of rAOM and 24 ears (17 children) with a confirmed history of cOME were tested at 3 years of age within 3 months of ventilation tube placement. The parameters of the FRT were compared between these groups using a two-tailed Student's t test and the frequencies of ears evidencing eustachian tube dilation with swallowing were compared between groups using a χ^2 test.

Results.—Passive resistance and one measure of active function were significantly higher in the rAOM group. The frequency of tubal dilation was not significantly different between groups. There were no differences in any of the FRT measures between cOME ears that did and did not have acute otitis media by history.

▶ Otitis media (OM) is a very common diagnosis from pediatric emergency departments. Poor eustachian tube function has been suggested as the reason for OM. This study evaluated the forced response test (inflation-deflation test, Valsalva, sniffing, the 9-step test) on function of the eustachian tube. This small pilot study found that passive function parameters were lower in the recurrent acute OM. Chronic OM had relatively normal function parameters. Unfortunately, all these noninvasive tests that could potentially be performed in the

ED were not an ideal set because of its high variability. The search for that ideal test in determining chronic OM versus recurrent OM continues.

E. C. Quintana, MD, MPH

Is a Lumbar Puncture Necessary When Evaluating Febrile Infants (30 to 90 Days of Age) With an Abnormal Urinalysis?

Paquette K, Cheng MP, McGillivray D, et al (McGill Univ, Montréal, Québec, Canada)
Pediatr Emerg Care 27:1057-1061, 2011

Objectives.—Guidelines for the management of febrile infants aged 30 to 90 days presenting to the emergency department (ED) suggest that a lumbar puncture (LP) should be performed routinely if a positive urinalysis is found during initial investigations. The aim of our study was to assess the necessity of routine LPs in infants aged 30 to 90 days presenting to the ED for a fever without source but are found to have a positive urine analysis.

Methods.—We retrospectively reviewed the records of all infants aged 30 to 90 days, presenting to the Montreal Children's Hospital ED from October 2001 to August 2005 who underwent an LP for bacterial culture, in addition to urinalysis and blood and urine cultures. Descriptive statistics and their corresponding confidence intervals were used.

Results.—Overall, 392 infants were identified using the microbiology laboratory database. Fifty-seven patients had an abnormal urinalysis. Of these, 1 infant (71 days old) had an *Escherichia coli* urinary tract infection, bacteremia, and meningitis. This patient, however, was not well on history, and the peripheral white blood cell count was low at 2.9×10^9/L. Thus, the negative predictive value of an abnormal urinalysis for meningitis was 98.2%.

Conclusions.—Routine LPs are not required in infants (30–90 days) presenting to the ED with a fever and a positive urinalysis if they are considered at low risk for serious bacterial infection based on clinical and laboratory criteria. However, we recommend that judicious clinical judgment be used; in doubt, an LP should be performed before empiric antibiotic therapy is begun (Table 1).

▶ The evaluation and management of febrile infants, age 30 to 90 days, remains a moving target. While several guidelines and recommendations exist, a standardized approach is not available. The authors of this study attempted to apply a common sense approach to the management of the febrile infant (30 to 90 days of age) with a presumed urinary tract infection (UTI). Following the Rochester criteria, as described in detail in the article, all febrile patients had urine, blood, and cerebrospinal fluid (CSF) cultures performed. Patients with presumed UTIs based on the urinalysis were extremely unlikely to have concomitant bacterial meningitis (1.8%). More importantly, only 4 of the included 392 patients had positive CSF cultures, resulting in 388 negative lumbar puncture results. All 4 patients with meningitis has grossly altered physical examinations with lethargy, dehydration, hypotension, and other

TABLE 1.—Characteristics of Infant With Meningitis

Characteristics	Patient 1	Patient 2	Patient 3	Patient 4
Age, d	71	49	41	33
Clinical	38.5°C (rectally), mottled skin, cool extremities, irritability, lethargy, and decreased feeding	39.7°C (R), hypotension responsive to bolus, lethargy, petechial rash	38.6°C (R), shortness of breath, grunting; resuscitated and intubated in ED	38.6°C (R), somnolent, fussy, dehydrated, and decreased feeding
Peripheral WBC count, $\times 10^9$/L	2.9	3.0	1.3	14.8
Blood culture	E. coli	N. meningitidis group B	Group B Streptococcus	Negative
Urinalysis	Leukocyte esterase positive, nitrite positive, 6 RBCs/HPF, 4 WBCs/HPF	Negative	Negative	Negative
Urine culture	E. coli >10^8/L	Negative	Negative	Negative
CSF culture	E. coli	N. meningitidis group B	Negative after antibiotics (LP: WBCs, 1592; 68% neutrophils; proteins, 2.38 mmol/L)	E. coli

RBC indicates red blood cells.

abnormalities (Table 1). Understanding the consequences of missed bacterial meningitis, this low prevalence of disease calls into question the reflexive decision to tap all well-appearing febrile infants, especially in the presence of a UTI.

E. C. Bruno, MD

Month-by-Month Age Analysis of the Risk for Serious Bacterial Infections in Febrile Infants With Bronchiolitis
Yarden-Bilavsky H, Ashkenazi-Hoffnung L, Livni G, et al (Schneider Children's Med Ctr, Petah Tiqva, Israel)
Clin Pediatr (Phila) 50:1052-1056, 2011

Objective.—This study's aim was to assess the risk of serious bacterial infections (SBI) in each of the first 3 months in hospitalized febrile infants with bronchiolitis.

Patients and Methods.—The risk of SBI was compared between hospitalized infant with or without bronchiolitis by age in months.

Results.—A total of 1125 febrile infants aged ≤3 months were admitted during the study period, 948 without and 177 with bronchiolitis. The incidence of SBI was significantly lower among infants with bronchiolitis compared with those without (4% vs 12.2%, *P* < .001). However, within the subgroup of neonates with bronchiolitis aged ≤28 days, the incidence of SBI was 9.7% and was not significantly lower than in neonates without bronchiolitis.

Conclusion.—The risk of SBI among febrile infants with bronchiolitis is significantly lower compared with febrile infants without bronchiolitis, but only after the neonatal period in which the risk for urinary tract infection was relatively high (9.7%) (Table 2).

▶ Prospectively, this observational study assesses the risk for serious bacterial infection (SBI) in each of the first 3 months of life in febrile infants with or without bronchiolitis. The participating patients were divided into 2 groups by the presence or absence of bronchiolitis. The diagnosis of SBI, namely meningitis, bacteremia, and urinary tract infection (UTI), was based on the growth of a known pathogenic bacteria in culture. SBIs were detected in 116 of the 948 infants without bronchiolitis (12.2%; UTI in 92, bacteremia with UTI in 7, isolated bacteremia in 8, and pneumonia in 9) compared with 7 of the 177 infants with bronchiolitis (4%; all UTI). This difference was statistically significant (*P* < .001). Among the 7 children in the bronchiolitis group with UTI, 6 were respiratory syncytial virus (RSV)-positive and 1 RSV-negative. The SBI rate in subgroup + RSV was similar to that for the entire bronchiolitis group. No statistically significant difference was noted between infants with or without bronchiolitis in the neonatal age group (9.7% vs 15.7%, *P* = .6). Within the subgroup of infants aged 29 to 60 days, those with bronchiolitis had a significantly lower rate of SBI than those without bronchiolitis (3.2% vs 10%, *P* = .03). A trend to less SBI in those with bronchiolitis was noted also for the age group of 61 to 90 days (1.9% vs 11.1%); however, because of

TABLE 2.—Incidence of SBI in Infants With or Without Bronchiolitis

| SBI | ≤28 Days | | | 29-60 Days | | | 61-90 Days | | |
	With Bronchiolitis (n = 31)	Without Bronchiolitis (n = 344)	P	With Bronchiolitis (n = 94)	Without Bronchiolitis (n = 487)	P	With Bronchiolitis (n = 52)	Without Bronchiolitis (n = 117)	P
UTI	3	44		3	40		1	8	
UTI with bacteremia	—	4		—	1		—	2	
Bacteremia	—	4		—	3		—	1	
Pneumonia	—	2		—	5		—	2	
Meningitis	—	—		—	—		—	0	
Total, n (%)	3 (9.7)	54 (15.7)	.6	3 (3.2)	49 (10)	.03	1 (1.9)	13 (11.1)	.066

Abbreviations: SBI, serious bacterial infections; UTI, urinary tract infection.

low numbers of hospitalized infants in this age group, this difference did not reach significance ($P = .066$) (Table 2). Of interest, the only type of SBI in infants with bronchiolitis in all age groups was UTI, especially in the neonate (≤28 days old). Based on this study, the following recommendations have been suggested: routine full-fever evaluation with empiric antibiotic treatment may not be justified in nontoxic febrile infants aged 90 days or younger with acute bronchiolitis. In the group of neonates aged 28 days or younger, we recommend obtaining blood and urinary cultures, whereas in those aged 29 to 90 days, obtaining only urine culture is more appropriate. Still, further larger prospective studies are needed.

E. C. Quintana, MD, MPH

National Ambulatory Antibiotic Prescribing Patterns for Pediatric Urinary Tract Infection, 1998–2007
Copp HL, Shapiro DJ, Hersh AL (Univ of California, San Francisco; Univ of Utah, Salt Lake City)
Pediatrics 127:1027-1033, 2011

Objective.—The goal of this study was to investigate patterns of ambulatory antibiotic use and to identify factors associated with broad-spectrum antibiotic prescribing for pediatric urinary tract infections (UTIs).

Methods.—We examined antibiotics prescribed for UTIs for children aged younger than 18 years from 1998 to 2007 using the National Ambulatory Medical Care Survey and National Hospital Ambulatory Medical Care Survey. Amoxicillin-clavulanate, quinolones, macrolides, and second- and third-generation cephalosporins were classified as broad-spectrum antibiotics. We evaluated trends in broad-spectrum antibiotic prescribing patterns and performed multivariable logistic regression to identify factors associated with broad-spectrum antibiotic use.

Results.—Antibiotics were prescribed for 70% of pediatric UTI visits. Trimethoprim-sulfamethoxazole was the most commonly prescribed antibiotic (49% of visits). Broad-spectrum antibiotics were prescribed one third of the time. There was no increase in overall use of broadspectrum antibiotics ($P = .67$); however, third-generation cephalosporin use doubled from 12% to 25% ($P = .02$). Children younger than 2 years old (odds ratio: 6.4 [95% confidence interval: 2.2—18.7, compared with children 13—17 years old]), females (odds ratio: 3.6 [95% confidence interval: 1.6—8.5]), and temperature ≥100.4°F (odds ratio: 2.9 [95% confidence interval: 1.0—8.6]) were independent predictors of broadspectrum antibiotic prescribing. Race, physician specialty, region, and insurance status were not associated with antibiotic selection.

Conclusions.—Ambulatory care physicians commonly prescribe broad-spectrum antibiotics for the treatment of pediatric UTIs, especially for febrile infants in whom complicated infections are more likely. The doubling in use of third-generation cephalosporins suggests that opportunities exist to promote more judicious antibiotic prescribing because most pediatric UTIs are susceptible to narrower alternatives.

▶ This retrospective observational study tried to determine the antibiotic use trends for urinary tract infections (UTIs) in children using national data (National Ambulatory Medical Care Survey and National Hospital Ambulatory Medical Care Survey). The study included the following physician specialties: pediatrics, family practice, and emergency medicine. The number of UTIs was approximately 1.5 million per year, with less than 1% requiring hospital admission. Seventy-seven percent of parenteral antibiotic used was a third-generation cephalosporin (ceftriaxone, 95%). Trimethoprim-sulfamethoxazole was the most commonly prescribed outpatient antibiotic (49%). Of note, most UTIs are caused by *Escherichia coli*, which has a low resistance to first-generation cephalosporins (3.5%—6.5% in females and males, respectively) in contrast to trimethoprim-sulfamethoxazole (20%—40% resistance). Children less than 2 years old and those with fever admitted to the hospital were more likely to receive broad-spectrum antibiotics. Not surprisingly, children younger than 2 years old, those with fever ≥100.4°F, and girls were independent predictors of broad-spectrum antibiotic use. Unfortunately, this study did not address the appropriateness of using narrower-spectrum antibiotics for UTIs.

E. C. Quintana, MD, MPH

Neonatal scalp abscess: is it a benign disease?
Weiner EJ, McIntosh MS, Joseph MM, et al (Drexel Univ College of Medicine, Philadelphia, Pennsylvania; Univ of Florida Health Science Ctr, Jacksonville; et al)
J Emerg Med 40:e97-e101, 2011

Background.—Neonatal scalp abscesses are a rare but potentially very serious condition.

Objectives.—This report serves to demonstrate meningitis as a potential complication of neonatal scalp abscess. In addition, we review the current

TABLE 1.—Summary of Cases

Case Number	Age of Patient (Days)	Fetal Scalp Electrode	Fever	Head Imaging	Wound Culture	CSF Culture	Antibiotics Used	Length of Stay (Days)
1	5	Yes	No	Cranial ultrasound	Coag-negative *staph*	*Enterococcus*	Ampicillin	14
2	6	Yes	No	Skull radiograph	Negative	Negative	Nafcillin	11
3	5	Yes	No	No	Negative	Negative	Ampicillin & Cefotaxime. Amoxicillin-clavulanate	5
4	6	Yes	Equivocal	Cranial ultrasound	Coag-negative *staph*	Negative	Clindamycin Cefotaxime	3
5	9	No (but vacuum assisted)	Yes	Cranial ultrasound	Coag-negative *staph*	Negative	Cefazolin Clindamycin	6
6	5	Yes	No	Cranial ultrasound	*E. coli*	Negative	Clindamycin Cefotaxime	5

CSF = cerebrospinal fluid; Coag-negative *staph* = coagulase-negative *staphylococci*.

literature on the subject and comment on the most appropriate evaluation and treatment.

Case Report.—We describe six cases of neonatal scalp abscesses with one complication of enterococcal meningitis.

Conclusion.—The emergency practitioner should recognize that a neonate with a scalp abscess needs to be evaluated for potential serious complications and treated empirically to cover for organisms of vaginal origin (Table 1).

▶ This article presented a case series of neonates presenting with neonatal scalp abscesses. Neonatal scalp abscess can occur infrequently (up to 5.4%) due to invasive fetal monitoring during labor and delivery period. The typical involved organisms are polymicrobial and vaginal bacteria. Although most of the lesions are localized and self-limited, serious complications of osteomyelitis, bacteremia, and septicemia need to be considered. In this case series, 1 patient had bacterial meningitis. It is important to note the management of these cases highlights a complete sepsis evaluation, including lumbar puncture, empiric intravenous antibiotics, and admission. The empirical use of antibiotics, after incision and drainage, should provide coverage for both aerobic and anaerobic microorganisms, remembering to add antibiotics that cross the blood—brain barrier in cases of meningitis (Table 1).

E. C. Quintana, MD, MPH

Pediatric emergency department-based rapid HIV testing: adolescent attitudes and preferences
Haines CJ, Uwazuoke K, Zussman B, et al (Drexel Univ College of Medicine, Philadelphia, PA)
Pediatr Emerg Care 27:13-16, 2011

Objective.—The objective of this study was to describe adolescent attitudes/preferences toward rapid HIV testing in a pediatric emergency department (PED).

Methods.—An anonymous survey was completed by adolescents who presented to an urban PED. The survey was completed while they participated in a rapid HIV prevention/testing program. Survey questions included demographics, HIV risk factors/knowledge, prior testing experience, and attitudes/preferences toward rapid HIV testing.

Results.—One hundred fourteen adolescents between the ages of 14 and 21 years were surveyed. Most respondents (69%) reported that the emergency department was a very high preference location for testing. Eighty percent of adolescents agreed that they were more likely to get tested for HIV if a rapid test was available. Most participants strongly agreed that it was important to receive pretest and posttest counseling for HIV. In addition, 38% strongly agreed that they preferred a same-sex counselor, whereas 9% strongly agreed that they preferred a same-ethnicity counselor. Eighty-one percent reported that they planned to get retested for HIV in the next 6 to 12 months.

Conclusions.—This study offers valuable new insights into adolescent attitudes and preferences for rapid HIV testing in a PED. Adolescents gave high ratings to the location, testing, and counseling process. Our data support the importance of structured counseling, which is contrary to current published perspectives of counseling efficacy. In addition, we found that the PED was a highly preferred location for rapid HIV testing, which supports the need for increased development of prevention and testing programs in this setting.

▶ Access to HIV testing has increased over the past few years. Emergency departments (ED) are an ideal location for testing; however, few do routine screening. This study surveyed adolescents who were being screened for HIV during their ED visit. During the study period,17% refused HIV testing because of sexual inactivity or lack of interest (47%). Their results were not surprising. Sixty-seven percent of adolescents stated that they were more likely to agree to HIV testing if a rapid test was available rather than requesting one. Seventy-eight percent gained better understanding of their risks of contracting HIV and the ease of HIV testing in the ED. Their preference indicated that adolescents would likely prefer to be screened by their primary care physician or in the ED rather than at school or another clinic location. Eighty-one percent planned to be screened again in 6 to 12 months. Further ED-based testing programs with structured counseling are warranted for the future in the pediatric ED.

E. C. Quintana, MD, MPH

Prospective Longitudinal Study of Signs and Symptoms Associated With Primary Tooth Eruption
Ramos-Jorge J, Pordeus IA, Ramos-Jorge ML, et al (Universidade Federal de Minas Gerais, Brazil; Universidade Federal dos Vales do Jequitinhonha e Mucuri, Diamantina, Brazil)
Pediatrics 128:471-476, 2011

Objective.—To assess the association between primary tooth eruption and the manifestation of signs and symptoms of teething in infants.

Methods.—An 8-month, longitudinal study was conducted with 47 non-institutionalized infants (ie, receiving care at home) between 5 and 15 months of age in the city of Diamantina, Brazil. The nonrandomized convenience sample was based on the registry of infants in this age range provided by the Diamantina Secretary of Health. Eligible participants were infants with up to 7 erupted incisors and no history of chronic disease or disorders that could cause an increase in the signs and symptoms assessed in the study. Tympanic and axillary temperature readings and clinical oral examinations were performed daily. A daily interview with the mothers was conducted to investigate the occurrence of 13 signs and symptoms associated with teething presented by the infants in the previous 24 hours.

Results.—Teething was associated with a rise in tympanic temperature on the day of the eruption ($P = .004$) and with the occurrence of other signs and symptoms. Readings of maximal tympanic and axillary temperatures were 36.8°C and 36.6°C, respectively. The most frequent signs and symptoms associated with teething were irritability (median: 0.60; $P < .001$), increased salivation (median: 0.50; $P < .001$), runny nose (median: 0.50; $P < .001$), and loss of appetite (median: 0.50; $P < .001$).

Conclusions.—Irritability, increased salivation, runny nose, loss of appetite, diarrhea, rash, and sleep disturbance were associated with primary tooth eruption. Results of this study support the concept that the occurrence of severe signs and symptoms, such as fever, could not be attributed to teething.

▶ How many times during a shift have you heard from caregivers that teething is to blame for many symptoms in infants, including fever? Finally, some light has been shed into this issue. This prospective study involved children from 5 to 15 months old over an 8-month period. Daily data collection was performed to measure temperature and possible signs and symptoms until 1 week after the eruption of the last incisor. Diagnosis of tooth eruption was performed with photographic analysis and the help of a pediatric dentist. Mothers were interviewed regarding the occurrence of increased salivation, rash, runny nose, diarrhea, loss of appetite, cold, irritability, fever, smelly urine, constipation, vomiting, colic, and seizures. Sleep disturbances, increased salivation, loss of appetite, and irritability were greatly reported on the day of and the day after tooth eruption. This study found a correlation between tooth eruption and diarrhea ($P < .001$). No specific symptoms could reliably predict teething. Most importantly, fever was not associated with teething ($P = .042$, $P = .065$, $P = .212$ for day before, day of, and day after eruption, respectively). No other clinically important symptom was associated with teething either. Although this may be a challenging myth to break to your caregiver, it is important that other causes for the presence of fever and severe symptoms are appropriately evaluated.

E. C. Quintana, MD, MPH

Risk factors for contamination of catheterized urine specimens in febrile children
Wingerter S, Bachur R (Harvard Med School, Boston, MA)
Pediatr Emerg Care 27:1-4, 2011

Background.—Urinary tract infections are the most common serious bacterial infection in febrile infants. Bladder catheterization is the preferred method of obtaining urine for culture in young children. Contamination of urine can be recognized when nonpathogens or multiple pathogens are isolated; preliminary culture results may lead to unnecessary antibiotics pending final identification. Some low-colony count (<50,000 colony-forming units per milliliter) cultures may represent contamination or asymptomatic bacteriuria.

Objective.—Identify clinical factors that lead to contamination of catheterized urine specimens.

Methods.—Physicians and nurses in an urban pediatric emergency department completed a survey after performing bladder catheterization of febrile children 36 months or younger. Contamination was defined by multiple pathogens, nonpathogens, or colony counts less than 10,000 colony-forming units per milliliter.

Results.—One hundred eighty-five children were studied. The median age was 8.4 months (interquartile range, 2.4-14.4 months). Sixty-eight percent were girls. Forty-six percent of boys were circumcised. Of the 185 children, 18 (10%) had true UTI. Fourteen percent of cultures were contaminated. Univariate analysis of potential predictors identified age younger than 6 months (odds ratio [OR], 6.8; 95% confidence interval [CI], 2.6-17.9), difficult catheterization (OR, 3.6; 95% CI, 1.5-8.6), and uncircumcised boys (OR, 5.7; 95% CI, 1.2-29.4). The contamination rate in uncircumcised boys younger than 6 months was 43% (95% CI, 26-66). Volume of urine, sex, and catheter size were not predictive of contamination.

Conclusions.—Children younger than 6 months and uncircumcised boys are at increased risk of contaminated specimens from bladder catheterization. Suprapubic aspiration or use of a fresh, sterile catheter with each repeated attempt at catheterization may lead to less contamination in these patients.

▶ Urinary tract infections are a common bacterial infection in pediatrics. Urinalysis and culture are an essential part of the evaluation of febrile children. The risks factors for contamination of catheterized urine specimen were evaluated in this study. Questionnaire questions to nurses catheterizing included patient's gender, circumcision status (if male), ease of catheterization, size of catheter, and urine volume. Fourteen percent of urine cultures were contaminated with all having negative urinalysis. Univariate analysis found that potential predictors of contamination were not surprising. They were age younger than 6 months old, difficulty catheterization, and uncircumcised boys.

Several limitations were noted in this study. The various level of expertise and experience in performing this procedure was not clarified. Also, the subjectiveness of the criteria of catheterization ease could vary from person to person, which is also subjective to expertise. Further criteria would be needed to determine which aspects make a catheterization difficult or not. Still, this is an interesting finding to keep in mind when approaching bladder catheterization in febrile children.

E. C. Quintana, MD, MPH

The Low Rate of Bacterial Meningitis in Children, Ages 6 to 18 Months, With Simple Febrile Seizures

Hom J, Medwid K (New York Univ School of Medicine)

Acad Emerg Med 18:1114-1120, 2011

Objectives.—This evidence-based review examines the risk of bacterial meningitis as diagnosed by lumbar puncture (LP) in children presenting to the emergency department (ED) with a simple febrile seizure. The study population consists of fully immunized children between ages 6 and 18 months of age with an unremarkable history and normal physical examination.

Methods.—MEDLINE, EMBASE, and Cochrane Library databases were searched for studies that enrolled children who presented with simple febrile seizure to the ED and had LP performed to rule out meningitis. The primary outcome measure was the risk of bacterial meningitis based on findings of the LP. The secondary outcome was the rate of cerebrospinal fluid (CSF) pleocytosis in children who were pretreated with antibiotics.

Results.—Two studies enrolling a total of 150 children met the inclusion and exclusion criteria. The overall rate of meningitis was 0% (95% confidence interval [CI] = 0.0% to 3.0%). The rate of CSF pleocytosis in children who were pretreated with antibiotics was 2.5% (95% CI = 0.0% to 14.0%).

Conclusions.—The sample size of the studies included in this review is too small to draw any definitive conclusion. However, their findings suggest that that the risk of bacterial meningitis in children presenting with simple febrile seizure is very low (Table 3).

▶ Febrile seizure is a common presentation in the pediatric emergency department. This MEDLINE search studied bacterial meningitis, diagnosed by lumbar puncture (LP) findings, and the rate of cerebrospinal fluid (CSF) pleocytosis in children who were pretreated with antibiotics. Two studies with an aggregate of 461 patients met the inclusion criteria. The rate of bacterial meningitis was 0 of 150 (Table 3). The secondary outcome was the rate of pleocytosis in children pretreated with antibiotics. Of the 78 children pretreated with antibiotics, only 40 had an LP performed. Only one of the 40 children, or 2.5%, had pleocytosis (Table 4 in the original article). The risk of bacterial meningitis in children who are partially treated with antibiotics becomes a diagnostic challenge. The updated 2011 guideline recommends that the clinician has the option to perform an LP only in children ages 6 to 12 months, when they are missing immunizations or have an indeterminate immunization status. The biggest limitation in this study is that it is a small sample size to draw any significant conclusions, but it was a suggestion that the rate of bacterial meningitis in children who presented with their simple febrile seizure and had a lumbar puncture performed is very low.

E. C. Quintana, MD, MPH

TABLE 3.—Performance and CSF Analysis of the LP

Reference	Rate of LP Performed With CSF Obtained (95% CI) in <12 Months of Age	Rate of LP Performed With CSF Obtained (95% CI) in 12–18 Months of Age	Total Rate of LP Performed With CSF Obtained (95% CI)	CSF Pleocytosis	Rate of Bacterial Meningitis in Patients With LP (95% CI)
Shaked et al., 2009[11]	28/56, 50.0% (37.3–62.7)*	N/A	28/56, 50.0% (37.3–62.7)	0	0/28, 0% (0.0–14.3)
Kimia et al., 2009[12]	60/100, 60.0% (50.2–69.1)	34/305, 11.2% (8.1–15.2)	94/405, 23.2% (19.4–27.6)†	10‡	0/94, 0% (0.0–4.7)

CSF = cerebral spinal fluid; LP = lumbar puncture; N/A = not applicable.
Editor's Note: Please refer to original journal article for full references.
*Ten of 18 children (55.6%) in the 6- to 9-month age group had an LP. Eighteen of 56 children (32.1%) in the 10- to 12-month age group had an LP.
†Study sample: ages 6 to 18 months; four patients had failed LP attempt and seven patients had LP deferred because of parental refusal.
‡The authors performed a correction for traumatic LP. [Corrected CSF white blood cell count = CSF white blood cell count − (CSF red blood cell count/500)]. The CSF correction was calculated on four patients, of whom two patients still showed CSF pleocytosis.

Urinary Tract Infection: Clinical Practice Guideline for the Diagnosis and Management of the Initial UTI in Febrile Infants and Children 2 to 24 Months
Subcommittee on Urinary Tract Infection, Steering Committee on Quality Improvement and Management
Pediatrics 128:595-610, 2011

Objective.—To revise the American Academy of Pediatrics practice parameter regarding the diagnosis and management of initial urinary tract infections (UTIs) in febrile infants and young children.

Methods.—Analysis of the medical literature published since the last version of the guideline was supplemented by analysis of data provided by authors of recent publications. The strength of evidence supporting each recommendation and the strength of the recommendation were assessed and graded.

Results.—Diagnosis is made on the basis of the presence of both pyuria and at least 50 000 colonies per mL of a single uropathogenic organism in an appropriately collected specimen of urine. After 7 to 14 days of antimicrobial treatment, close clinical follow-up monitoring should be maintained to permit prompt diagnosis and treatment of recurrent infections. Ultrasonography of the kidneys and bladder should be performed to detect anatomic abnormalities. Data from the most recent 6 studies do not support the use of antimicrobial prophylaxis to prevent febrile recurrent UTI in infants without vesicoureteral reflux (VUR) or with grade I to IV VUR. Therefore, a voiding cystourethrography (VCUG) is not recommended routinely after the first UTI; VCUG is indicated if renal and bladder ultrasonography reveals hydronephrosis, scarring, or other findings that would suggest either high-grade VUR or obstructive uropathy and in other atypical or complex clinical circumstances. VCUG should also be performed if there is a recurrence of a febrile UTI. The recommendations in this guideline do not indicate an exclusive course of treatment or serve as a standard of care; variations may be appropriate. Recommendations about antimicrobial prophylaxis and implications for performance of VCUG are based on currently available evidence. As with all American Academy of Pediatrics clinical guidelines, the recommendations will be reviewed routinely and incorporate new evidence, such as data from the Randomized Intervention for Children With Vesicoureteral Reflux (RIVUR) study.

Conclusions.—Changes in this revision include criteria for the diagnosis of UTI and recommendations for imaging.

▶ The American Academy of Pediatrics provided an updated clinical practice guideline (CPG) addressing the diagnosis and management of urinary tract infections (UTI) in febrile infants and children. Although the CPG provides direction for all phases of the entity, several portions of the document are applicable to the practice of emergency medicine. Patients considered to have a UTI as the cause of the febrile illness must have a catheterized or suprapubic aspiration specimen (Level A recommendations), unless the toddler is potty trained.

Bagged urine specimens are unacceptable, and emergency physicians (EPs) should undergo a Quixotic-like crusade to eliminate the urine bags entirely. Even if uninformed pediatric colleagues request the bagged specimens, the practice is dated and provides misinformation.

Additionally, the CPG supports the EP's clinical judgment. If the EP feels that a urinalysis with a few white blood cells does not explain the febrile illness, close follow-up without antimicrobial intervention is within the standard of care. The authors looked to define the diagnosis of UTI, requiring both a urinalysis that suggests UTI (pyuria and/or bacteriuria) and a urine culture with 50 000 colony-forming units per mL of a specific uropathogen. EPs will continue to make the presumptive diagnosis of UTI, send the urine for culture, provide appropriate antimicrobials, and recommend close follow-up to obtain culture results and ensure clinical improvement.

E. C. Bruno, MD

Neuroscience

Neurodiagnostic Evaluation of the Child With a Simple Febrile Seizure
Subcommittee on Febrile Seizures
Pediatrics 127:389-394, 2011

Objective.—To formulate evidence-based recommendations for health care professionals about the diagnosis and evaluation of a simple febrile seizure in infants and young children 6 through 60 months of age and to revise the practice guideline published by the American Academy of Pediatrics (AAP) in 1996.

Methods.—This review included search and analysis of the medical literature published since the last version of the guideline. Physicians with expertise and experience in the fields of neurology and epilepsy, pediatrics, epidemiology, and research methodologies constituted a subcommittee of the AAP Steering Committee on Quality Improvement and Management. The steering committee and other groups within the AAP and organizations outside the AAP reviewed the guideline. The subcommittee member who reviewed the literature for the 1996 AAP practice guidelines searched for articles published since the last guideline through 2009, supplemented by articles submitted by other committee members. Results from the literature search were provided to the subcommittee members for review. Interventions of direct interest included lumbar puncture, electroencephalography, blood studies, and neuroimaging. Multiple issues were raised and discussed iteratively until consensus was reached about recommendations. The strength of evidence supporting each recommendation and the strength of the recommendation were assessed by the committee member most experienced in informatics and epidemiology and graded according to AAP policy.

Conclusions.—Clinicians evaluating infants or young children after a simple febrile seizure should direct their attention toward identifying the cause of the child's fever. Meningitis should be considered in the differential diagnosis for any febrile child, and lumbar puncture should be performed if there are clinical signs or symptoms of concern. For any infant between 6 and 12 months of age who presents with a seizure and fever, a lumbar puncture is an option when the child is considered deficient in *Haemophilus influenzae* type b (Hib) or *Streptococcus pneumoniae* immunizations (ie, has not received scheduled immunizations as recommended), or when immunization status cannot be determined, because of an increased risk of bacterial meningitis. A lumbar puncture is an option for children who are pretreated with antibiotics. In general, a simple febrile seizure does not usually require further evaluation, specifically electroencephalography, blood studies, or neuroimaging.

▶ This article represents the long-awaited revision to the American Academy of Pediatrics' (AAP) 1996 Clinical Practice Guideline (CPG) addressing the management of pediatric patients who experience a simple febrile seizure. The new recommendations suggest that the health care profession perform minimal interventions when possible. Although the article includes discussions related to not performing routine blood studies, electroencephalography, or neuroimaging, the crux of the statement is the position on lumbar punctures (LPs). The authors analyzed literature that became available after the publication of the first CPG and concluded that fewer interventions, specifically LPs, were necessary when evaluating a patient aged 6 to 60 months who experiences a simple febrile seizure. This modification is of critical importance, because a significant portion of the AAP's membership likely violates the recommendations in the 1996 guideline. The seizure must meet the definition of "simple," the patient must be current on the advised immunization schedule, and the patient must not be on antibiotics, since the medications can mask the meningismus that could be present in an intracranial infection. The publishing and subsequent reviews of the revised CPG will presumably result in fewer LPs but may strengthen the treating physician's stance when entreating parents and caregivers for the permission to perform the LP on the child.

E. C. Bruno, MD

Practice variability in the management of complex febrile seizures by pediatric emergency physicians and fellows
Sales JW, Bulloch B, Hostetler MA (Phoenix Children's Hosp, AZ)
CJEM 13:145-149, 2011

Objective.—Febrile seizures are the most common type of childhood seizure and are categorized as simple or complex. Complex febrile seizures (CFSs) are defined as events that are focal, prolonged (>15 minutes), or recurrent. The management of CFS is poorly defined. The objective of this study was to determine the degree of variability in the emergency department evaluation of children with CFSs.

Methods.—An online survey questionnaire was developed and sent to physicians identified via the listserv of the emergency medicine section of the American Academy of Pediatrics and the pediatric emergency medicine discussion list. The questionnaire consisted of five hypothetical case vignettes describing children under 5 years of age presenting with a CFS. Following review of the first four vignettes, participants were asked if they would (1) obtain blood and urine for evaluation; (2) perform a lumbar puncture; (3) perform neurologic imaging while the child was in the emergency department; (4) admit the child to the hospital; or (5) discharge with follow-up as an outpatient, with either the primary care provider or a neurologist. The final vignette determined if antiepileptic medication would be prescribed by the physician on discharge.

Results.—Of the 353 physicians who participated, 293 (83%) were pediatric emergency medicine attending physicians and 60 (17%) were pediatric emergency medicine fellows. Overall, 54% of participants indicated that they would obtain blood for evaluation, 62% would obtain urine, 34% would perform a lumbar puncture, and 36% would perform neurologic imaging. The overall hypothetical admission rate for the case vignettes was 42%.

Conclusions.—This study indicates that extensive variability exists in the emergency department approach to patients with CFS. Our findings suggest that optimal management for CFS remains unclear and support the potential benefit of future prospective studies on this subject.

▶ Management of complex febrile seizures remains an area of controversy. A treating physician's primary concern is the identification of those patients who seize because of an intracranial infection. Emergency physicians, both general emergency medicine and pediatric emergency medicine, are responsible for the diagnostic approach to these patients and are subject to "Monday-morning quarterbacking" by the inpatient and primary pediatricians if an adverse event occurs. The authors of this study surveyed pediatric emergency physicians, using case vignettes, to determine practice patterns in the management of patients with complex febrile seizures. The narrative included patients of varied ages with events that represented complex febrile seizures in children who otherwise appeared well. The responses to the survey demonstrated no consistent pattern in regard to diagnostic testing (blood, urine, or cerebrospinal fluid), radiographic evaluations, and dispositions. Patients were rarely started on antiepileptic medications (5%). Without a standard approach to these patients, a conservative strategy may be best.

E. C. Bruno, MD

Procedures

Bedside Ultrasound in the Diagnosis of Pediatric Clavicle Fractures

Chien M, Bulloch B, Garcia-Filion P, et al (Phoenix Children's Hosp, AZ)
Pediatr Emerg Care 27:1038-1041, 2011

Objective.—The objective of the study was to determine the diagnostic accuracy of pediatric emergency physicians in diagnosing clavicle fractures by bedside ultrasound (US).

Methods.—This was a prospective study of pediatric emergency department (ED) patients with suspected clavicle fractures conducted in a tertiary-care, freestanding pediatric hospital. A convenience sample of patients younger than 17 years underwent bedside US for detection of clavicle fracture by pediatric emergency physicians with limited US training. Ultrasound findings were compared with standard radiographs, which were considered the criterion standard. Pain scores using the validated color analog scale (0-10) were determined before and during US. Total length of stay in the ED, time to US, and time to radiograph were recorded.

Results.—Fifty-eight patients were enrolled, of which 39 (67%) had fracture determined by radiograph. Ultrasound interpretation gave a sensitivity of 89.7% (95% confidence interval [CI], 75.8%−97.1%) and specificity of 89.5% (95% CI, 66.9%−98.7%). Positive and negative predictive values were 94.6% (95% CI, 81.8%−99.3%) and 81.0% (95% CI, 58.1%−94.5%), respectively. Positive and negative likelihood ratios were 8.33 and 0.11, respectively. Pain scores averaged 4.7 before US and 5.2 during US ($P = 0.204$). There was a statistically significant difference between mean time to US (76 minutes) and mean time to radiograph (107 minutes) ($P < 0.001$).

Conclusions.—Pediatric emergency physicians with minimal formal training can accurately diagnose clavicle fractures by US. In addition, US itself is not associated with an increase in pain and may reduce length of stay in the ED (Fig 1, Table 1).

▶ One of the more useful and easily used applications is the detection of skeletal fractures with bedside ultrasound scan (US). Adult literature has been extensive in this regard when compared with pediatric studies in the use of US to detect skeletal fractures. By using US, ideally there would be decrease of stay (not having to wait for radiology), less radiation exposure, and less pain. The first examination was conducted with the patient in the supine position with the face rotated opposite the examined side and the arm held still. The transducer was placed parallel to the long axis of the clavicle and perpendicular to the plane of the body on the nonaffected clavicle. The normal clavicle presented as a continuous S-shaped echodense structure. Subsequently, the examination was carried out on the affected clavicle. A sign of fracture manifested as a discontinuity of bone echogenicity, steps, or axial deviation and was denoted simply as yes or no for evidence of fracture (Fig 1). Pain scores using the validated color analog scale (0−10) for patients older than 5 years

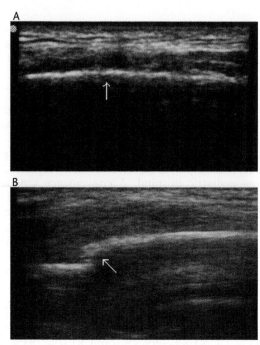

FIGURE 1.—Ultrasound images of normal (A) and fractured (B) clavicle. Arrows point to region of normal clavicle and region of discontinuity. (Reprinted from Chien M, Bulloch B, Garcia-Filion P, et al. Bedside ultrasound in the diagnosis of pediatric clavicle fractures. *Pediatr Emerg Care.* 2011;27:1038-1041, with permission from Lippincott Williams & Wilkins.)

TABLE 1.—Performance Metrics of Bedside US to Identify Clavicle Fractures

	Radiograph +	Radiograph −
Ultrasound +	35	2
Ultrasound −	4	17

Sensitivity, 89.7% (CI, 75.8%−97.1%); specificity, 89.5% (CI, 66.9%−98.7%); PPV, 94.6% (CI, 81.8%−99.3%); NPV, 81.0% (CI, 58.1%−94.5%); +LR, 8.53; −LR, 0.11.

were determined at baseline just before and during the procedure. No pain medications were given. This study found that US interpretation gave a sensitivity of 89.7% and specificity of 89.5%; positive predictive value and negative predictive value were 94.6% and 81.0%, respectively. Positive and negative likelihood ratios were 8.33 and 0.11, respectively (Table 1). Most importantly, there was an agreement of 90% between the ultrasound and radiographic findings. There was a statistically significant difference between mean time to US (76 [SD, 46] minutes) and mean time to radiograph (107 [SD, 48] minutes) ($P < .001$). Pain scores in children older than 5 years were available in 35 of 58 patients and averaged 4.7 (SD, 2.3) before US and 5.2 (SD, 0.39) during US ($P = .204$). This showed that there wasn't a significant increase of pain by doing US. This is a consideration for using bedside US for evaluation of clavicular fractures.

E. C. Quintana, MD, MPH

Bedside ultrasound in the diagnosis of skull fractures in the pediatric emergency department

Ramirez-Schrempp D, Vinci RJ, Liteplo AS (Boston Univ School of Medicine/ Boston Med Ctr, MA)

Pediatr Emerg Care 27:312-314, 2011

Bedside ultrasound has become a diagnostic tool that is commonly used in the emergency department. In trained hands, it can be used to diagnose multiple pathologies. In this case series, we describe the utility of ultrasound in diagnosing skull fractures in pediatric patients with scalp hematomas.

▶ Diagnostic imaging is the choice for those children at high risk with head trauma. It is very sensitive for diagnosing skull fractures and intracranial bleed. Obtaining head CT in all asymptomatic patients is costly and increases exposure to potential radiation. This study evaluates ultrasound as an alternative to CT scanning and x-rays. This case series demonstrated that a bedside ultrasound with a high-frequency linear probe can be used to evaluate any skull fractures under areas of hematomas. Fractures would appear as dark effects under bony cortex, or angulated bone fractures would be visualized. All patients were under 2 years old with hematomas ranging from 3 to 4 cm after falls and head trauma. Ultrasound was able to find evidence of skull fracture, which was confirmed with head CT (Figs 1 and 2 in the original article). Although this was a small case series, it demonstrated that ultrasound is a useful tool in the emergency department. It is a reproducible, noninvasive technique that lacks the potentially harmful radiation exposure. Further studies are warranted.

E. C. Quintana, MD, MPH

Detection of hypoventilation by capnography and its association with hypoxia in children undergoing sedation with ketamine

Langhan ML, Chen L, Marshall C, et al (Yale Univ School of Medicine, New Haven, CT)

Pediatr Emerg Care 27:394-397, 2011

Objectives.—Hypopneic hypoventilation, a decrease in tidal volume without a change in respiratory rate, is not easily detected by standard monitoring practices during sedation but can be detected by capnography. Our goal was to determine the frequency of hypopneic hypoventilation and its association with hypoxia in children undergoing sedation with ketamine.

Methods.—Children who received intravenous ketamine with or without midazolam for sedation in a pediatric emergency department were prospectively enrolled. Heart rate, respiratory rate, pulse oximetry, and end-tidal carbon dioxide (ET(CO2)) levels were recorded every 30 seconds.

Results.—Fifty-eight subjects were included in this study. Fifty percent of subjects had recorded ET(CO2) values less than 30 mm Hg without a rise in respiratory rate. Twenty-eight percent of subjects experienced a decrease in pulse oximetry less than 95%. Patients who experienced a persistent decrease in ET(CO2) at least 30 seconds in length were much more likely to have a persistent decrease in pulse oximetry than those with normal or transient decreases in ET(CO2) (relative risk, 6.6; 95% confidence interval, 1.4-30.5). Decreases in ET(CO2) occurred on an average of 3.7 minutes before decreases in pulse oximetry.

Conclusions.—Hypopneic hypoventilation as detected by capnography is common in children undergoing sedation with ketamine with or without midazolam. Hypoxia is frequently preceded by low ET(CO2) levels. Further studies are needed to determine if the addition of routine monitoring with capnography can reduce the frequency of hypoxia in children undergoing sedation.

▶ Moderate sedation is commonly used in many pediatric procedures. Capnography offers the advantage of providing an approximate of arterial carbon dioxide in the respiratory cycle. Nasal oral cannulas offer an easy, noninvasive option to detect hypoventilation by detecting a decrease in respiratory rate (elevated EtCO2) and decrease in tidal volume with a normal respiratory rate (lower EtCO2). This prospective observational study determined that 50% of patients had EtCO2 less 30 mm Hg without increase of respiratory rate. Fifty-five percent had persistent episodes for 2 or more consecutive 30-second events. Thirty-one percent with low EtCO2 were more likely to have persistent low pulse oximeter. The relative risk of hypoxia with low EtCO2 was 6.6. Decreases of EtCO2 preceded low pulse oximetry by a mean of slightly less than 4 minutes (range: 1–10 minutes). This study showed that hypopneic hypoventilation with Et CO2 less than 30 mm Hg without an increase in respiratory rate is a common event in children with moderate sedation. More studies are needed to determine whether capnography can reduce the incidence of hypoxia in the pediatric ED moderate sedation.

E. C. Quintana, MD, MPH

Management of uncomplicated nail bed lacerations presenting to a children's emergency department

Al-Qadhi S, Chan KJ, Fong G, et al (Hosp for Sick Children, Toronto, Ontario, Canada)
Pediatr Emerg Care 27:379-383, 2011

Objective.—This study examined the mechanisms of injury and the pattern of care for children who presented to the emergency department with uncomplicated nail bed lacerations.

Methods.—A retrospective chart review was conducted from January 2004 to December 2007 for all children younger than 18 years who presented to a tertiary children's hospital with an uncomplicated nail bed laceration.

Results.—There were 84 cases of uncomplicated nail bed injuries for more than a 4-year period. Sixty percent of the subjects were males. The mean age was 5.3 (SD, 4.1) years. Most injuries occurred at home (58%), and the most common mechanism of injury was a door (67%). Approximately 40% of patients were treated by emergency physicians. There was no significant difference in acute and chronic complications or in the length of stay in the emergency department, between patients treated by emergency physicians and by plastic surgeons.

Conclusions.—Most nail bed injuries in children occur at home, and the door seems to be the major mechanism of injury. Approximately 57% of these are children younger than 5 years. Only 42% of uncomplicated nail bed lacerations are treated by emergency physicians, yet there is no significant difference in outcomes between plastic surgeons and emergency physicians. Our study suggests that there is a role in public education for primary prevention, and with proper training, pediatric emergency physicians can treat uncomplicated nail bed lacerations.

▶ Nail bed injuries are a fairly common occurrence in fingertip injuries. Primary repair of nail bed has been the standard of care for nail bed injuries. Using retrospective chart review, this study evaluated uncomplicated nail bed injuries and management. In this study, both simple and stellate nail bed lacerations were considered uncomplicated (Fig 1 in the original article). The mean age was 5.3 years with a male predominance. Door-related injuries occurring at home were by far the most common mechanism of nail bed injuries. Although the length of stay was 51 minutes shorter for emergency medicine (EM) physicians managing nail bed injuries compared with plastic surgeons, it was not statistically significant. Forty-two percent of patients were managed by EM physicians, 83% were referred to plastic surgery for follow-up, and 84% kept their follow-up appointments. The study did not show any difference in acute or chronic complications between plastic surgeons or EM physicians. The acute complications found for EM physicians were 1 subungual hematoma, 1 suture breakdown, and 1 poor dressing. The acute complications for plastic surgeons were 2 infections. The chronic complications for EM physicians were 1 nail deformity, whereas the plastic surgeons had 1 chronic infection as their complication (Table 1 in the original article). Hence, training of simple nail bed repair should be provided to all EM physician fellows/trainees.

E. C. Quintana, MD, MPH

Outcomes After Rigid Bronchoscopy in Children With Suspected or Confirmed Foreign Body Aspiration: A Retrospective Study

Maddali MM, Mathew M, Chandwani J, et al (Royal Hosp, Seeb, Muscat, Sultanate of Oman; Sultan Qaboos Univ, Muscat, Sultanate of Oman)

J Cardiothorac Vasc Anesth 25:1005-1008, 2011

Objective.—To identify the determinants of immediate outcome after rigid bronchoscopy for suspected or confirmed foreign body (FB) aspiration. The outcome may be affected by the duration of bronchoscopy, the type of FB, the time between inhalation and removal of the FB, and the type of anesthetic induction. Arterial desaturation, bronco-laryngospasm, and the need for tracheal reintubation as complications were investigated.

Design.—A retrospective study.

Setting.—A single tertiary care center.

Participants.—One hundred seventy-five children who underwent rigid bronchoscopy.

Interventions.—None.

Measurements and Main Results.—Age, duration after suspected or witnessed inhalation before bronchoscopy, and the type of FB had no relationship to the occurrence of complications. The prolongation of bronchoscopy beyond 30 minutes was associated with a significant increase in complications as was the use of intravenous rather than inhalation induction of anesthesia.

Conclusions.—Reducing the bronchoscopy time may not be an option, but an awareness of the risk of complications may prompt a more intense postanesthesia monitoring strategy (Tables 3 and 4).

▶ Rigid bronchoscopy under general anesthesia is the method of choice for diagnosis and removal for foreign body (FB) aspiration. This study evaluated the complications and outcomes from rigid bronchoscopy. FBs were categorized in 2 groups: organic and inorganic. Organic FBs included nuts (ie, peanuts, almonds, cashews, and pistachios), seeds (ie, melon, olive, bean, and sunflower), and food particles (ie, pieces of carrot, chickpeas, and dates). The inorganic category included toy parts (ie, whistles, light bulbs, plastic, and metal pins), pencil pieces, sharps (ie, scarf pins and needles), prayer beads, coins, and gravel. There were no small batteries. One hundred seventy-five were admitted for suspected (35) or witnessed (123) FB aspiration in children less than 3 years old. Age was not a factor on the complication rate. More patients had a history of possible FB aspiration exceeding 24 hours (98) than those seen within 24 hours (77), but there was no difference in the complication rate between the 2 groups ($P = 0.093$) (Table 3). Twenty-five patients had inhalation anesthesia induction only, and they had fewer complications ($P = 0.033$) (Table 3). The overall postprocedure anesthesia duration was 14.4 ± 6.6 minutes (mean standard deviation). Patients whose bronchoscopy exceeded 30 minutes had a significantly higher complication rate ($P = 0.0002$) and a higher incidence of tracheal reintubation ($P = 0.0006$) (Table 4). Despite complications, the overall length of hospital stay was 1.7 ± 1.6 days. High-risk patients as in this series

TABLE 3.—Anesthetic Information of Patients in Relation to Complications and Types of FB

	Postprocedural Complications No (%)
Age group	
≤3 years (n = 115)	56 (48.7)
>3 years (n = 60)	27 (45.0)
p value	0.642*
Duration of aspiration	
≤24 h (n = 77)	31 (40.3)
>24 h (n = 98)	52 (53.1)
p value	0.093
Anesthetic technique	
Inhalation (n = 25)	7 (28.0)
Intravenous (n = 150)	76 (50.7)
p value	0.033*

	Duration of Bronchoscopy (min) Mean ± SD	Time >30 min (%)
Age group		
≤3 years (n = 115)		72 (62.6)
>3 years (n = 60)		42 (70.0)
p value		0.330*
Type of FB		
None (n = 35)	31.4 ± 17.5	19 (54.3)
Organic (n = 88)	38.1 ± 24.4	63 (71.6)
Inorganic (n = 52)	36.9 ± 26.3	32 (61.5)
p value	0.366†	0.155*

Abbreviation: SD, standard deviation.
*Chi-square test.
†Analysis of variance.

TABLE 4.—Postprocedure Complications in Relation to the Duration of Bronchoscopy, the Incidence of Reintubation, and the Length of Hospital Stay

Postprocedure Complications and Tracheal Intubation	Desaturation No (%)	Bronchospasm/Laryngospasm No (%)
Overall (175)	80 (45.7)	3 (1.7)
Reintubation	76 (43.4)	—
Organic (n = 88)*	43 (48.9)	2 (2.3)
Reintubation†	43 (48.9)	—
Inorganic (n = 52)*	23 (44.2)	1
Reintubation‡	19 (36.5)	—
Duration of Bronchoscopy	Complications	Incidence of Reintubation
≤30 min (n = 61)	17 (27.9)	14 (23.0)
>30 min (n = 114)	66 (57.9)	62 (54.4)
p value‡	0.0002	0.0006
Length of hospital stay in days	(mean ± SD)	
All cases	1.7 ± 1.6	
Organic	1.6 ± 1.4	
Inorganic	1.7 ± 1.6	

*p = 0.595.
†p = 0.156.
‡Chi-square test.

(ie, those with a bronchoscopy duration lasting more than 30 minutes and those undergoing anesthetic induction with intravenous agents) merit close observation for complete recovery from anesthetic agents, a brief duration of postprocedure artificial ventilation with gradual weaning, tracheal toileting, bronchodilator nebulization, humidified gases, and watching for a gas leak around the endotracheal tube to ensure that there would be no laryngeal edema.

E. C. Quintana, MD, MPH

Pulmonary

Coprescription of Antibiotics and Asthma Drugs in Children

De Boeck K, Vermeulen F, Meyts I, et al (Univ Hosp of Leuven, Belgium; et al)
Pediatrics 127:1022-1026, 2011

Background.—In children, antibiotics as well as asthma drugs are frequently prescribed. We investigated the effects of the codispensing of antibiotics and asthma drugs to children.

Methods.—Using a health insurance database, we examined dispensing and codispensing of antibiotics and asthma drugs for the period of a 1 year in 892 841 Belgian children aged <18 years.

Results.—For a 1-year period, an antibiotic was dispensed to 44.21% of children: 73.05% aged <3 years; 49.62% aged 3 to 7 years; and 34.21% aged 8 to <18 years. An asthma drug was dispensed to 16.04% of children: 44.81% aged <3 years; 17.90% aged 3 to 7 years; and 7.64% aged 8 to <18 years. Overall, an antibiotic was dispensed without an asthma drug to 38.62% of children versus with an asthma drug to 73.50% of children (*P* < .0001). More frequent dispensing of antibiotics to children who received an asthma drug (odds ratio: 1.90; 95% confidence interval: 1.89—1.91) occurred in all age categories (*P* < .0001). In 35.64% of children with an asthma drug dispensed, an antibiotic was dispensed on the same day.

Conclusions.—In all age groups, dispensing of antibiotics is more likely in children who have an asthma drug dispensed in the same year. In all age groups, codispensing of antibiotics and asthma drugs is a common practice. Efforts to decrease antibiotic use in children could be improved by focusing on children who are being treated with asthma drugs.

▶ This observational study from Belgium evaluated the frequency of dispensing prescriptions for both asthma medications and antibiotics. Regardless of age, most children who were given a prescription for asthma medication, received an antibiotic prescription, especially in the younger-than-3-years age group (odds ratio, 1.90). About a third of those subjects received both asthma and antibiotic prescriptions on the same day. Sixty-four percent of the dispensed antibiotics was amoxicillin, followed by macrolides (14.2%) and cephalosphorins (12.2%). Unfortunately, other investigators have reported the use of antibiotics for upper respiratory infections that are clearly of a viral origin and trigger wheezing in children with reactive airway disease. When presented with a child with respiratory symptoms, it is important to distinguish between those who are febrile and have signs and symptoms consistent with a lower airway bacterial infection for which antibiotics may be the treatment from those who would benefit just from a beta-agonist medication.

This study was strong for several reasons. Its observations remained consistent through the period of 2 years, without any statistically significant variation from year to year. Its study size gave it significant strength.

E. C. Quintana, MD, MPH

Exhaled nitric oxide levels during treatment of pediatric acute asthma exacerbations and association with the need for hospitalization
Nelson KA, Lee P, Trinkaus K, et al (Children's Hosp of Boston, MA)
Pediatr Emerg Care 27:249-255, 2011

Objectives.—To examine how exhaled nitric oxide (eNO) levels measured before and after treatment of asthma exacerbations relate to emergency department (ED) disposition.

Methods.—We enrolled children 6 to 17 years old treated for asthma exacerbations in a pediatric ED. Using an offline single-breath eNO sampling technique, we collected replicate initial samples before treatment and replicate final samples when disposition was decided. We determined correlations and coefficients of variability of eNO values (parts per billion, ppb) of samples and compared by disposition (hospitalization or discharge) mean initial and final eNO levels and initial-to-final change.

Results.—Eighty-one subjects had initial and final eNO values; 24 subjects with more severe presentations had final values only. Replicate eNO samples were correlated (initial r = 0.98, final r = 0.99) and had low coefficients of variability (initial, 0.059 ± 0.057; final, 0.061 ± 0.070). For subjects with initial and final values, initial eNO levels were similar by disposition (mean difference, −8.0 ppb; 95% confidence interval [CI], −24.8 to 8.9 ppb), as were final levels (mean difference, −2.8 ppb; 95% CI, −23.8 to 18.2 ppb). Overall, final eNO was higher than initial (36.3 ± 29.7 vs 31.5 ± 23.9 ppb), but only 63% of subjects had any increase. Change in eNO was similar by disposition (mean difference, 4.6 ppb; 95% CI, −3.4 to 12.6). For more severe subjects with final eNO only, eNO was similar by disposition (P = 0.47).

Conclusions.—For children aged 6 to 17 years with asthma exacerbations, eNO levels can be reliably measured. However, eNO levels measured before treatment or when disposition was determined did not distinguish children needing hospitalization.

▶ Exhaled nitric oxide (eNO) is easily measured from a single breath noninvasively to determine airway inflammation. These eNO levels are elevated in patients with chronic asthma. This study wanted to evaluate whether levels of eNO would determine disposition on patients with an acute asthma exacerbation in the pediatric emergency department (ED). The measurements occurred at initial evaluation (before receiving any medications) and final evaluation (soon after disposition decision was made). Initial or final eNO levels did not consistently discriminate hospitalization from discharge based on receiver operator curve. Sixty-three percent had increased final eNO levels (initial mean eNO 32 vs final mean eNO 36.3 ppb). The hospitalization rate was similar according to eNO change direction ($P = 0.33$).

There were some limitations on this study. There is a group of asthmatic patients who were deemed to be so severe that patients didn't have an initial eNO. The patients were only from a single site so there is a question of external validity, which may not be applied to a different population and other different settings. However, this may be the beginning of exploring noninvasive respiratory measurements to determine disposition of acute asthma exacerbations in the pediatric ED.

E. C. Quintana, MD, MPH

Safety and clinical findings of BiPAP utilization in children 20 kg or less for asthma exacerbations
Williams AM, Abramo TJ, Shah MV, et al (Monroe Carell Jr Children's Hosp at Vanderbilt, Nashville)
Intensive Care Med 37:1338-1343, 2011

Purpose.—To investigate safety and clinical findings of bilevel positive airway pressure (BiPAP) utilization in children 20 kg or less for asthma exacerbations.

Methods.—Retrospective and prospective descriptive analysis of 165 enrolled subjects with moderate and severe asthma exacerbations who weighed 20 kg or less and who received BiPAP treatment at a large, urban children's hospital pediatric emergency department (PED).

Results.—Age was 0.6—8.27 years (mean 3.7 years, SD 1.6 years). None exhibited worsening hypoxia, pneumothorax, or death. Four progressed to intubation after significant period on BiPAP. Overall, BiPAP subjects showed improvement in pediatric asthma score (PAS). BiPAP initiation PAS range was 8—15 (mean 12.1, SD 1.6); BiPAP termination or 4 h PAS mean was 6.3 (SD 2.2); delta PAS showed improvement mean 5.8 (SD 2.4). Seventy-one had trial off BiPAP in PED for clinical improvement; seven were restarted. PED BiPAP duration range was 30—720 min (mean 210 min, SD 158 min); total hospitalization BiPAP duration was 1—90 h. Ninety-nine (60%) subjects were admitted to the PICU and continued BiPAP for 0—47 h (mean 6.6 h, SD 8.6 h). Fifty-seven (35%) required ward admission; none were transferred to PICU. Nine (5%) were discharged home from the PED; none returned within 72 h.

Conclusions.—BiPAP utilization in acute pediatric asthma exacerbations for patients 20 kg or less is safe and may improve clinical outcomes. These findings warrant future prospective investigation of BiPAP efficacy in pediatric asthma patients.

▶ Pediatric patients with significant respiratory distress can incite anxiety in the emergency physician (EP) responsible for their care. This visceral response is further exacerbated by the even younger asthmatic patients. After management with standard interventions including bronchodilators and corticosteroids fail to produce marked clinical improvement, EPs will look for additional interventions to stave off intubation. One consideration, as in adults, is the use of bilevel positive airway pressure (BiPAP). This study evaluated clinical response to BiPAP in patients with severe asthma exacerbations. The authors demonstrated that BiPAP was safe in patients less than 20 kg, showing no increase in death or pneumothorax. These results are encouraging, providing the treating EP with another weapon in the arsenal against pediatric asthma. The BiPAP device is readily accessible in many emergency departments in the United States, but it is unclear whether appropriately sized equipment is available for use in non-pediatric emergency medicine—dedicated facilities.

E. C. Bruno, MD

Steroids and bronchodilators for acute bronchiolitis in the first two years of life: systematic review and meta-analysis
Hartling L, Fernandes RM, Bialy L, et al (Univ of Alberta, Edmonton, Canada; Inst of Molecular Medicine, Lisbon, Portugal; et al)
BMJ 342:d1714, 2011

Objective.—To evaluate and compare the efficacy and safety of bronchodilators and steroids, alone or combined, for the acute management of bronchiolitis in children aged less than 2 years.

Design.—Systematic review and meta-analysis.

Data sources.—Medline, Embase, Central, Scopus, PubMed, LILACS, IranMedEx, conference proceedings, and trial registers.

Inclusion Criteria.—Randomised controlled trials of children aged 24 months or less with a first episode of bronchiolitis with wheezing comparing any bronchodilator or steroid, alone or combined, with placebo or another intervention (other bronchodilator, other steroid, standard care).

Review Methods.—Two reviewers assessed studies for inclusion and risk of bias and extracted data. Primary outcomes were selected by clinicians a priori based on clinical relevance: rate of admission for outpatients (day 1 and up to day 7) and length of stay for inpatients. Direct meta-analyses were carried out using random effects models. A mixed treatment comparison using a Bayesian network model was used to compare all interventions simultaneously.

Results.—48 trials (4897 patients, 13 comparisons) were included. Risk of bias was low in 17% (n=8), unclear in 52% (n=25), and high in 31% (n=15). Only adrenaline (epinephrine) reduced admissions on day 1 (compared with placebo: pooled risk ratio 0.67, 95% confidence interval 0.50 to 0.89; number needed to treat 15, 95% confidence interval 10 to 45 for a baseline risk of 20%; 920 patients). Unadjusted results from a single large trial with low risk of bias showed that combined dexamethasone and adrenaline reduced admissions on day 7 (risk ratio 0.65, 0.44 to 0.95; number needed to treat 11, 7 to 76 for a baseline risk of 26%; 400

patients). A mixed treatment comparison supported adrenaline alone or combined with steroids as the preferred treatments for outpatients (probability of being the best treatment based on admissions at day 1 were 45% and 39%, respectively). The incidence of reported harms did not differ. None of the interventions examined showed clear efficacy for length of stay among inpatients.

Conclusions.—Evidence shows the effectiveness and superiority of adrenaline for outcomes of most clinical relevance among outpatients with acute bronchiolitis, and evidence from a single precise trial for combined adrenaline and dexamethasone.

▶ The management of bronchiolitis in children remains a moving target. Researchers have attempted multiple interventions, including corticosteroids, nebulized medications (epinephrine, beta-agonists, and hypertonic saline), antibiotics, and supplemental oxygenation, with mixed results. Significant variations endure. Accumulating the existing research, the authors of this meta-analysis labored to identify a standard of care in the management of bronchiolitis in pediatric patients aged 0 to 24 months. The assessment of racemic epinephrine use to prevent admission revealed a number needed to treat of 15 (range 4-20). They were unable to demonstrate a significant harm with the use of epinephrine. Although not statistically significant, the combination of dexamethasone and racemic epinephrine trended toward decreased admission rate when compared with placebo alone. The review goes on to reiterate the paucity of conclusive evidence and wide variations in practice regarding the use of corticosteroids and bronchodilators in the treatment of bronchiolitis. Supportive care, including deep nasal suctioning and supplemental oxygenation, and a trial of bronchodilators are probably reasonable steps in the patient with mild to moderate disease, but when severity of illness worsens, the previously discussed armamentarium is likely pressed into service.

E. C. Bruno, MD

Surgery

Abusive Head Trauma During a Time of Increased Unemployment: A Multicenter Analysis

Berger RP, Fromkin JB, Stutz H, et al (Children's Hosp of Pittsburgh of UPMC, PA; et al)
Pediatrics 128:637-643, 2011

Objective.—To evaluate the rate of abusive head trauma (AHT) in 3 regions of the United States before and during an economic recession and assess whether there is a relationship between the rate of AHT and county-level unemployment rates.

Methods.—Clinical data were collected for AHT cases diagnosed in children younger than 5 years from January 1, 2004 until June 30, 2009, by hospital-based child protection teams within 3 geographic regions. The recession was defined as December 1, 2007 through June 30, 2009. Quarterly unemployment rates were collected for every county in which an AHT case occurred.

Results.—During the 5½-year study period, a total of 422 children were diagnosed with AHT in a 74-county region. The overall rate of AHT increased from 8.9 in 100 000 (95% confidence interval [CI]: 7.8—10.0) before the recession to 14.7 in 100 000 (95% CI: 12.5—16.9) during the recession ($P < .001$). There was no difference in the clinical characteristics of subjects in the prerecession versus recession period. There was no relationship between the rate of AHT and county-level unemployment rates.

Conclusions.—The rate of AHT increased significantly in 3 distinct geographic regions during the 19 months of an economic recession compared with the 47 months before the recession. This finding is consistent with our understanding of the effect of stress on violence. Given the high morbidity and mortality rates for children with AHT, these results are concerning and suggest that prevention efforts might need to be increased significantly during times of economic hardship.

▶ Abuse head trauma can potentially have permanent neurologic as well as behavioral and social sequelae. Prior studies have evaluated the relationship between the child abuser and the head trauma victims; however, there hasn't been a study evaluating the effect of the alleged perpetrator's gender on the victim, victims' outcomes, and perpetrators' legal outcomes. Forty-eight cases were reviewed. All data were collected from a multidisciplinary child protection consultation team and child protection agencies. Thirty-four were identified as a primary suspect by either child protection service or criminal investigation. There were 17 women and 17 men. There was no statistical difference in victim's age, delay in medical care, or length of hospitalization between the identified perpetrators (IP) versus nonidentified perpetrators (NIP). Retinal hemorrhages, acute presentation, and confession were statistically significant with IP. In the NIP group, there were multiple caregivers and positive family court findings of abuse or neglect in 57% of them. Although most victims were male with a mean age of 7 months, there was no gender difference in mortality. Ninety-one percent presented with acute symptoms, such as arrest, seizures, or unresponsiveness. Ninety-four percent had intracranial hemorrhage on CT, and almost 53% had both primary and secondary brain injuries. Primary brain injuries were defined as mechanical forces directly applied to external head and tissues, such as skull fracture, deformation, or subdural, subarachnoid, or intracranial hemorrhage. Secondary brain injuries were defined as complications due to vascular or metabolic changes from the initial trauma, such as cerebral edema, hypoxic damage, or herniations. Most of the victims had skeletal survey and retinal hemorrhages, and 17% had suspicious bruising on exam. Seventeen percent of victims died and were autopsied. Autopsy showed evidence of rotational acceleration-deceleration injury with 3 victims showing additional evidence of impact. Of the survivors, 53.6% had normal examination on discharge with 46% referred to rehabilitation.

Perpetrators were predominantly men with a median 27 years ($P = .001$). Females perpetrators were a median age of 34 years. Biological parents were the most common perpetrators, followed by the mother's boyfriend. The most common history offered on presentation was a short fall from less than 3 feet (47%). Eighty-eight percent male perpetrators confessed; most stated shaking their victims. Seventeen percent of female perpetrators confessed. Male perpetrators were more frequently convicted than female perpetrators ($P = .005$). In conclusion, there were statistically significant differences in perpetrator gender. Victims of male perpetrators had more severe symptoms, neurosurgical interventions, and poorer outcomes. Similarly, they were more likely to confess and be convicted than their female counterparts.

E. C. Quintana, MD, MPH

Acute scrotum in children: an 18-year retrospective study
Yang C Jr, Song B, Liu X, et al (Children's Hosp of Chongqing Med Univ, China)
Pediatr Emerg Care 27:270-274, 2011

Purpose.—This study aimed to compare clinical manifestations, physical examination findings, laboratory, and radiographic dates in pediatric patients with different pathological diagnoses of acute scrotum as well as to accurately establish the true incidence of various pathological diagnoses of acute scrotum.

Methods.—The records of children hospitalized for acute scrotum from 1990 to 2008 were reviewed.

Results.—A total of 1228 cases were included in the study (103 with testicular torsion, 918 with torsion of the testicular appendix, 72 with tunica vaginalis inflammation, 46 with epididymitis and 89 with other pathological diagnoses). Duration of pain less than 6 hours, fever, vomiting, history of trauma or activities, absence of cremasteric reflex, and abnormal testicle direction were significantly associated with testicular torsion. Blue dot sign and tender nodule were found significantly associated with torsion of the testicular appendix. Ultrasound showed decreased or absent blood flow in 91.3% testicular torsion patients; enlarged epididymis was found in 91.1% and 91.3% patients with torsion of the testicular appendix and epididymitis, respectively; and scrotal wall edema and hydrocele were found significantly associated with tunica vaginalis inflammation. Our salvageability rate in testicular torsion was 30.1%.

Conclusions.—Overlap existed between testicular torsion and other acute scrotum. The clinical manifestations, physical examination findings, laboratory, and radiographic data were helpful in distinguishing acute scrotum. Doppler ultrasound is an indispensable imaging modality for the clinical assessment of patients with acute scrotum; in the presence of a clinical suspicion of testicular torsion, even with an apparently normal-color Doppler ultrasound, surgical exploration is still indicated.

▶ Evaluation for acute scrotum is fairly common in the emergency department. It needs appropriate early and prompt recognition, evaluation, and management. One hundred three patients (total patients, 1215) had a final diagnosis of testicular torsion. Eight of them were neonatal cases. A great majority of cases (918) were torsion of testicular appendix. Antibiotics and analgesics were given in 23.1% of those patients with appendiceal testicular torsion. Fifty-four percent of patients with testicular torsion who had received antibiotics and analgesics required orchiectomy for testis gangrene. Another larger group requiring orchiectomy had used herbal medications or were self-medicating (18.1%). The statistically significant clinical findings with testicular torsion were left testicle affected, duration of symptoms less than 6 hours, fever, vomiting, and history of trauma or activities (*P* < .001). Physical examination findings were absence of cremasteric reflex and abnormal testicle direction (*P* < .001) in testicular torsion, whereas blue dot sign and tender nodule were found in torsion of testicular appendix. Peak age for testicular torsion was 13 to 14 years and younger than 1 year old; in contrast, testicular appendiceal torsion peaked between 8 and 11 years old. Testicular torsion and epididymitis predominantly occurred in the left (*P* < .001), whereas appendiceal torsion was equally distributed. Ultrasound findings of lack of scrotal wall, testicular swelling or extratesticular nodule, or abnormal testicular texture were significantly associated with testicular torsion. Extratesticular node was significantly associated with appendiceal testicular torsion and epididymitis. As expected, decreased or lack of testicular blood flow was diagnostic in 93% of testicular torsion. Although clinical findings and laboratory tests were helpful in diagnosing testicular torsion, ultrasound scan was indispensable in the acute scrotum evaluation.

E. C. Quintana, MD, MPH

Delayed diagnosis of injuries in pediatric trauma: the role of radiographic ordering practices
Willner EL, Jackson HA, Nager AL (Children's Hosp Los Angeles, CA)
Am J Emerg Med 30:115-123, 2012

Objectives.—We sought to describe the use of radiographic studies in pediatric major trauma patients and determine the extent to which a selective, clinically guided use of imaging contributes to delayed diagnosis of injury (DDI).

Methods.—We conducted a retrospective chart review of 324 consecutive pediatric major trauma patients at our level 1 trauma center. One radiologist reviewed all imaging. *Delayed diagnosis of injury* was defined as detection after more than 12 hours. Equivalency testing was performed to compare radiology use in patients with and without DDI.

Results.—Twenty-six (8%) of 324 patients had 36 DDI; 27 (75%) of 36 were orthopedic injuries. Median time to DDI detection was 20.5 hours (interquartile range, 15-60.5). During initial evaluation, DDI patients had similar numbers of plain radiographs (3.5 vs 3, *P* = .54) but more computed tomographic (CT) scans (4 vs 3, *P* = .03) compared with patients without DDI. Sixteen percent of all patients received CT thorax; 55%, CT cervical spine; and 56%, CT abdomen. Only 1 clinically important DDI was detected solely on the basis of a later CT scan (0.3%; 95% confidence

TABLE 2.—DDI Patient Details

Age (y)	DDI	Hours to Diagnosis	How Detected?	Treatment Change	Mechanism	Admission Diagnoses	Initial GCS
14	Humerus fx	19	New study	Reduction and splinting	Auto vs ped	Parietal skull fx, AMS	7
10	L inferior pubic ramus fx	17	Reread	Orthopedics consult	Auto vs ped	Aortic dissection, orbital fx, pulmonary contusion, CHI, pneumothorax	10
4	Tiny L frontal hemorrhage	15	Reread	No change	Fall, >15 ft	Occipital skull fx, CHI	15
13	Ileum fx (from bullet)	20	Delay in reading	Antibiotics, orthopedics consult	GSW	GSW to abdomen	15
12	Displacement of tibia plateau fx	40	Orthopedic attending	Called back from home for CT scan and cast	Auto vs skateboard	Anterior cruciate ligament tear, tibia fx	15
3	Tiny L frontal hemorrhage	15	Reread	No change	Fall, >15 ft	Parietal skull fx, CHI, periorbital contusion	15
8	L clavicle posterior dislocation	29	New study	Operative reduction (second OR)	Auto vs ped	Radius and ulna fxs, neck pain	15
12	5th metacarpal fx	16	Reread	Cast	Auto vs bike	CHI, chin and lip lacerations	15
13	L clavicle fx	22	New study	Orthopedics consult, sling	Auto vs bike	CHI, neck pain, concussion	15
12	L superior and inferior pubic rami fxs	a	Reread	Unknown (transferred)	Auto vs ped	CHI	15
13	Occipital skull fx Tiny subdural	15	Reread	Neurosurgery consultation	MVC	CHI, multiple facial lacerations, neck pain	15
12	Mastoid bone/air cells fx	15	New study	Otolaryngology consult, audiology testing	Auto vs bike	Open femur fx, Occipital and parietal skull fxs	4
3	R pubic ramus fx	17	Reread	No change	Fall, >15 ft	CHI, flank abrasion, tooth fx	15
13	L scapula body fx	62	Reread (by orthopedist)	No change	Auto vs skateboard	AMS, frontal skull fx, facial fxs, tibia and clavicle fxs	6
4	L ileum fx, L4 transverse process fx	19, 45	New study	Orthopedics consult, TLSO spine brace	MVC	Abdominal contusion, CHI, cervical tenderness	15

13	Nasal bone fx	23	Reread	Plastic surgery consult, additional imaging	Motorcycle	Intraventricular hemorrhage, tibia and fibula fxs, pulmonary contusion, oral trauma	13
7	L superior and inferior pubic rami fxs	15	Reread	Orthopedics consult	Auto vs ped	CHI, intraventricular hemorrhage	3
3	1st + 3rd metatarsal and cuboid fxs	14	New study	Cast	Fall, >15 ft	Epidural bleed, parietal skull fx	14
3	R tibia fx	15	New study	Cast	Auto vs ped	Pulmonary contusions, multiple abrasions	15
13	Proximal humerus avulsion fx	60	New study	No change	Auto vs bike	R frontal cerebral contusion, pneumocephalus, leg laceration, AMS, CHI	11
3	Tibia fxs	24	New study	Cast	MVC	CHI, scalp laceration, anemia	15
6	Infratentorial/brainstem subdural, atlantoaxial distraction	278, 278	New study	Neurosurgery consult, hard cervical collar ×2 mo	MVC (ejected)	CHI, pulmonary contusion, pneumothorax, shock, respiratory failure	10
2	Tibia Fx, fibula fx	21	New study	Cast	Crush (gate)	CHI, facial abrasions	15
6	Nondisplaced ileum fx, 4th + 5th metacarpal fxs	240, 696	New study	Orthopedics consult	Auto vs ped	AMS, subdural hematoma, R temporal bone fx, pulmonary contusions	5
12	Small bowel mesentery tear, with subsequent bowel herniation	102	Clinical examination	Laparotomy, partial small bowel resection	MVC (ejected)	Hip dislocation, pelvic fx, splenic laceration	15
13	2nd rib fx, T1-T2 ligamentous injury[b]	600, 144	New study	Soft cervical collar ×2 mo	MVC	CHI, bilateral pneumothoraces, liver laceration, splenic laceration, subarachnoid hemorrhage	3

Fx indicates fracture; AMS, altered mental status; CHI, closed head injury; GSW, gunshot wound; R, right; L, left; OR, operating room. L4, fourth lumber vertebra.
[a]Unable to determine exact time.
[b]Stable injury detected on MRI; soft tissue swelling on CT.

interval, 0-1.5). No cervical spine, intrathoracic, or intraabdominal DDI was attributable to failure to obtain a CT during initial evaluation. Patients with DDI had higher injury severity scores, intubation rates, and pediatric intensive care unit admission rates than those without DDI.

Conclusions.—Patients with DDI had similar initial plain x-ray evaluations to patients without DDI, despite DDI patients being more severely injured. Delayed diagnosis of injury was not attributable to inadequate CT use. Most DDIs were orthopedic, highlighting the importance of a tertiary survey and a low threshold for skeletal radiographs (Table 2).

▶ This retrospective study evaluated delayed diagnosis of injury (DDI), which has been defined in the literature as detection of a previously unsuspected injury attributable to trauma greater than 12 or 24 hours after presentation. There are limited studies in the pediatric population. Twenty-six (8%) of 324 patients had 1 or more DDIs (Table 2). There were a total of 36 DDIs in the 26 patients identified. Seventy-five percent of DDIs were orthopedic, such as fracture or dislocation of any bone excluding face and skull. Almost 80% required a change in the treatment after detection. Twenty (55.6%; 95% confidence interval [CI], 38.1−72.1) of 36 DDIs were detected on a new radiographic study. Thirteen DDIs (36.1%; 95% CI, 20.8−53.8) were attributable to problems with radiographic interpretations. This study found that patients with and without DDI received statistically similar numbers of initial radiographic studies, including total number of studies and total number of plain x-rays. Patients with DDI received more total computed tomography scans (CTs) than did patients without DDI because of a higher proportion having abdominal/pelvic CTs and being more injured (higher ISS) and thus less likely to communicate any complaints. This fact could have been a barrier to the evaluation of subtle injury findings. The areas of most DDIs were extremities, pelvis, and clavicles; therefore, careful examination is warranted to those areas specifically.

E. C. Quintana, MD, MPH

Effect of age on cervical spine injury in pediatric population: a National Trauma Data Bank review
Mohseni S, Talving P, Branco BC, et al (Univ of Southern California, Los Angeles)
J Pediatr Surg 46:1771-1776, 2011

Background.—The objective of this study was to characterize the incidence, risk factors, and patterns of cervical spine injury (CSI) in different pediatric developmental ages.

Methods.—A retrospective review of the National Trauma Data Bank was conducted for the period of January 2002 through December 2006 to identify pediatric patients admitted following blunt trauma. Patients were stratified into 4 developmental age groups: infants/toddlers (age 0-3 years), preschool/young children (age 4-9 years), preadolescents (age 10-13 years), and adolescents (age 14-17 years). Patients with a CSI were identified by the *International Classification of Diseases, Ninth Revision* codes. Demographics, clinical injury data, level of CSI, and outcomes were abstracted and analyzed.

Results.—A total of 240,647 patients met the inclusion criteria. Of these, 1.3% (n = 3,035) sustained a CSI. The incidence of CSI in the stratified age groups was 0.4% in infants/toddlers, 0.4% in preschool/young children, 0.8% in preadolescents, and 2.6% in adolescents. The level of CSI (upper [C1-C4] vs lower [C5-C7]) according to the age groups was as follows: infants and toddlers, 70% vs 25%; preschool/young children, 74% vs 17%; preadolescents, 52% vs 37%; and adolescents, 40% vs 45%, respectively. The adjusted risk for CSI increased 2-fold in preadolescents and 5-fold in adolescents.

Conclusion.—The incidence of pediatric CSI increases in a stepwise fashion after 9 years of age. We noted an increase in lower CSI and a decrease in upper CSI after the age of 9 years. The incidence of upper CSI compared with lower CSI was higher in preadolescents (52% vs 37%) and almost equal in adolescents (40% vs 45%).

▶ This study characterized the incidence, risk factors, and patterns of cervical spine injuries from the national trauma databank in pediatric patients. Sixty-four percent were male (*P* = .002). The incidence was 0.4% in infants/toddlers, 0.4% in preschoolers/young children, 0.8% in preadolescents, and 2.6% in adolescents. Hypotension, Glasgow Coma Score less 8, and an Injury Severity Score greater than 16 at admission were all risk factors associated with cervical spine injury. The risk for cervical spine injury is increased 2-fold in preadolescents and 5-fold in adolescents (*P* < .001) compared with infants and toddlers. The incidence of lower cervical injuries increased with increasing age after 9 years old (45% in adolescents, *P* < .001). This study demonstrated that the transition from the pediatric to adult cervical spine injury pattern seemed to occur around the age of 9, with the concomitant vertebral ossification and maturity. The incidence of upper cervical spine injuries was high in preadolescents versus younger children (57% vs 37%). There was a trend of increased mortality in the younger age groups (5.2% in infants/toddlers, *P* = .08). These findings may aid in the management of pediatric cervical spine injury.

E. C. Quintana, MD, MPH

Effectiveness of Biobrane for treatment of partial-thickness burns in children
Lesher AP, Curry RH, Evans J, et al (Med Univ of South Carolina, Charleston)
J Pediatr Surg 46:1759-1763, 2011

Purpose.—Wound care for partial-thickness burns should alleviate pain, decrease hospital length of stay, and be readily applied to a variety of wounds. The effectiveness of Biobrane (UDL Laboratories, Rockford,

IL) is compared with that of Beta Glucan Collagen (BGC; Brennan Medical, St. Paul, MN) in a retrospective cohort study.

Methods.—A retrospective chart review of all children treated at a tertiary care pediatric hospital between 2003 and 2009 identified patients with partial-thickness burns treated with Biobrane. These patients were compared with historical controls treated with BGC.

Results.—A total of 235 children between the ages of 4 weeks and 18 years with an average of 6.0% body surface area partial-thickness burns were treated with Biobrane. In a multivariate statistical analysis, patients treated with Biobrane healed significantly faster than those treated with BGC (Biobrane vs BGC: median, 9 vs 13 days; $P = .019$; hazard ratio, 1.68). In addition, patients who required inpatient treatment trended toward having shorter length of hospital stay in the Biobrane group (2.6 vs 4.1 days, $P = .079$).

Conclusion.—Partial-thickness burn care consists of early debridement and application of a burn wound dressing. Biobrane dressings result in faster healing compared with BGC and may decrease hospital length of stay for patients requiring inpatient admission.

▶ Partial thickness burns, which are described as superficial or deep, presenting with pain, fluid-filled blisters and redness, are common in children. This report described the experience of Biobrane (biosynthetic material promoting reepithelialization). Thirty-five percent of patients with partial thickness burns had this biosynthetic material as part of their burn management. There was a decrease of days to heal, although it was not statistically significant ($P = .019$). This is an initial study showing that we should consider, in appropriate cases, using biosynthetic wound dressing. Its ease of use and application and its flexibility makes it ideal for pediatrics.

E. C. Quintana, MD, MPH

Hypothermia is associated with poor outcome in pediatric trauma patients
Sundberg J, Estrada C, Jenkins C, et al (Vanderbilt Univ, Nashville, TN)
Am J Emerg Med 29:1019-1022, 2011

Objective.—The objective of the study was to determine if hypothermia in pediatric trauma patients is associated with increased mortality.

Methods.—We reviewed the charts of level 1 trauma patients aged 3 months to 17 years who presented between September 2006 and March 2008. We analyzed data for patients with temperatures recorded within 30 minutes of arrival to the pediatric emergency department. Logistic regression models were used to test for associations of hypothermia with death while adjusting for mode of transport, season of year, and presence of intracranial pathology as documented by an abnormal head computed tomographic scan.

Results.—Of the 226 level 1 trauma patients presenting during the study period, 190 met inclusion criteria. Twenty-one patients (11%) died. The odds ratio (OR) of a hypothermic patient dying was 9.2 times that of a normothermic patient when adjusting for seasonal variation (95% confidence interval [CI], 3.2-26.2; $P < 0.0001$). The OR of a hypothermic patient dying was 8.7 times that of a normothermic patient when adjusting for mode of transport (ground vs air) (95% CI, 3.1-24.6; $P < 0.0001$). Although it did not reach statistical significance, there was a trend toward an association between hypothermia and the presence of traumatic brain injury as evidenced by an abnormal head computed tomographic scan (OR = 2.4; 95% CI, 0.9-6.0; $P = .07$).

Conclusions.—Hypothermia is a risk factor for increased mortality in pediatric trauma patients. This pilot study warrants a more detailed, multicenter analysis to assess the impact of hypothermia in the pediatric trauma patient.

▶ Children are at increased risk of hypothermia for multiple reasons including a high body surface area to mass ratio and higher metabolic rate. Hypothermia, temperature less than 35°C has been described as a lethal factor in adult trauma. This study looked at any type of effects in the pediatric trauma, determining whether hypothermic pediatric trauma patients have a higher mortality rate. One hundred eight (57%) of the patients were transported from the scene, and 80 (42%) were interfacility transports. Sixty-three (33%) of the patients were transported by ambulance, and 127 (67%) were transported by air. Of the hypothermic patients whose injury time was recorded, the median time from injury to hospital arrival was 80 minutes. Eighty percent of patients had CT done. There was a trend between hypothermia and a positive head CT scan result (odds ratio = 2.4, $P = .07$, not statistically significant). The odds ratio of a hypothermic patient dying was 9.2 when adjusting for seasonal variation ($P < .0001$). The odds ratio of a hypothermic patient dying was 8.7 when adjusting for mode of transport (ground vs air; $P < .0001$). In conclusion, this study demonstrated that even when accounting for possible confounding variables such as season and mode of transport, hypothermia remains an independent risk factor associated with increased mortality.

E. C. Quintana, MD, MPH

Paediatric pelvic ring fractures and associated injuries
Leonard M, Ibrahim M, McKenna P, et al (Childrens Univ Hosp, Dublin, Ireland)
Injury 42:1027-1030, 2011

Introduction.—Paediatric pelvic fractures have been infrequently reviewed. The study was performed to highlight the unique features of pelvic fractures in children.

Patients and Methods.—A 14-year retrospective study was undertaken of all patients treated for a pelvic fracture at our institute.

Results.—Thirty-nine children were included. The mean Injury Severity Score (ISS) was 17.1 (range 4—75). Simple ring fractures were the most common type (46%), dominated by pedestrian versus motor vehicle trauma (58.9%). A pelvic fracture was evident on the initial plain radiographs of all 39 children. Further radiographic investigations (12 CTs and 1 MRI) were undertaken in 13 (33%) of the children. Additional posterior ring fractures were identified in 9. A total of 32 children (82%) sustained one or more associated injuries. Head injuries accounted for 25% and orthopaedic/skeletal injuries for 33% of all associated injuries. Fourteen children required a total of 24 acute surgical procedures. Mean out-patient clinical follow-up was for 27 months (range 3—85). There was one mortality in this series. Eight children (20%) suffered long term sequelae.

Conclusion.—Paediatric pelvic fractures differ from their adult counterpart in aetiology, fracture type, and associated injury pattern. They represent a reliable marker for severe trauma. Prospective studies are required to define optimal treatment guidelines, particularly in older children (Fig 3, Table 1).

▶ Pediatric pelvic fracture represents a reliable marker of multisystem trauma. The greater cartilaginous volume and bony plasticity of the pediatric pelvis provides an increased capacity for energy absorption prior to fracture. This 14-year retrospective study of all children admitted with a pelvic fracture in Ireland was evaluated. Over the study period, 39 children who had sustained a pelvic fracture were treated. The most common mechanism of injury was a pedestrian being struck by a motor vehicle, accounting for 23 of all cases. A pelvic fracture was evident on the initial plain radiographs (anterior—posterior, inlet, outlet views) of all 39 children. Further radiographic investigations (12 computed tomography scans

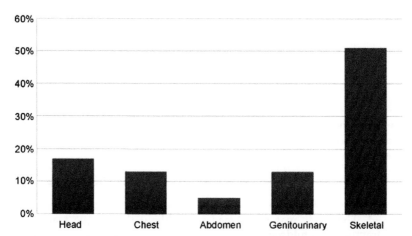

FIGURE 3.—Incidence of associated injuries per body region. (Reprinted from the Injury, International Journal of the Care of the Injured, Leonard M, Ibrahim M, McKenna P, et al. Paediatric pelvic ring fractures and associated injuries. *Injury.* 2011;42:1027-1030. Copyright 2011, with permission from Elsevier.)

TABLE 1.—Distribution of Associated Non-Pelvic Fractures

Bone Involved	Total	Percentage of Patients
Vertebrae	1	2.6
Clavicle	2	5.1
Humerus	3	7.7
Radius/ulna	2	2.6
Femur	11	23
Tibia/fibula	3	5.1

and 1 magnetic resonance imaging scan) of the pelvic injury were undertaken in 13 of the children. Most (18 of 39) had a simple ring fracture, 13 children sustained a type 4 ring disruption fracture, 6 had a type 2 iliac wing fracture, and only 2 had a type 1 bony avulsion. The 6 children who had long-term complications related to their pelvic injury were in the older age group (range 10–14), had sustained type 3 or 4 fractures, and had been treated nonoperatively. Associated injuries were very common. Head injuries accounted for 25% of these and consisted of 6 disfiguring facial (Fig 3) lacerations, 5 soft tissue injuries (extensive facial bruising, subconjuctival hemorrhage) 4 skull fractures, 3 parenchymal brain injuries, and 2 significant dental injuries. Injuries to the chest included 7 pulmonary contusions, 2 pneumothoraces, 1 hemothorax with a ruptured diaphragm, and 4 cases of multiple rib fractures. Genitourinary injuries comprised 2 ruptured bladders, 2 ruptured urethras, 2 subcapsular hematomas, 1 perinephric hematoma, 1 pelvic hematoma, 1 introitus laceration, and 1 levator ani tear. Injuries to the abdomen included 2 large abdominal contusions, 1 splenic laceration (requiring splenectomy), 1 liver laceration, 1 liver contusion, and 1 intramuscular hematoma. Associated orthopedic/skeletal injuries consisted of 22 fractures in 18 children (Table 1). This study should remind us that the injury patterns in pediatric pelvic trauma are quite different from those in adults.

E. C. Quintana, MD, MPH

Pediatric firearm injuries: a 10-year single-center experience of 194 patients
Senger C, Keijzer R, Smith G, et al (Univ of Alabama at Birmingham)
J Pediatr Surg 46:927-932, 2011

Background.—The objective was to investigate the relationship of high gun ownership and gun death rate on children and determine predictors influencing the incidence and outcome of pediatric firearm injuries in a major pediatric level 1 trauma center.

Methods.—We performed a retrospective review of our trauma registry to identify hospital admissions between April 1999 and March 2010. We extracted demographic and geographic data, seasonal variation, injury type, firearm type, and outcome.

Results.—We identified 194 firearm injuries. The incidence did not change during the past decade. Most occurred during the second half of the year (61.4%). Mean age was 12.2 ± 4.6 years (range, 0.4-19.2 years).

Unintentional shootings accounted for 100 injuries followed by assaults (n = 55) and innocent bystanders (n = 39). African American children were most often injured because of a violent cause (60.3%), whereas white children were shot unintentionally (80.1%). Powder-propelled firearms caused 82.5% of injuries. Overall, 17.5% of children required an operation, and 9.3% died.

Conclusions.—The overwhelming majority of children were injured after a gun went off unintentionally, whereas most African American children were shot violently. We identified certain seasonal and geographic clusters. These data can be used to target gun injury prevention programs.

▶ Firearm injuries are a major health risk of children in the United States, especially for those living in states where many own firearms. Children living in 1 of the 5 states with the highest gun availability (Louisiana, Alabama, Mississippi, Arkansas, and West Virginia) are more likely to die of a gunshot wound injury. In this study in Alabama, the mean age of patients with firearm injury was 12.2 years with an incidence peaked in 2005 (n = 25) and was lowest in 2001 (n = 12). No clear trend was identified in the number of patients admitted. Firearm injuries occurred more frequently in boys (n = 151) than in girls (n = 43) and 55.7% in African-American boys. Extremities were injured in 43.8%, followed by the head in 28.4% (the face was considered a separate category) and abdominal injuries in 20.1%. Younger kids were most likely to have a head injury caused by firearms, whereas older kids had injuries to extremities. The overall death rate was 9.3%, with highest mortality rates among children 0 to 4 years (20.0%) and in injuries involving the head (23.7%). African-American children were most often injured because of a violent cause (60.3%), whereas white children were more likely to be shot unintentionally (80.1%). Younger children were more likely injured by non–violence-based causes, whereas the risk of a violent cause (assault, innocent bystander) increased with age and was highest among 14- to 15-year-old adolescents (Fig 3a and b in the original article). Even though this information was from a single institution, it would not be surprising to extrapolate similar findings to other US emergency departments.

E. C. Quintana, MD, MPH

Pediatric Trauma Transport Performance Measures in a Mountain State: Adherence and Outcomes
Gleich SJ, Bennett TD, Bratton SL, et al (Univ of Utah, Salt Lake City)
J Trauma 71:1016-1022, 2011

Background.—Utah state trauma audit filters assess expeditious care at referring emergency departments for severely injured patients to avoid delays in transfer. We evaluated two state performance measures related to pediatric trauma care before arrival at the Level I trauma center.

Methods.—Analysis of the Primary Children's Medical Center (PCMC) trauma database for children with Injury Severity Scores (ISS) >15 from

2006 to 2009 was performed. Patient care was evaluated for referring hospital emergency department triage time of <2 hours and total transfer time of ≤6 hours for rural and ≤4 hours for urban place of injury.

Results.—Four hundred twelve patients with ISS >15 were admitted via interhospital transfer from within Utah. Approximately 50% of patients were triaged <2 hours, which increased to almost two thirds when restricted to those initially evaluated within 100 miles (helicopter range) of PCMC. Factors associated with delayed triaged included lower ISS, less severe head injury, greater distance from the trauma center, and primary chest/abdominal injuries. Death and poor outcome did not differ significantly by triage in <2 hours or ≥2 hours. Adherence with the total transfer time goal was 94% for rural and 76% for urban place of injury.

Conclusions.—There was substantial nonadherence with trauma performance measures for triage in <2 hours among pediatric trauma patients with ISS >15. Because of low rates of poor outcome, we are unable to determine whether adherence with state triage goals lessens morbidity or mortality.

▶ Trauma care is regionalized in many states; however, children injured in rural areas have less rapid access to specialized trauma care. The Utah system was evaluated for outcomes: referring hospital emergency department (ED) triage time (ED admit to discharge) less than 2 hours and total transfer time (ED admit to arrival at Primary Children's Medical Center [PCMC] ED). For children injured in rural areas, the total transfer time goal is 6 hours or less and, for urban areas, 4 hours or less. Among all trauma admissions, 45% of patients were transported to PCMC in Salt Lake City, UT, directly from the site of injury, and 55% were referred from another hospital within a multistate area (including Utah). Those children with triage times < 2 hours were more severely injured (median Injury Severity Scores, 20 vs 17), and a larger proportion had severe traumatic brain injury (Glasgow Coma Score ≤8; 36.2% vs 16.8%). In addition, the children with triage times < 2 hours were more likely to have injuries resulting from abuse (19.0% vs 8.9%). Children triaged < 2 hours were injured closer to PCMC (median distance, 68 miles vs 150 miles), were more likely to be transported by helicopter (71.9% vs 47.1%), and had less time elapsed after injury before arrival at PCMC (median time, 176 minutes vs 326 minutes). There were no differences between season of injury and time of day. Children triaged < 2 hours were more likely to require intensive care unit admission (84.2% vs 60.2%), to have a poor outcome (9.5% vs 4.2%), and to die (9.5% vs 2.1%). They also were more likely to undergo mechanical ventilation, intracranial pressure monitoring, and invasive arterial pressure monitoring. As expected, those initially treated at hospitals further from PCMC had delayed triage (OR, 1.01 per mile). Those transported via helicopter (OR, 0.52) and children with severe traumatic brain injury (OR, 0.39) were less likely to have delayed triage, whereas patients with injury to the trunk (OR, 1.85) were more likely to have delayed triage. Another interesting finding in our analysis was that children who were most severely injured in their chest and abdomen as opposed to their head, spine, or extremities had significantly greater odds of delayed triage.

E. C. Quintana, MD, MPH

Primary Repair of Facial Dog Bite Injuries in Children
Wu PS, Beres A, Tashjian DB, et al (Baystate Med Ctr, Springfield, MA; McGill Univ Health Centre, Montreal, Quebec, Canada; Baystate Children's Hospital, Springfield, MA)
Pediatr Emer Care 27:801-803, 2011

Objectives.—The management of dog bite wounds is controversial, and current data on risk of infection are variable and inconsistent. Furthermore, the use of prophylactic or empiric antibiotics for the treatment of these wounds is debatable. We investigate the rate of wound infections and other complications after primary repair of pediatric facial dog bite injuries.

Methods.—We reviewed 87 consecutive patients aged 18 years or younger who had facial dog bite injuries from January 2003 to December 2008. Variables examined were age, sex, setting of repair, number of sutures used for repair, whether surgical drains were used, and antibiotic administration. End points measured were incidence of wound infection, need for scar revision, and any wound complications.

Results.—The mean age of patients was 6.8 years, and the majority were women (53%). All facial injuries were primarily repaired at the time of presentation either in the emergency department (ED; 46%), operating room (OR; 51%), or an outpatient setting (3%). All patients received an antibiotic course, none of the patients developed wound infection, and no subsequent scar revisions were performed. Three patients repaired in the OR underwent placement of a total of 4 closed-suction drains. The mean (SD) age of patients repaired in the OR was significantly younger than those repaired in the ED (5.7 [3.9] vs 8.0 [4.5] years, respectively; $P < 0.01$). The number of sutures used were greater for patients repaired in the OR than in the ED (66.4 [39.6] vs 21.7 [12.5], respectively; $P < 0.01$).

Conclusions.—Intuitively, younger patients and patients with greater severity injuries are more likely to undergo repair in the OR, and this was supported by our data. Overall, we found that primary repair of pediatric facial dog bite injuries, including complex soft-tissue injuries, is safe when performed in conjunction with antibiotic administration; however, further cross-specialty studies are needed to fully characterize these end points in a larger population.

▶ Most animal bites in pediatrics are attributable to dogs. We have been taught that dog bites are contaminated because of the mixed flora of the dog's mouth. The management has been variable regarding primary closure on head and face. This study retrospectively evaluated the safety of primary repair with low incidence of infection and good cosmetic repair. There was no gender difference. Younger patients needed repair in the operating room versus emergency department repair (statistically significant at $P = .0097$). None of the patients presented had neurovascular, bony, or ophthalmologic involvement or injuries that required repair or debridement. All patients received antibiotics, and none had subsequent any cellulitis on follow-up. In conclusion, primary repair of dog bites with administration of antibiotics resulted in low incidence of infection and good cosmetic results in this study of not-severe dog bites.

E. C. Quintana, MD, MPH

Risk Factors for Blunt Cerebrovascular Injury in Children: Do They Mimic Those Seen in Adults?
Kopelman TR, Berardoni NE, O'Neill PJ, et al (Maricopa Med Ctr, Phoenix, AZ)
J Trauma 71:559-564, 2011

Background.—Eastern Association for the Surgery of Trauma guideline for the evaluation of blunt cerebrovascular injury (BCVI) states that pediatric trauma patients should be evaluated using the same criteria as the adult population. The purpose of our study was to determine whether adult criteria translate to the pediatric population.

Methods.—Retrospective evaluation was performed at a Level I trauma center of blunt pediatric trauma patients (age <15 years) presenting over a 5-year period. Data obtained included patient demographics, presence of adult risk factors for BCVI (Glasgow coma scale ≤8, skull base fracture, cervical spine fracture, complex facial fractures, and soft tissue injury to the neck), presence of signs/symptoms of BCVI, method of evaluation, treatment, and outcome.

Results.—A total of 1,209 pediatric trauma patients were admitted during the study period. While 128 patients met criteria on retrospective review for evaluation based on Eastern Association for the Surgery of Trauma criteria, only 52 patients (42%) received subsequent radiographic evaluation. In all, 14 carotid artery or vertebral artery injuries were identified in 11 patients (all admissions, 0.9% incidence; all screened, 21% incidence). Adult risk factors were present in 91% of patients diagnosed with an injury. Major thoracic injury was found in 67% of patients with carotid artery injuries. Cervical spine fracture was found in 100% of patients with vertebral artery injuries. Stroke occurred in four patients (36%). Stroke rate after admission for untreated patients was 38% (3/8) versus 0.0% in those treated (0/2). Mortality was 27% because of concomitant severe traumatic brain injury.

Conclusion.—Risk factors for BCVI in the pediatric trauma patient appear to mimic those of the adult patient.

▶ This retrospective study from trauma service admissions evaluated adult risk factors for blunt cerebrovascular injury (BCVI) as risk factors for pediatric BCVI. The adult risk factors are basilar skull fracture, Glasgow Coma score (GCS) ≤ 8, cervical spine fracture, or more than 1 risk factor. Patients were found to have carotid artery or vertebral artery injuries (0.9% incidence). Adult BCVI incidence

TABLE 2.—Presence of BCVI in Pediatric Patients With Identified Adult Risk Factors

Adult Risk Factor	Number of Patients	Number With BCVI (%)
Basilar skull fracture	41	7 (17)
GCS score ≤8	16	5 (31)
Soft tissue neck injury	3	1 (33)
Cervical spine fracture	13	3 (23)
LeForte II/III facial fracture	0	—
Neurologic signs or symptoms concerning for BCVI	2	2 (100)
More than one risk factor	20	4 (20)
Total	52	11 (21)

is about 1%. The mean age of BCVI was 8 years. Male gender and collision of motorized vehicle were common factors in most injuries. Most injuries were partial thickness damage to vessels with bilateral injuries in 33% of patients (carotid artery). No patient had anterior and posterior vascular concomitant injuries. In the adult population, the highest risk for BCVI is cervical spine fracture followed by basilar skull fracture. Conversely, in the pediatric population, basilar skull fracture was the most commonly associated injury with BCVI, followed by GCS ≤ 8 (Table 2). Additionally, ecchymosis or seat belt mark to neck may be more significant with BCVI. These findings should be kept in mind during pediatric trauma management when BCVI is under consideration.

E. C. Quintana, MD, MPH

Trauma

Elevated Cardiac Troponin I Level in Cases of Thoracic Nonaccidental Trauma

Bennett BL, Mahabee-Gittens M, Chua MS, et al (Cincinnati Children's Hosp Med Ctr, OH)
Pediatr Emerg Care 27:941-944, 2011

Background.—Injury patterns in nonaccidental trauma (NAT) often include injury to the chest. However, signs and symptoms of cardiac insult are often nonspecific and may be missed. Evaluation with serum cardiac troponin I (CTnI), a specific indicator of myocardial injury, could improve the comprehensive evaluation of patients with suspected NAT.

Objective.—The objective of this study was to describe the patient characteristics and results of CTnI testing in children with thoracic NAT.

Methods.—Children presenting to the emergency department were included if CTnI was obtained and they had at least one of the following: history of blunt trauma to the chest, bruising or abrasions to the chest, or fractures of the ribs, sternum, or clavicles. A serum CTnI level above 0.04 ng/mL was considered elevated.

Results.—Ten patients (6 males) with an age range from 2 months to 4 years (mean [SD], 20 [20] months) were identified during the 17-month study period. All patients were evaluated with NAT. Cardiac troponin I level was elevated in 7 (70%) of 10 patients with levels between 2 and 50 times the upper limit of normal.

Conclusions.—This report is the first to document elevation of CTnI levels in cases of thoracic NAT. The elevation of the level of this specific biomarker may be indicative of sufficient chest trauma to result in the heart being injured, independent of the presence of cardiac decompensation or shock from other causes. Prospective evaluation of the forensic and clinical use of CTnI in this population is warranted.

▶ Pediatric nonaccidental trauma remains a visceral response-inducing clinical scenario. The treating emergency physician is responsible for identification of life-threatening injuries and ensuring that subsequent injuries are prevented. Significant chest trauma may be part of this clinical situation, and evaluation of cardiac enzymes may be part of the workup. The authors of this retrospective review looked to determine if serum cardiac troponin I (CTnI) is an appropriate marker to identify myocardial injury. They report that CTnI is elevated in 70% of pediatric patients presenting with nonaccidental chest trauma. While this is purported to be the first documentation of elevated troponin in nonaccidental trauma, some faults in the report are present. First, the retrospective nature of the review imports selection bias, as the treating physician is more likely to order the CTnI in patients with more concerning injuries. Second, the study only contained 10 patients. This topic is primed for a prospective, multicenter trial in which all pediatric patients with nonaccidental chest trauma have cardiac enzyme diagnostic testing.

E. C. Bruno, MD

Elevated Cardiac Troponin I Level in Cases of Thoracic Nonaccidental Trauma

Bennett BL, Mahabee-Gittens M, Chua MS, et al (Cincinnati Children's Hosp Med Ctr, OH)
Pediatr Emerg Care 27:941-944, 2011

Background.—Injury patterns in nonaccidental trauma (NAT) often include injury to the chest. However, signs and symptoms of cardiac insult are often nonspecific and may be missed. Evaluation with serum cardiac troponin I (CTnI), a specific indicator of myocardial injury, could improve the comprehensive evaluation of patients with suspected NAT.

Objective.—The objective of this study was to describe the patient characteristics and results of CTnI testing in children with thoracic NAT.

Methods.—Children presenting to the emergency department were included if CTnI was obtained and they had at least one of the following: history of blunt trauma to the chest, bruising or abrasions to the chest, or fractures of the ribs, sternum, or clavicles. A serum CTnI level above 0.04 ng/mL was considered elevated.

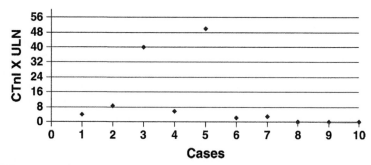

FIGURE 1.—Cardiac troponin I level as a multiple of the upper limit of normal (ULN). (Reprinted from Bennett BL, Mahabee-Gittens M, Chua MS, et al. Elevated cardiac troponin I level in cases of thoracic nonaccidental trauma. *Pediatr Emerg Care*. 2011;27:941-944, with permission from Lippincott Williams & Wilkins.)

Results.—Ten patients (6 males) with an age range from 2 months to 4 years (mean [SD], 20 [20] months) were identified during the 17-month study period. All patients were evaluated with NAT. Cardiac troponin I level was elevated in 7 (70%) of 10 patients with levels between 2 and 50 times the upper limit of normal.

Conclusions.—This report is the first to document elevation of CTnI levels in cases of thoracic NAT. The elevation of the level of this specific biomarker may be indicative of sufficient chest trauma to result in the heart being injured, independent of the presence of cardiac decompensation or shock from other causes. Prospective evaluation of the forensic and clinical use of CTnI in this population is warranted (Fig 1).

▶ This is a retrospective chart review of children with suspected nonaccidental chest trauma with serum cardiac troponin I. Cardiac troponin I level was elevated in 7 of 10 (70%) patients with levels between 2 and 50 times the upper limit of normal (Fig 1). No cardiac abnormalities were noted with cardiac auscultation. The initial electrocardiogram (EKG) of 1 patient had low voltages and signs of right heart strain with resolution of these findings 24 hours later. Two patients (20%) had other signs of cardiac involvement (hypotension, EKG changes) in addition to the elevation in cardiac troponin I level. This study found that using troponin I is advantageous to chest x-ray or chest computed tomography in determining cardiac contusion. A normal EKG finding does not exclude cardiac insult. It is important to remember that the relatively compliant chest wall in children allows intrathoracic injury to occur without external or radiographic signs of injury. The potential importance of troponin I is regarding forensic evidence. Troponin I could not only be used for clinical management but for showing that cardiac damage has occurred similar to skin bruising on a child maltreatment case.

E. C. Quintana, MD, MPH

Is the Broselow Tape a Reliable Indicator for Use in All Pediatric Trauma Patients?: A Look at a Rural Trauma Center

Knight JC, Nazim M, Riggs D, et al (West Virginia Univ, Morgantown)
Pediatr Emerg Care 27:479-482, 2011

Objective.—The purpose of this study was to determine the effectiveness of the Broselow tape in the evaluation of pediatric trauma patients.

Methods.—The trauma registry of a rural level I trauma center was examined. All pediatric trauma patients 16 years or younger were reviewed from 2002 to 2006, totaling 2358 patients. The Broselow tape measures to 146.5 cm. Patients whose height correlated with the tape and had their heights and weights in the medical record were included. The constant variable was the heights by which the estimated weights of the Broselow tape were compared with the actual weights of the patients.

Results.—A total of 657 patients matched this height and had both heights and weights in their record. Most children (349/657; 53.1%) fell outside the predicted weight range, and of these, 77.1% of the actual weights were greater than those predicted by the Broselow scale. This is observed across all age groups. In patients with heights less than 75 cm, two thirds of patients' weights correlated with the Broselow estimated weight; however, those that deviated did so by 2 to 3 color intervals larger. This deviation was statistically significant in all groups.

Conclusions.—In our population, the Broselow tape is an ineffective tool to predict weight in more than 50% of pediatric trauma patients.

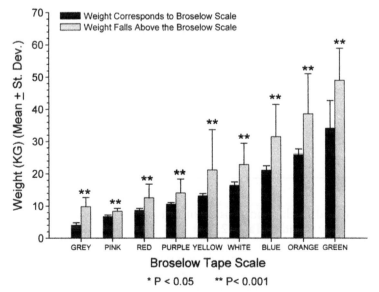

FIGURE 2.—Correlation and noncorrelation of the patient population. (Reprinted from Knight JC, Nazim M, Riggs D, et al. Is the broselow tape a reliable indicator for use in all pediatric trauma patients?: A look at a rural trauma center. *Pediatr Emerg Care.* 2011;27:479-482, Lippincott Williams & Wilkins.)

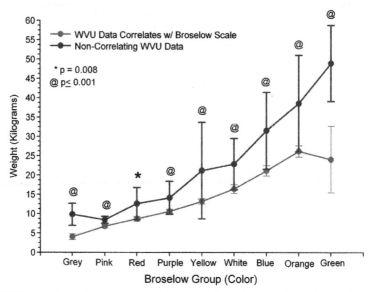

FIGURE 3.—Noncorrelation patients and degree of deviation from Broselow scale. (Reprinted from Knight JC, Nazim M, Riggs D, et al. Is the broselow tape a reliable indicator for use in all pediatric trauma patients?: A look at a rural trauma center. *Pediatr Emerg Care.* 2011;27:479-482, Lippincott Williams & Wilkins.)

TABLE 2.—Evaluation of the Validity of Broselow Correlation in Trauma Patients

Color	Estimated Weight (kg)	Patients With Correlating Weights, Mean (SD), n	Patients With Weight Above the Broselow, Mean (SD), n
Gray	3–5	4.0 (0.76), 22	9.8 (2.86),[†] 7
Pink	6–7	6.73 (0.47), 11	8.4 (0.89),[†] 5
Red	8–9	8.65 (0.61), 17	12.6 (4.18),[*] 7
Purple	10–11	10.61 (0.50), 18	14.12 (4.26),[†] 25
Yellow	12–14	13.2 (0.70), 39	21.19 (12.5),[†] 37
White	15–18	16.41 (1.13), 44	22.88 (6.63),[†] 40
Blue	19–23	21.14 (1.35), 56	31.53 (9.96),[†] 34
Orange	24–29	26.2 (1.47), 41	38.6 (12.49),[†] 54
Green	30–36	34.08 (8.6), 60	49.0 (9.86),[†] 60

[*]$P < 0.01$.
[†]$P \leq 0.001$.

This may lead to the underdosing of emergency medications and blood products (Figs 2 and 3, Table 2).

▶ Pediatric pharmacology and fluid resuscitation is dependent on weight-based dosing. Many times in acutely ill pediatric patients, weighing the patient is not possible. Both physician and parent weight estimation is mostly inaccurate. Recently, the accuracy of the Broselow tape has come into question, largely secondary to the growing problem of obesity in the pediatric population.

Most (349 of 657; 53.1%) fell outside the predicted weight range (Fig 2). Of these, 77.1% of the actual weights were greater than those predicted by the Broselow scale, and 22.9% (80 of 349) were less. In the patient groups with heights greater than 75 cm (29.5 in, purple region), 46.0% of patients' actual weights correlated with the Broselow estimated weight (Table 2). In patients with heights less than 75 cm, two-thirds of patients' weights correlated with the Broselow estimated weight; however, those that deviated did so by 2 to 3 color intervals greater (Fig 3). This deviation was statistically significant in all groups. This study showed that Broselow tape-guided resuscitations would potentially be compromised and prolonged secondary to underdosing. Further studies are needed to determine if actual versus ideal weight should be used for critically ill resuscitations.

E. C. Quintana, MD, MPH

Miscellaneous

A Randomized Controlled Trial of Home Injury Hazard Reduction: The HOME Injury Study

Phelan KJ, Khoury J, Xu Y, et al (Univ of Cincinnati, OH)
Arch Pediatr Adolesc Med 165:339-345, 2011

Objective.—To test the efficacy of installing safety devices in the homes of young children on total injury rates and on injuries deemed a priori modifiable by the installation of these devices.

Design.—A nested, prospective, randomized controlled trial.

Setting.—Indoor environment of housing units.

Participants.—Mothers and their children from birth to 3 years old participating in the Home Observation and Measures of the Environment study. Among 8878 prenatal patients, 1263 (14.2%) were eligible, 413 (32.7%) agreed to participate, and 355 were randomly assigned to the intervention (n = 181) or control (n = 174) groups.

Intervention.—Installation of multiple passive measures (eg, stair gates, cabinet locks, and smoke detectors) to reduce exposure to injury hazards. Injury hazards were assessed at home visits by teams of trained research assistants using a validated survey.

Main Outcome Measure.—Modifiable and medically attended injury (ie, telephone calls, office visits, and emergency visits for injury).

Results.—The mean age of children at intervention was 6.3 months. Injury hazards were reduced in the intervention homes but not in the control homes at 1 and 2 years ($P < .004$). There was no difference in the rate for all medically attended injuries in intervention children compared with controls: 14.3 injuries (95% confidence interval [CI], 9.7-21.1 injuries) vs 20.8 injuries (95% CI, 14.4-29.9 injuries) per 100 child-years ($P = .17$); but there was a significant reduction in the rate of modifiable medically attended injuries in intervention children compared with controls: 2.3 injuries (95% CI, 1.0-5.5 injuries) vs 7.7 injuries (95% CI, 4.2-14.2 injuries) per 100 child-years ($P = .03$).

Conclusion.—An intervention to reduce exposure to hazards in homes led to a 70% reduction in the rate of modifiable medically attended injury. *Trial Registration.*—clinicaltrials.gov. Identifier: NCT00129324.

▶ An ounce of prevention is equal to a pound of cure. This is an old maxim that drives a lot of the work in injury prevention.

The study design differed from several previous studies of home-safety efforts. Equipment was chosen on the basis of injury patterns well documented previously (eg, stair gates, cabinet locks, smoke detectors) and were installed by technicians so that the subjects were not required to do the task. Also, all of the equipment was paid for by the study so that there was no inequality of subjects from different economic status as has occurred in prior studies.

In this study, the authors were able to show that this safety intervention in the home significantly reduced the rate of injuries among children under 3 years of age. This amounted to approximately 70% fewer contacts or visits to medical providers for children in households with installed safety gear. What we do not know is the significance of these injuries. A related question is how many of these injuries were managed by a phone call for instructions or reassurance versus those that needed emergency care. It would help to know more about these 2 issues before the cost-benefit perspective of these interventions can be established.

N. B. Handly, MD, MSc, MS

A simple modified bicarbonate regimen for urine alkalinization in moderate pediatric salicylate poisoning in the emergency department
Ong Gy (KK Women's and Children's Hosp, Singapore)
Pediatr Emerg Care 27:306-308, 2011

A 4-year-old Indian girl was seen in our emergency department for unintentional ingestion of topical medication oil with subsequent salicylate poisoning. Serum levels were 52 mg/dL at 12 hours after ingestion. She was started on urine alkalization therapy to enhance salicylate elimination. This was achieved by a bicarbonate bolus of 1 mEq/kg for an hour and a continuous bicarbonate-potassium-dextrose combination infusion. The infusion regimen was modified from adult recommendations to tailor for pediatric physiological requirements in a young child. This consisted of a combination solution of dextrose 5%-sodium bicarbonate-potassium chloride with similar sodium content as half-strength (0.45%) saline and supplemental potassium, which is crucial for effective urine alkalinization. The combination fluid was administered at a rate 1.5 times her maintenance fluid requirement to achieve a urine output of 1.5 to 2 mL/kg per hour and a urine pH of 7.5 to 8.5. This regimen was well tolerated with good outcome. Many pediatricians and toxicologists achieve urine alkalinization by giving multiple bicarbonate boluses and have separate hydration fluids with dextrose and supplemental potassium. These regimens may involve complex calculations and multiple infusions that may lead to increased risk of calculation and medication errors especially in the busy emergency department setting. This case report highlights the use of a simple modified urine alkalinization regimen for moderate salicylate poisoning in a young child in the emergency department.

▶ Salicylate poisoning is a rare occurrence in pediatrics; however, the morbidity and mortality is high. Salicylate ingestion is rapidly absorbed from the stomach, and toxicity can occur with any free salicylate fractions. Alkaline urine greatly increases elimination in the urine. Alkalinization in pediatrics can be tricky because it can lead to hypokalemia, hypoglycemia, and dehydration. This case presented the management of unintentional ingestion of salicylates from a topical ointment for musculoskeletal pains. This patient had ingested 5 mL in 2 separate doses. She showed hyperpnea and recurrent vomiting as her salicylate toxicity symptoms. Salicylate level was confirmed at 52 mg/dL. She had prolonged prothrombin time at time of presentation, an indication of significant salicylate ingestion/toxicity. Rather than using multiple bicarbonate boluses, this case report (modified "adult version") used the following regimen: in 500 mL D5W, add 40 mEq of sodium bicarbonate (2 ampulla) and add 10 to 20 mEq of potassium (10–20 mL of 7.45% KCl). This solution will contain 72 mEq/L of sodium with 18 to 36 mEq K with dextrose, which can be run at 1.5 to 2 times maintenance to keep urine output 1.5 to 2 mL/kg/h and urine pH of 7.5 to 8.5. This formula is somewhat similar to the adult's formula of using 3 ampulla of sodium bicarbonate in 1 L D5W. Further studies are warranted to determine efficacy and safety of the modified "adult version" in children.

E. C. Quintana, MD, MPH

Child Passenger Safety: An Evidence-Based Review
Barraco RD, Child Passenger Safety Workgroup of the EAST Practice Management Guideline Committee (Lehigh Valley Health Network, Allentown, PA; et al)
J Trauma 69:1588-1590, 2010

Child restraints are clearly effective in injury prevention and reduction of injury severity at all ages examined, particularly high-back belt positioning booster seats. Rear seat position is also effective, especially when used in conjunction with child restraints. Legislation is also effective in improving compliance and even reducing injury. There are some data showing that primary laws are the most effective form of legislation. Further research is required on the effectiveness of legislation on injury and mortality (Table A1).

▶ Motor vehicle crashes are among the top causes of death for children younger than 14 years. Proper use of restraints can reduce injuries and fatalities. This study evaluated evidence based on literature search on restraint and

TABLE A1.—Car Safety Seats: A Guide for Families 2009

Age	Type of Seat	General Guideline
Infants	Infant seats and rear-facing convertible seats	All infants should always ride rear-facing until they are at least 1 yr of age and weigh at least 20 pounds.
Toddlers/Preschoolers	Convertible seats	It is best to ride rear-facing as long as possible. Children 1 yr of age and at least 20 pounds can ride forward-facing.
School-aged children	Booster seats	Booster seats are for older children who have outgrown their forward-facing car safety seats. Children should stay in a booster seat until adult belts fit correctly (usually when a child reaches about 4 feet 9 inches in height and is between 8 and 12 yr of age).
Older children	Seat belts	Children who have outgrown their booster seats should ride in a lap and shoulder belt in the back seat until 13 yr of age.

By American Academy of Pediatrics, 2009. Available at: http://www.aap.org/healthtopics/carseatsafety.cfm.

legislation effectiveness. Unrestrained children < 4 years old had a higher relative risk for fractures (RR = 4.4), concussions (RR = 2.7), open wounds (RR = 2.5), and hospitalization (RR = 2.5) compared with restrained children. Compared with children in proper restraints, the risk of injury was 3-fold in unrestrained children. Inappropriate use of restraints (ie, using seat belts when child needed child safety seats) was double of those using appropriate restraints. Studies showed that age-appropriate restrained children had a significant reduction in severe injuries, including solid and hollow visceral injuries, except for the back. Lap belts only were associated with an increased spinal cord injury when compared with 3-point restraints. Facial fractures increased in inappropriately restrained children, especially seating in front seat (RR = 1.6 and 1.8, respectively). Backless booster seats were found to be no different from seatbelts in injury risk. The center rear seat was the safest, with a reduction up to 24% for fatal injuries compared with the outboard seats. There was a wide range of magnitude of decrease in injury and death (10% to 50%) with the enactment of child restraint legislation.

The emergency department is an ideal environment to discuss age-appropriate car restraints, especially when pediatric patients present with any complaint related to a motor vehicle accident. Keeping car seat guidelines close for "consultation" is key in an appropriate discussion (Table A1).

E. C. Quintana, MD, MPH

Development of a Screening Tool for Pediatric Sexual Assault May Reduce Emergency-Department Visits
Floyed RL, Hirsh DA, Greenbaum VJ, et al (Emory Univ School of Medicine, Atlanta, GA; Children's Healthcare of Atlanta, GA)
Pediatrics 128:221-226, 2011

Objective.—To define the characteristics of a novel screening tool used to identify which prepubertal children should potentially receive an initial evaluation for alleged sexual assault in a nonemergent setting.

Methods.—Electronic medical records were retrospectively reviewed from 2007 to 2008. Visits with a chief complaint or diagnosis of alleged sexual assault for patients aged 12 years or younger were identified. Complete records, those with no evaluation before pediatric emergency-department arrival, and those with child advocacy center follow-up were included. Records were reviewed to answer the following: (1) Did the incident occur in the past 72 hours, and was there oral or genital to genital/anal contact? (2) Was genital or rectal pain, bleeding, discharge, or injury present? (3) Was there concern for the child's safety? (4) Was an unrelated emergency medical condition present? An affirmative response to any of the questions was considered a positive screen (warranting immediate evaluation); all others were considered negative screens. Those who had positive physical examination findings of anogenital trauma or infection, a change in custody, or an emergency medical condition were defined as high risk (having a positive outcome).

Results.—A total of 163 cases met study criteria; 90 of 163 (55%) patients had positive screens and 73 of 163 (45%) had negative screens. No patients with negative screens were classified as high risk. The screening tool has sensitivity of 100% (95% confidence interval: 93.5—100.0).

Conclusions.—This screening tool may be effective for determining which children do not require emergency-department evaluation for alleged sexual assault.

▶ This article from Emory University attempts to develop a simple screening tool that can be used to determine which children do not require immediate emergency department evaluation for alleged sexual assault and instead can be referred to another venue where nonemergent assessment is available. The evaluation of alleged sexual assault is a labor-intensive and documentation-intensive endeavor that is fraught with legal implications and emotional overlay with which few physicians feel comfortable. When you add the fact that the victim is a child, these trepidations are magnified. If this tool can be validated in further studies, it could prove very useful indeed.

E. A. Ramoska, MD, MPHE

Emergency Department Laboratory Evaluations of Fever Without Source in Children Aged 3 to 36 Months

Simon AE, Lukacs SL, Mendola P (Natl Ctr for Health Statistics, Hyattsville, MD; Kennedy Shriver Natl Inst of Child Health and Human Development, Rockville, MD)
Pediatrics 128:e1368-e1375, 2011

Objective.—This article describes ordering of diagnostic tests, admission rates, and antibiotic administration among visits to US emergency departments (EDs) by children aged 3 to 36 months with fever without source (FWS).

Methods.—The 2006–2008 National Hospital Ambulatory Medical Care Survey–Emergency Department was used to identify visits by 3- to 36-month-old children with FWS. Percentages of visits that included a complete blood count (CBC), urinalysis, blood culture, radiograph, rapid influenza test, admission to hospital, and ceftriaxone and other antibiotic administration were calculated. Multivariate logistic regression was used to identify factors associated with ordering of a CBC and urinalysis.

Results.—No tests were ordered in 58.6% of visits for FWS. CBCs were ordered in 20.5% of visits and urinalysis in 17.4% of visits. Even among girls with a temperature of ≥39°C, urinalysis was ordered in only 40.2% of visits. Ceftriaxone was given in 7.1% and other antibiotics in 18.3% of visits; 5.2% of the children at these visits were admitted to the hospital. In multivariate analysis, increased temperature, being female, and higher median income of the patient's zip code were associated with increased odds of having a CBC and urinalysis ordered. Being 24 to 36 months of age was associated with lower odds of receiving both a CBC and a urinalysis.

Conclusions.—Most US emergency department visits for FWS among children aged 3 to 36 months, physicians do not order diagnostic tests. Being female, having a higher fever, and higher median income of the patient's zip code were associated with ordering CBCs and urinalysis.

▶ Prior to advances in vaccinations, febrile patients aged 3 to 36 months fell between the 0- to 3-month sepsis workup up and the 36-month and older more adult-like workup. The authors of this retrospective review looked to identify what the average emergency physician is doing in the evaluation of febrile patients aged 3 to 36 months without a source for said fever. Rather than previously used scenario-based data gathering, the researchers reviewed a national database to ascertain practice patterns in this clinical condition. They determined that fever without a source represents more than 20% of emergency department visits for patients age 3 to 36 months. Treating physicians ordered no tests in more than 50% of patients. Considering the propensity of urinary tract infections in female patients, it is disheartening that treating emergency physicians (EPs) ordered a urinalysis only 40% of the time. The results demonstrate that emergency physicians are using their clinical acumen to treat these patients.

Fevers in immunized patients are typically viral and therefore need a "tincture of time" in addition to antipyretics and supportive care. EPs should substantiate the vaccination schedule and verify follow-up before discharging these patients without a more thorough evaluation. Readers should be aware that controversy exists regarding the management of the patients younger than 3 months.

E. C. Bruno, MD

Health Effects of Energy Drinks on Children, Adolescents, and Young Adults
Seifert SM, Schaechter JL, Hershorin ER, et al (Univ of Miami, FL)
Pediatrics 127:511-528, 2011

Objective.—To review the effects, adverse consequences, and extent of energy drink consumption among children, adolescents, and young adults.

Methods.—We searched PubMed and Google using "energy drink," "sports drink," "guarana," "caffeine," "taurine," "ADHD," "diabetes," "children," "adolescents," "insulin," "eating disorders," and "poison control center" to identify articles related to energy drinks. Manufacturer Web sites were reviewed for product information.

Results.—According to self-report surveys, energy drinks are consumed by 30% to 50% of adolescents and young adults. Frequently containing high and unregulated amounts of caffeine, these drinks have been reported in association with serious adverse effects, especially in children, adolescents, and young adults with seizures, diabetes, cardiac abnormalities, or mood and behavioral disorders or those who take certain medications. Of the 5448 US caffeine overdoses reported in 2007, 46% occurred in those younger than 19 years. Several countries and states have debated or restricted energy drink sales and advertising.

Conclusions.—Energy drinks have no therapeutic benefit, and many ingredients are understudied and not regulated. The known and unknown pharmacology of agents included in such drinks, combined with reports of toxicity, raises concern for potentially serious adverse effects in association with energy drink use. In the short-term, pediatricians need to be aware of the possible effects of energy drinks in vulnerable populations and screen for consumption to educate families. Long-term research should aim to understand the effects in at-risk populations. Toxicity surveillance should be improved, and regulations of energy drink sales and consumption should be based on appropriate research.

▶ The popularity of using energy drinks has been exponentially increasing over the last few years. There are many flavors, colors, and brands to please anyone out there. They are ubiquitous in any markets. They usually contain high concentration of caffeine, taurine, vitamins, sugar, and some herbal supplements marketed to give energy, help with weight loss, and improve athletic performance and stamina, just to mention a few of their advertisements. Heavy caffeine consumption associated with these drinks has been associated with seizures, mania, stroke, and sudden death. The effects in pediatrics have been limited. This study found that more than 28% of children older than

12 years are drinking these energy drinks regularly. In college students, the use of energy drinks was greater than 51%, at least once weekly. US poison control centers have not tracked overdoses due to energy drinks specifically because they are under the classification of caffeine overdose. Just recently, US poison control centers added them as a separate category. Germany has tracked its incidence since 2002 with reported outcomes including, but not limited to, liver and kidney failure, respiratory disorders, agitation, seizures, psychotic conditions, rhabdomyolysis, heart failure, and death. Similar reports have been documented from Ireland and New Zealand. The reports suggest that these energy drinks may have serious adverse health effects. Other ingredients (herbals and vitamins) that are unregulated and understudied could increase the harmful effects in children's physiology and growth. Further research is needed to define safe doses, if any, in pediatrics.

E. C. Quintana, MD, MPH

Pediatric Injuries Attributable to Falls From Windows in the United States in 1990–2008
Harris VA, Rochette LM, Smith GA (The Res Inst at Nationwide Children's Hosp, Columbus, OH)
Pediatrics 128:455-462, 2011

Objective.—To examine the epidemiological features of pediatric injuries related to falls from windows.

Methods.—By using the National Electronic Injury Surveillance System, emergency department (ED) data for pediatric injury cases associated with window falls in 1990–2008 were reviewed.

Results.—An estimated 98 415 children (95% confidence interval [CI]: 82 416–114 419) were treated in US hospital EDs for window fall–related injuries during the 19-year study period (average: 5180 patients per year [95% CI: 4828–5531]). The mean age of children was 5.1 years, and boys accounted for 58.1% of cases. One-fourth (25.4%) of the patients required admission to the hospital. The annual injury rate decreased significantly during the study period because of a decrease in the annual injury rate among 0- to 4-year-old children. Children 0 to 4 years of age were more likely to sustain head injuries (injury proportion ratio [IPR]: 3.22 [95% CI: 2.65–3.91]) and to be hospitalized or to die (IPR: 1.65 [95% CI: 1.38–1.97]) compared with children 5 to 17 years of age. Children who landed on hard surfaces were more likely to sustain head injuries (IPR: 2.05 [95% CI: 1.53–2.74]) and to be hospitalized or to die (IPR: 2.23 [95% CI: 1.57–3.17]) compared with children who landed on cushioning surfaces.

Conclusions.—To our knowledge, this is the first study to investigate window fall–related injuries treated in US hospital EDs by using a nationally representative sample. These injuries are an important pediatric public

TABLE 1.—Characteristics of Injuries Attributable to Falls From Windows Among Children 0 to 17 Years of Age Treated in US EDs in 1990—2008

Characteristic	No., Estimate (95% CI)	%
Gender		
Male	57 134 (47 551—66 718)	58.1
Female	41 232 (34 311—48 153)	41.9
Age		
0—4 y	63 730 (52 151—75 308)	64.8
5—17 y	34 685 (29 209—40 162)	35.2
Window height		
First story	22 017 (17 440—26 594)	30.8
Second story	44 850 (35 726—53 974)	62.7
Third story or higher	4665 (2979—6352)	6.5
ED disposition		
Treated/examined and released	73 131 (61 059—85 204)	74.4
Hospitalized	24 968 (17 833—32 103)	25.4
Fatal injury	a	0.2
Body region injured		
Head and face	45 975 (37 571—54 379)	48.6
Trunk	16 688 (13 631—19 745)	17.6
Upper extremity	9914 (7868—11 960)	10.5
Lower extremity	17 510 (14 202—20 817)	18.5
Other	4511 (3156—5865)	4.8
Diagnosis		
Head injury	25 484 (19 263—31 704)	26.2
Fracture	15 290 (12 206—18 373)	15.7
Laceration	7391 (5960—8822)	7.6
Soft-tissue injury	39 777 (33 182—46 371)	40.9
Other	9273 (7124—11 422)	9.6
Risky behavior		
No	84 587 (70 316—98 858)	85.9
Yes	13 828 (10 897—16 760)	14.1

[a]National estimates of frequencies were not possible because of the sample size of <20 cases.

health problem, and increased prevention efforts are needed, including development and evaluation of innovative prevention programs (Table 1).

▶ Falls from windows occur frequently, especially in large urban populations. Previous studies have found that preschool-aged children have the highest risk of falling, boys fall more frequently than girls, window falls have high morbidity rates, and falls show seasonal trends, with peaks during warmer months. This study is among children treated in US hospital emergency departments (EDs) during a 19-year period, 1990 to 2008. An estimated 98 415 children were treated in US hospital EDs for injuries attributable to a fall from a window, with an average of 5180 patients yearly. Fifty-eight percent were boys with a mean age of 5.1 years old. Boys had an average annual injury rate of 8.3 injuries per 100 000 children, and girls had a rate of 6.3 injuries per 100 000 children. There was a statistically significant linear decrease in the annual injury rate during the 19-year study period (−0.155 cases per 100 000 children per year; $P = .003$). One-story falls accounted for 30.8% (22 017 cases), 2-story falls accounted for 62.7% (44 850 cases), and ≥3-story falls accounted for 6.5% (4665 cases). Eighty-eight percent of cases stated that the window had a screen in place before the fall. Unfortunately, in 75.7% of cases, there were no documented landing surfaces. Forty-eight percent involved injuries of the head or face, 18.5% injuries of the lower extremities, 17.6% injuries of the trunk, 10.5% injuries of the upper extremities, and 4.8% other injuries. Children 0 to 4 years of age were 1.65 times more likely to injure the head or face, needing hospitalization or leading to death. Children 5 to 17 years of age were more likely to sustain injuries to the upper extremities than children 0 to 4 years old. Compared with lower heights, patients who fell from ≥3 stories were more likely to sustain fractures and to be hospitalized or to die. Patients who fell from 1 story had greater proportions of lacerations and soft tissue injuries and were more likely to be examined or treated and released from the ED (Table 1). Patients who landed on hard surfaces were more likely to sustain head injuries and to be hospitalized or to die. Among children 5 to 17 years of age, patients who engaged in risky behavior were more likely to sustain injuries to the lower extremities. This study shows the importance of prevention measures, such as window guards or locks and placing furniture away from windows.

E. C. Quintana, MD, MPH

Pediatric Submersion Events in Portable Above-Ground Pools in the United States, 2001–2009
Shields BJ, Pollack-Nelson C, Smith GA (The Res Inst at Nationwide Children's Hosp, Columbus, OH; Independent Safety Consulting, Rockville, MD)
Pediatrics 128:45-52, 2011

Objective.—The goal of this study was to describe the epidemiology of pediatric submersion events occurring in portable pools in the United States.

Methods.—A retrospective analysis of fatal and nonfatal submersion events involving children younger than 12 years in portable pools was conducted using injury and fatality data compiled by the US Consumer Product Safety Commission from 2001 through 2009.

Results.—There were 209 fatal and 35 nonfatal submersion cases reported to the commission from 2001 through 2009. The majority (94%) involved children younger than 5 years, 56% involved boys, 73% occurred in the child's own yard, and 81% occurred during the summer months. The number of submersion events increased rapidly from 2001 to 2005 and then leveled off from 2005 to 2009.

Conclusions.—The use of portable pools in residential settings poses a significant risk of submersion-related morbidity and mortality to children, especially in the <5-year-old age group. No single strategy will prevent all submersion deaths and injuries; therefore, layers of protection are recommended. Industry is advised to engage in development of protective devices that are effective and affordable for portable pools, including isolation fencing, pool alarms, and safety covers. A strong and pervasive consumer education campaign is needed to make consumers aware of the dangers of

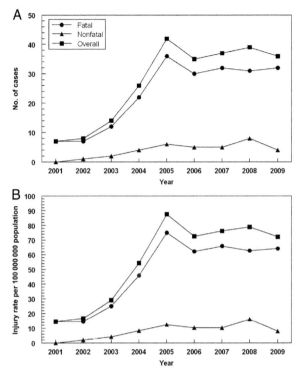

FIGURE 1.—**A,** Number of submersion events for children younger than 12 years, according to year and type of event (fatal, nonfatal, and overall) in the United States in 2001–2009. **B,** Injury rate per 100 000 000 US resident population younger than 12 years, according to year and type of event (fatal, nonfatal, and overall) in the United States in 2001–2009. (Reprinted from Shields BJ, Pollack-Nelson C, Smith GA. Pediatric Submersion Events in Portable Above-Ground Pools in the United States, 2001–2009. *Pediatrics* 2011;128:45-52. Copyright © 2011, with permission from the American Academy of Pediatrics.)

portable pools, because these small, inexpensive, consumer-installed pools may not generate the same sense of risk as an in-ground pool (Fig 1).

▶ One of the leading causes of unintentional death in children is drowning, especially in boys younger than 5 years. This study evaluated submersion events in portable pools (eg, wading pools, inflatable pools). From a total of 244 cases, 86% were fatal involving children younger than 12 years old. Forty-two percent were 1 year old, and 56% were boys. The number of submersion cases increased from 2001 to 2005 (*P* = .02), although there was no increase of rate in subsequent years (2005–2009) (Fig 1). As expected, most incidents occurred during the summer months of June, July, and August without any statistically significant difference in the days of the week. There was no significant difference in water depth. The pool was located in the patient's backyard in 73% of the cases. Thirty-nine percent of submersion cases were unsupervised. Submersion duration was not documented in most cases (80%) with a range of 1 minute to more than 2 hours. CPR was initiated by parents or bystanders in less than 20% of all cases. Prevention of these events would be challenging because most owners of portable pools would be against fencing. Current recommendations for in-ground pool fencing are fencing at least 4 feet high, nonclimbable, no opening under the fence or between uprights greater than 4 inches, and self-latching gates that open away from the pool. Prevention requires multiple strategies.

E. C. Quintana, MD, MPH

Physicians' Perceptions of Background Noise in a Pediatric Emergency Department
Ratnapalan S, Cieslak P, Mizzi T, et al (The Hosp for Sick Children, Toronto, Ontario, Canada)
Pediatr Emerg Care 27:826-833, 2011

Objective.—The objectives of this study were to measure noise levels in a tertiary care pediatric emergency department (ED) and to identify attending staff physicians' and first-year residents' perceptions of background noise levels and its impact on communication and teaching.

Methods.—A mixed methodology was used in this study. A sound level meter measuring 30 to 140 dB was placed in the ED for a week. All consenting staff physicians and first-year residents were surveyed using a semistructured questionnaire during the study period to assess their perceptions of background noise and its impact. Descriptive statistics were used for quantitative analysis. Narrative answers were coded and analyzed using the method of meaning condensation to assess the impact of background noise on both communication and teaching.

Results.—The average noise level in the ED is 68.73 dB for a 24-hour period. The number sound peaks higher than 80 dB, with an average of 309 dB/d (minimum, 193 dB; maximum, 461 dB). Only 35% of staff physicians' surveys and 22% of residents' surveys identified the noise levels to be uncomfortable. However, background noise in the ED was perceived as stressful, affecting interaction, communication, and teaching between residents and staff physicians. Staff physicians and residents stated that they feel helpless when it is too noisy and did not have good strategies to reduce background noise in the ED.

Conclusions.—The high background noise levels in a pediatric ED are perceived as stressful and interfering with communication and teaching. Noise levels in EDs should be measured, and noise reduction strategies should be implemented because physicians are not consistent in identifying excessive noise levels.

▶ How often do patients and/or caregivers complain that the emergency department (ED) is too noisy? This study evaluated our perceptions of noise in the pediatric ED. The noise meter recorded readings were an average of 68 dB, which was higher than the recommended 40- to 45-dB daytime hospital noise and 35-dB nighttime hospital noise. A maximum of 115-dB for 15 seconds was recorded. There was no difference during patient volume or day of the week regarding noise level. Eighty percent of staff physicians noted that pediatric ED was noisy; moreover, all residents considered it noisier than the adult ED. Sixty-five percent surveyed had to shout to be heard during their shifts. As expected, the survey found that daytime and evening shifts were noisier, with sign-out times the noisiest. Forty percent of staff physicians had to ask for quiet because of noise during their shift. Even though only 11% of residents reported that noise interfered with their teaching, it is possible that most teaching is done by observation or demonstration or that the resident did not admit its hindrance. This is something to keep in mind during your next ED shift.

E. C. Quintana, MD, MPH

Use of Skeletal Surveys to Evaluate for Physical Abuse: Analysis of 703 Consecutive Skeletal Surveys
Duffy SO, Squires J, Fromkin JB, et al (Wright State Univ, Dayton, OH; Children's Hosp of Pittsburgh of UPMC, PA)
Pediatrics 127:e47-e52, 2011

Objectives.—The goals were to assess the use of the skeletal survey (SS) to evaluate for physical abuse in a large consecutive sample, to identify characteristics of children most likely to have unsuspected fractures, and to determine how often SS results influenced directly the decision to make a diagnosis of abuse.

Methods.—A retrospective, descriptive study of a consecutive sample of children who underwent an SS at a single children's hospital over 4 years was performed. Data on demographic characteristics, clinical presentation, SS results, and effects of SS results on clinical diagnoses were collected. A positive SS result was defined as a SS which identified a previously unsuspected fracture(s).

Results.—Of the 703 SSs, 10.8% yielded positive results. Children <6 months of age, children with an apparent life-threatening event or seizure, and children with suspected abusive head trauma had the highest rates of positive SS results. Of children with positive SS results, 79% had ≥1 healing fracture.

Conclusions.—This is the largest study to date to describe the use of the SS. Almost 11% of SS results were positive. The SS results influenced directly the decision to make a diagnosis of abuse for 50% of children with positive SS results. These data, combined with the high morbidity rates for missed abuse and the large proportion of children with healing fractures detected through SS, suggest that broader use of SS, particularly for high-risk populations, may be warranted (Table 3).

▶ Child maltreatment is a concerning and potentially deadly pediatric presentation in our emergency departments (EDs) that warrants careful consideration. Fractures are common evidence of physical abuse. The skeletal survey (SS) has been used as a tool for detecting clinically unsuspected fractures. The SS is recommended by the American Academy of Pediatrics for all children < 2 years old

TABLE 3.—Positive SS Results According to Age

Age	SS Performed	No (%) Positive SS Results
0–5.9 mo	292	48 (16.4)
6–11.9 mo	165	12 (7.2)
12–23.9 mo	135	9 (7.3)
24–59 mo	105	6 (5.7)
>60 mo	6	1 (16.7)

and in selected children between 2 and 5 years old with suspected physical abuse. This retrospective, descriptive study evaluated all consecutive SSs in an attempt to decrease selection biases. Ninety-seven percent of SSs were done in the ED with a median patient age of 8 months. Eighty-four percent of patients were < 2 years old, and 57% were boys. The most common reason for ED presentation was trauma followed by injury. The most common reason for SS was a recognized fracture, followed by features of child abuse, suspected abusive head trauma, and social concerns. Ten percent of SSs yielded positive results with a higher rate in children younger than 6 months of age ($P < 0.00$) (Table 3). Most had a single fracture, followed by 2 fractures (24%), and 3 or more fractures (21%). The most common location of unsuspected fractures was the ribs. Overall, 79% of all children for whom age data (ie, acute vs nonacute/healing) were available had one or more healing fracture. Children with presentations of apparent life-threatening event/apnea, seizure, or head trauma had higher rates of positive SS results than those who presented for other reasons. Children with recognized fractures were not more likely to have positive SS than children who had an SS done with other concerns. Despite the retrospective limitations of this study, this large study yielded results that would suggest using more SSs, especially in children younger than 6 months.

E. C. Quintana, MD, MPH

8 Emergency Medical Service Systems

Airway

Rocuronium versus Succinylcholine in Air Medical Rapid-Sequence Intubation

Hiestand B, Cudnik MT, Thomson D, et al (Wake Forest Univ, Winston-Salem, NC; The Ohio State Univ, Columbus; David P. Thomson, Inc, Manlius, NY)

Prehosp Emerg Care 15:457-463, 2011

Background.—It is not known how rocuronium compares with succinylcholine in its effect on intubation success during air medical rapid-sequence intubation (RSI).

Objective.—To examine the impact of succinylcholine use on the odds of successful prehospital intubation.

Methods.—We performed a retrospective analysis of a critical care transport service administrative database containing patient encounters from 2004 to 2008. Rotor transports of patients ≥18 years old, requiring airway management (intubation or backup airway: laryngeal mask airway, Combitube, or cricothyrotomy), and receiving either rocuronium or succinylcholine were included in the analysis. Patients receiving both drugs were excluded. Multiple imputation was used to account for records that were missing data elements. A propensity score based on patient and encounter characteristics was calculated to control for the effect of clinical factors on the choice of drug by air medical personnel. Logistic regression was used to assess the impact of succinylcholine use on the odds of first-attempt intubation. Ordinal logistic regression was used to assess the impact of succinylcholine on the number of attempts required to intubate (1, 2, or ≥3 or backup airway).

Results.—A total of 1,045 patients met the criteria for analysis; 761 (73%) were male, and the median age was 41 years (interquartile range 26−56). Eight hundred seventy-six (84%) were transported from the scene, and 484 (46%) received succinylcholine. Six hundred twelve (59%) were intubated on the first attempt, 322 (31%) required two attempts, 69 required three or more attempts (7%), and 42 required a backup airway (4%). After propensity score adjustment, succinylcholine was associated with a higher incidence of first-attempt intubation (odds ratio 1.4, 95% CI 1.1–1.8), as well as improved odds for requiring fewer attempts to intubate (odds ratio 1.5, 95% CI 1.2–1.9), as compared with rocuronium.

Conclusions.—Rapid-sequence intubation was more successful with fewer attempts in patients intubated by air medical crews with succinylcholine as opposed to rocuronium. Prospective, randomized studies are needed to confirm these findings and to explore the impact of succinylcholine on the outcomes of air medical–transported patients.

▶ This study attempted to compare the use of 2 paralytic agents, succinylcholine and rocuronium, in helicopter emergency medical services (HEMS). The information that could be gleaned from a study of this nature can be useful in providing a compendium of differential characteristics that could be used in the revision and development of future HEMS protocols. However, the data collection and experimental design of this study, although extensive, leaves many ambiguities and unaddressed issues that weaken the final conclusion.

The design of this data collection lacks specific inclusion and exclusion criteria on various levels. Various mitigating circumstances that occur may have affected the data but are not quantified or correlated to the final outcome. Pharmacological characteristics of the 2 drugs do not appear to be well correlated with the conclusion drawn. The definitions created for a particular event were not specific, such as what was considered an airway attempt or a successful first-pass intubation without a rescue airway attempt. How did the medics choose between rocuronium and succinylcholine? What were the conditions that led to the decision to use one drug over the other? The authors needed to use a propensity score and imputation in their data calculations and interpretation, which may have left variables inappropriately interpolated into the final conclusions.

Another concern is that there are no final outcome data reported on the patients. Did the decision to use one drug over the other have any effect on the patients' final outcomes? How is it that using succinylcholine is actually better than rocuronium? Could it have been the medics skill set and knowledge, or was it the medical condition of the patient that dictated the need of intubation and affected the decision of which drug was used?

The idea behind the study has practical value. However, the data need to be reevaluated, and the data collection and experimental design need to be reevaluated and appropriately modified to capture the parameters necessary to draw a meaningful conclusion.

B. M. Minczak, MS, MD, PhD, PH-MD

Cardiovascular

Prehospital triage in the ambulance reduces infarct size and improves clinical outcome

Postma S, Dambrink J-HE, de Boer M-J, et al (Diagram, Zwolle, Netherlands; Isala Klinieken, Zwolle, Netherlands; et al)

Am Heart J 161:276-282, 2011

Background.—We evaluated the effect of prehospital triage (PHT) in the ambulance on infarct size and clinical outcome and studied its relationship to the distance of patient's residence to the nearest percutaneous coronary intervention (PCI) center.

Methods.—All consecutive ST-segment elevation myocardial infarction patients who were transported to the Isala klinieken from 1998 to 2008 were registered in a dedicated database. Of these, 2,288 (45%) were referred via a spoke center and 2.840 (55%) via PHT.

Results.—PHT patients were more often treated within 3 hours after symptom onset (46.2% vs 26.8%, $P < .001$), more often had a post-procedural thrombolysis in myocardial infarction (TIMI) 3 flow (93.0% vs 89.7%, $P < .001$) had a smaller infarct size (peak creatine kinase $2,188 \pm 2,187$ vs $2,575 \pm 2,259$ IU/L, $P < .001$) and had a lower 1-year mortality (4.9% vs 7.0%, $P = .002$). After multivariate analysis, PHT was independently associated with ischemic time less than 3 hours (OR 2.45, 95% CI 2.13-2.83), a peak creatine kinase less than the median value (OR 1.19, 95% CI 1.04-1.36) and a lower 1-year mortality (OR 0.67, 95% CI 0.50-0.91). The observed differences between PHT patients and the spoke group were more pronounced in the subgroup of patients living >38 km from the PCI center.

Conclusion.—PHT in the ambulance is associated with a shorter time to treatment, a smaller infarct size and a more favorable clinical outcome, especially with longer distance from the patient's residence to the nearest PCI center. Therefore, PHT in the ambulance may reduce the negative effect of living at a longer distance from the PCI center.

▶ This observational study from the Netherlands was conducted over a 10-year period. It suggests that using prehospital triage (PHT; ie, having trained paramedics perform a prehospital electrocardiogram and having a computer interpret whether it shows an ST elevation myocardial infarction) is associated with a decreased time to diagnosis, a decreased time to percutaneous coronary intervention (PCI), and a lower 1-year mortality rate. The number needed to treat is 48. Moreover, more patients in the PHT group were treated in accordance with American College of Cardiology/American Heart Association and European Society of Cardiology guidelines compared with patients who presented to an outside spoke center hospital and had to be transferred to the PCI center.

Although the total ischemic time (ie, the treatment from symptom onset to balloon inflation) was always significantly lower in the PHT group compared with the spoke-center referral group, regardless of the distance from the PCI center (a difference of 68 min in the < 38 km group and 81 min in the > 38 group), the mortality benefit was only statistically significant in the subgroup of patients who lived more than 38 km (23.6 miles) from the PCI center.

This study suggests that using PHT by ambulance personnel will reduce time to PCI. A mortality rate benefit is incurred for patients living a greater distance from the PCI center (38 km in this study). Whether this approach is cost-effective when compared with alternate strategies, such as using fibrinolytics prior to referral, remains an open question.

E. A. Ramoska, MD, MPHE

Prehospital Troponin T Testing in the Diagnosis and Triage of Patients with Suspected Acute Myocardial Infarction

Sørensen JT, Terkelsen CJ, Steengaard C, et al (Aarhus Univ Hosp, Denmark; Aarhus Univ Hosp, Skejby, Denmark; et al)
Am J Cardiol 107:1436-1440, 2011

Prehospital electrocardiographic (ECG) diagnosis has improved triage and outcome in patients with acute ST-elevation myocardial infarction. However, many patients with acute myocardial infarction (AMI) present with equivocal ECG patterns making prehospital ECG diagnosis difficult. We aimed to investigate the feasibility and ability of prehospital troponin T (TnT) testing to improve diagnosis in patients with chest pain transported by ambulance. From June 2008 through September 2009, patients from the central Denmark region with suspected AMI and transported by ambulance were eligible for prehospital TnT testing with a qualitative point-of-care test (cutpoint 0.10 ng/ml). Quantitative TnT was measured at hospital arrival and after 8 and 24 hours (cutpoint 0.03 ng/ml). A prehospital electrocardiogram was recorded in all patients. Prehospital TnT testing was attempted in 958 patients with a 97% success rate. In 258 patients, in-hospital TnT values were increased (≥0.03 ng/ml) during admission. The prehospital test identified 26% and the first in-hospital test detected 81% of patients with increased TnT measurements during admission. A diagnosis of AMI was established in 208 of 258 patients with increased TnT. The prehospital test identified 30% of these patients, whereas the first in-hospital test detected 79%. Median times from symptom onset to blood sampling were 83 minutes (46 to 167) for the prehospital sample and 165 minutes (110 to 276) for the admission sample. In conclusion, prehospital TnT testing is feasible with a high success rate. This study indicates that prehospital implementation of quantitative tests, with lower detection limits, could identify most patients with AMI irrespective of ECG changes.

▶ This study, from Aarhus University Hospital in Denmark, looked at a convenience sample of 958 patients with suspected acute myocardial infarction and tried to determine whether prehospital testing of troponin T (TnT) was feasible and useful. It definitely was feasible; they completed the test in the ambulance in 928 patients (97%). However, the test was not very useful. The initial prehospital TnT was only positive in 63 of the 202 patients who were ultimately diagnosed with an AMI (sensitivity = 31%). Moreover, a negative TnT test did not guarantee that the patient would not be diagnosed with an AMI. The negative predictive value was only 84%.

These results certainly make sense. Cardiac biomarkers, when measured early in the evolution of an AMI, are not very good at picking out which patients will ultimately be diagnosed with an AMI. The diagnostic accuracy of biomarkers in the emergency department is not very good; by measuring them even earlier (in the prehospital setting), it stands to reason that their diagnostic use will not be improved.

E. A. Ramoska, MD, MPHE

Serial Prehospital 12-Lead Electrocardiograms Increase Identification of ST-segment Elevation Myocardial Infarction

Verbeek PR, Ryan D, Turner L, et al (Univ of Toronto, Ontario, Canada)
Prehosp Emerg Care 16:109-114, 2011

Background.—Many prehospital protocols require acquisition of a single 12-lead electrocardiogram (ECG) when assessing a patient for ST-segment elevation myocardial infarction (STEMI). However, it is known that ECG evidence of STEMI can evolve over time.

Objectives.—To determine how often the first and, if necessary, second or third prehospital ECGs identified STEMI, and the time intervals associated with acquiring these ECGs and arrival at the emergency department (ED).

Methods.—We retrospectively analyzed 325 consecutive prehospital STEMIs identified between June 2008 and May 2009 in a large third-service emergency medical services (EMS) system. If the first ECG did not identify STEMI, protocol required a second ECG just before transport and, if necessary, a third ECG before entering the receiving ED. Paramedics who identified STEMI at any time bypassed participating local EDs, taking patients directly to the percutaneous coronary intervention (PCI) center. Paramedics used computerized ECG interpretation with STEMI diagnosis defined as an "acute MI" report by GE/Marquette 12-SL software in ZOLL E-series defibrillator/cardiac monitors (ZOLL Medical, Chelmsford, MA). We recorded the time of each ECG, and the ordinal number of the diagnostic ECG. We then determined the number of cases and frequency of STEMI diagnosis on the first, second, or third ECG. We also measured the interval between ECGs and the interval from the initial positive ECG to arrival at the ED.

Results.—STEMI was identified on the first prehospital ECG in 275 cases, on the second ECG in 30 cases, and on the third ECG in 20 cases (cumulative percentages of 84.6%, 93.8%, and 100%, respectively). For STEMIs identified on the second or third ECG, 90% were identified within 25 minutes after the first ECG. The median times from identification of STEMI to arrival at the ED were 17.5 minutes, 11.0 minutes, and 0.7

minutes for STEMIs identified on the first, second, and third ECGs, respectively.

Conclusions.—A single prehospital ECG would have identified only 84.6% of STEMI patients. This suggests caution using a single prehospital ECG to rule out STEMI. Three serial ECGs acquired over 25 minutes is feasible and may be valuable in maximizing prehospital diagnostic yield, particularly where emergent access to PCI exists.

▶ This study was conducted to determine whether acquiring several sequential electrocardiograms (ECGs) in patients with chest pain during a prehospital encounter with paramedics would increase the likelihood of detecting/ diagnosing the presence of an ST segment elevation myocardial infarction (STEMI). These investigators performed a retrospective review of the data derived from the CODE STEMI program used by the 2-tiered, third service emergency medical system (EMS) in Toronto, Canada. Conducting this study accomplished several things. First, this study provided data supporting the presumptive premise that led to the development of this protocol, that is, acquiring several ECGs would increase the chances of detecting an STEMI. This protocol called for the acquisition of an initial ECG on arrival at the bedside of the patient. If there was evidence of an STEMI, a receiving hospital capable of providing percutaneous coronary intervention (PCI) was notified by the medics and the catheterization laboratory was activated. The patient was then immediately transported to the PCI center for treatment. If the first ECG did not provide evidence of an STEMI, the protocol called for the acquisition of a second ECG when the patient was loaded into the ambulance. As before, if the ECG demonstrated evidence of an STEMI, the PCI center was activated and the patient was expediently transported. If yet again the ECG was nondiagnostic of an STEMI, a third ECG was obtained on arrival at the hospital. If the ECG was now read as positive, the patient was promptly transported to the PCI center. If the receiving hospital did not have PCI capability, the patient was not offloaded, but the ambulance transported the patient to a facility that was capable of performing the procedure immediately. All pertinent issues for executing this protocol were prearranged with the facilities involved.

When a patient is experiencing chest pain due to compromised coronary blood flow, time-dependent pathophysiological changes are occurring within the myocardium. Despite this compromise in coronary blood flow during the early phase of cardiac ischemia, electrophysiological evidence of an STEMI may be absent, rendering the ECG normal or nondiagnostic. As myocardial ischemia progresses, the damage to the myocardium increases, followed by changes in the ECG. By obtaining several ECGs during the time course of this process, the chances of detecting an STEMI increase. This can be inferred from the ordinal data in this study, which demonstrates cumulative percentages of 84.6%, 93.8%, and 100.0% of detection of an STEMI by the first, second, and third ECG acquisition, respectively. Thus, performing serial ECGs appears to increase the specificity for detecting STEMI significantly. Hence, there are fewer missed opportunities for detecting the STEMI. Second, this study demonstrated that "time to balloon" can be decreased by performing these serial ECGs, because there are fewer delays in initiating the PCI center response. This is because of the prehospital activation of the catheterization laboratory, which saves time by having the laboratory prepare for the procedure while the patient is en route to the hospital. Getting the patient to PCI promptly has been demonstrated to preserve cardiac function and improve the survival rates of the patients who received the needed intervention early on. Remember, "time is muscle." Third, the information provided by this work may decrease and/or prevent the devastating outcomes that can occur as a result of failure to diagnose or outright miss during diagnosing an STEMI.

As an aside, recent American Heart Association Guidelines (2010) suggest that EMSs acquire an ECG on a patient with chest pain as soon as possible in the evaluation. However, there are no recommendations for obtaining additional ECGs during the prehospital evaluation. In the hospital setting, performing serial ECGs is recommended in patients who are having continuous chest pain/pressure or in patients who continue to have signs and symptoms highly suggestive of an acute coronary syndrome.

This study also illustrated the importance of considering the pathophysiology of a time-dependent disease process when developing an algorithm or protocol. By being familiar with the process, the appropriate parameters can be measured at the appropriate times and sampling frequencies in order to increase the diagnostic value or yield of the evaluating test or procedure.

Regarding the limitations of this study, the CODE STEMI protocol called for sequential acquisition of ECGs at specified time points in the prehospital EMS encounter, which the authors of the study referred to as landmarks. If instead additional sequential ECGs were to be obtained when the patients had changes in the signs and symptoms of their chest pain or pressure, there is the possibility that additional STEMIs may have been detected. However, if the patients had persistent pain or pressure, without a perceptible change noted by the patient, some of the EMS providers may not have considered doing an ECG, thus leading to underutilization of ECG acquisition.

Finally, with the regionalization of health care systems and the development of chest pain centers, PCI centers, these data provide evidence that "bypassing" a facility incapable of providing PCI may be appropriate in the future.

B. M. Minczak, MS, MD, PhD, PH-MD

Severity of Cardiovascular Disease Patients Transported by Air Ambulance

Hata N, Shinada T, Kobayashi N, et al (Chiba Hokusoh Hosp, Japan)
Air Med J 30:328-332, 2011

Introduction.—Although helicopters have been used in an air ambulance system for the past decade in Japan, the appropriate selection of patients for this transport mode has not been investigated. The present study investigates which patients could potentially benefit the most from helicopter emergency medical service (HEMS).

Methods.—We investigated the extent of circulatory and respiratory support required in the intensive care unit (ICU) and ultimate outcomes of 2340 patients with cardiovascular disease admitted to 1 institution between October 2001 and December 2009. Two hundred and seventy were transported by HEMS (HEMS group), and 2070 were transported by other means (non-HEMS group).

Results.—Temporary cardiac pacing, ventilator management, intra-aortic balloon pumping, percutaneous cardiopulmonary support, electrical defibrillation, and therapeutic hypothermia were more frequently required by patients in the HEMS group vs. the non-HEMS group (10.4%, 28.1%, 17.0%, 5.2%, 10.0% and 3.4% vs. 8%, 17.9%, 10.9%, 2.3%, 4.5% and 0.4%, respectively). The mortality rate was higher in the HEMS group than in the non-HEMS group in the ICU (9.6% vs. 5.3%).

Conclusion.—Disease was more clinically severe and the outcome was poorer among patients with cardiovascular diseases transported by HEMS than by other means.

▶ Making the decision of who to fly and when to fly often presents a dilemma to the physician taking care of a critically ill patient. Aside from issues pertinent to aviation, such as time, distances involved, weather, and staff availability for the flight, the health care provider must consider the nature of the disease and the effects the transfer may have on the final outcome and prognosis of the patient. This study attempts to answer the question of which patients would benefit the most from the use of helicopter emergency medical service (HEMS).

In an attempt to answer this question, patients were divided into 2 groups: those who were brought to the hospital by HEMS ($n = 270$) and those brought to the hospital by non-HEMS ($n = 2070$). The variables and parameters analyzed were the extent of cardiovascular and respiratory support needed for patients admitted to the intensive care unit (ICU) and the final outcome of these patients.

The conclusions drawn by the investigators from the data provided suggest that patients with cardiovascular diseases such as acute coronary syndrome, acute heart failure, aortic diseases, pulmonary embolism, life-threatening arrhythmias, and infectious heart diseases who were transported by HEMS required more extensive circulatory and respiratory support. However, the discussion that is provided does not provide a clear correlation between the use of HEMS and the final outcomes. The fact that HEMS was used to transported patients who were more critically ill does not mean that the transport precipitated an adverse effect on these patients. There was some mention of a study in which a catecholamine surge was noted in patients who were transported by air and that those investigators noted a potential association of this surge with the presence of arrhythmias, but this group of authors speculates that this finding may be caused by the severity of the patients' condition, not the use of HEMS.

One concern I have is that these investigators are attempting to draw conclusions based on findings from observations of disproportionate, ill-matched groups, without appropriate statistical analysis. An actual cause and effect is not clearly established.

Therefore, currently the use of HEMS for critically ill patients appears to be appropriate, and although this group occasionally needs more medical intervention, it is unlikely that the need for additional care was precipitated by the actual mode of transport.

B. M. Minczak, MS, MD, PhD, PH-MD

Sustained Ventricular Fibrillation in an Alert Patient: Preserved Hemodynamics with a Left Ventricular Assist Device
Patel P, Williams JG, Brice JH (Univ of North Carolina School of Medicine, Chapel Hill; Univ of North Carolina, Chapel Hill)
Prehosp Emerg Care 15:533-536, 2011

Emergency medical services (EMS) encountered an alert patient with sustained ventricular fibrillation with preserved hemodynamics via a left ventricular assist device (LVAD). Multiple firings of the patient's implantable defibrillator were the only sign that this patient was experiencing the usually fatal ventricular arrhythmia. Initial attempts at rhythm conversion with amiodarone and 200-J biphasic shocks were unsuccessful. The patient was finally defibrillated to normal sinus rhythm after a 360-J biphasic shock. This case conference highlights the increasing prevalence of LVADs. These devices are used not only as a bridge to cardiac transplantation, but also as definitive therapy for patients in end-stage cardiac failure. Ventricular fibrillation has been shown to be well tolerated in patients with LVADs, and we discuss a standard of care for these patients. The occurrence of sustained ventricular fibrillation in patients with ventricular assist devices represents a challenging situation for EMS and emergency department providers and one that will be increasingly encountered in the future.

▶ Physicians involved in providing medical oversight to various levels of prehospital emergency medical systems (EMS) should read this case report and promptly conduct a thorough review, then, if needed, initiate a revision of current protocols in use by EMS personnel. This case stresses the need for EMS medical directors to keep up with and systematically review prehospital patient care reports looking for potential dilemmas in the provision of advanced cardiac care in the prehospital arena. Furthermore, this report demonstrates the utility and value of EMS physicians maintaining medical oversight and regular involvement in the education and training of crews under their purview.

Current advances in biomedical engineering, computer software, and the miniaturization and improvement of batteries and mechanical components has led to an increase in prevalence of sophisticated medical equipment outside the hospital, specifically in the homes of cardiac patients. In fact, many patients now have devices actually implanted within their bodies. It is common for heart patients with serious pathophysiological conditions to be out in the community walking about with pacemakers, automatic implanted cardiac defibrillators (AICDs), halter monitors, and various event monitors. Many cardiac patients now have automated external defibrillators (AEDs) in their homes, and family members are trained in cardiopulmonary resuscitation (CPR). Even more amazingly, some patients who have end-stage cardiac failure and may soon need a heart transplant are released from the hospital with a mechanical ventricular assist device. The most common device now in use is the left ventricular assist device or LVAD, which provides continuous blood flow from the left ventricle into the aorta, thus enhancing left ventricular output in the failing heart. There is a possibility that in the near future, many more devices like this will be prevalent in the community.

The presence of these devices can significantly alter the presentation of a patient. For instance, the EMS personnel called to evaluate and treat a patient with an AICD/pacer and an LVAD will face a significant challenge. Current American Heart Association (AHA) guidelines stress the importance of providing "high-quality" CPR for patients who have succumbed to sudden cardiac arrest and have no pulse. The emphasis is on assessing the patient and initiating chest compressions in a pulseless patient without unnecessary delays. Patients who have an LVAD and have no pulse do not need chest compressions. Furthermore, the AHA recommends that once a defibrillator or an AED is present, the patient's rhythm should be assessed, and if ventricular fibrillation (VF) is present, the rescuer should defibrillate the patient. These LVAD patients may be hemodynamically stable and not need any intervention at all unless their condition deteriorates.

A patient who has end-stage cardiac failure and has an AICD and LVAD may require assistance and call for help via 911. Upon arrival, the EMS personnel may find the patient pulseless and in sustained VF. When the medics attempt to determine the patient's blood pressure, they will not be able to use the indirect method of sphygmomanometry and auscultation because of the continuous blood flow provided by the LVAD. In addition, pulse oximetry will not be obtainable. Yet the patient may be awake, alert, oriented, and have no specific cardiac symptoms. The appropriate treatment may be nothing more than expedient transport to the appropriate facility. Thus, the appropriate evaluation and treatment of the patient must be conducted within the context of the situation. Therefore, a prerequisite for a positive patient outcome is having a thorough working understanding of the equipment and its effects on the patient.

Provision of continuing medical education with concomitant modification and timely updates of protocols will help improve the capabilities of the EMS crew in evaluating and effectively stabilizing the patient. EMS systems and hospitals having the availability of direct medical command to assist in guiding EMS personnel through these dilemmas may find that this, in addition to the updated protocols, is useful in modifying care in unexpected situations.

Emergency medicine physicians may find it useful to review the current literature and case reports so that they will be prepared to assess and treat patients with these devices when they present to the emergency department. Furthermore, there will be a better understanding of the care indicated for the patient after he or she has been treated in the field prior to arriving at the hospital.

Current practice suggests that more of these ventricular assist devices will appear in the prehospital setting given the prevalence of heart failure cases significantly exceeds the number of heart transplants because of the lack of readily available donor hearts. In addition, LVADs are proving to be an effective treatment modality for end-stage heart disease, and their use will probably increase. Other devices are in development or undergoing trials and may be coming to an emergency department near you.

B. M. Minczak, MS, MD, PhD, PH-MD

Syncope in the emergency department: comparison of standardized admission criteria with clinical practice
Daccarett M, Jetter TL, Wasmund SL, et al (Univ of Utah, Salt Lake City)
Europace 13:1632-1638, 2011

Aims.—Syncope is a major health care problem that accounts for many emergency department (ED) and hospital admissions. This study was conducted to investigate the short-term risk of serious events in patients presenting to the ED with syncope and to compare guideline-based admission criteria with those adopted in clinical practice.

Methods and Results.—A single-centre retrospective analysis was performed on ED visits between January and June 2009. We used the ICD-9 code 780.2 for syncope as the primary diagnosis. The prevalence of serious events within 7 days of the index presentation was evaluated. In addition, admissions and discharges were classified as being appropriate or inappropriate based on standardized guideline-based criteria integrated in a new Faint-Algorithm developed at the University of Utah. Two hundred and fifty-four ED visits met the inclusion criteria. One hundred and thirty-six patients were discharged home and the remaining 118 were admitted. The prevalence of serious events in the discharged and admission groups were 5 and 10, respectively, ($P = $ NS). According to the Faint-Algorithm, the number of inappropriate discharges and admissions were 8 out of 136 and 69 out of 118, respectively. Using the Faint-Algorithm, only 57 patients instead of 118 patients should have been admitted resulting in a 52% reduction in admission rate. Furthermore, in the remaining 197 patients who should have been discharged, the prevalence of serious events was not significantly different than that observed in the 136 patients who were actually discharged (3% vs. 4%).

Conclusion.—There are significant numbers of inappropriate discharges and admissions in patients presenting with syncope. The standardized guideline-based criteria integrated in the new Faint-Algorithm provide promise but require further prospective evaluation (Tables 1 and 4).

▶ Syncope is defined as a sudden, transient, self-limited loss of consciousness with a loss of postural tone. Syncope accounts for 1% to 3% of all patients presenting to emergency departments and up to 6% of all hospital admissions. Each year more than 1.4 million people are evaluated for syncope in the United States alone, with a cost of more than $2 billion per year.

Every year there are several new articles describing different ways to determine which patients can be discharged from the emergency department with a low complication rate and which ones definitely need to be admitted. The general belief from most physicians, both emergency and admitting, is that

TABLE 1.—Faint-Algorithm Admission Criteria (Adapted From 2009 ESC Guidelines on Syncope)

Reason for Admission	Diagnostic Criteria
Cardiac-arrhythmic causes	
(1) Sinus bradycardia <40 beats/min or pauses >3 s	12-lead standard ECG
(2) Mobitz II or 2:1 second-degree or third-degree atrioventricular block	
(3) Alternating left and right bundle branch block	
(4) Sustained supraventricular tachycardia	
(5) Sustained ventricular tachycardia	
(6) Pacemaker (ICD) malfunction with cardiac pauses.	
(7) LBBB or RBBB+left/right axis deviation	
(8) Long-QT pattern	
(9) Brugada pattern	
(10) ARVD pattern	
(11) WPW pattern	
Cardiac-Ischaemic causes	
(12) Cardiac ischaemia	Chest pain *and* troponin abnormal
Cardiovascular and pulmonary structural causes	
(13) Prolapsing atrial myxoma, tumour	Echocardiogram (items 13–19 and 21)
(14) Severe aortic stenosis	
(15) Respiratory insufficiently defined as shortness of breath and O_2 saturation <70%	
(16) Acute aortic dissection	
(17) Pericardial tamponade	
(18) Severe hypertrophic obstructive cardiomyopathy (HOCM)	
(19) Severe prosthetic valve dysfunction	
(20) Sustained (≥2 measurements at >5 min) supine systolic hypotension ≤80 mmHg	Systolic blood pressure measurement (item 20)
(21) Severe systolic dysfunction (e.g. >40%)	
(22) History of myocardial infarction with mild LV dysfunction (LVEF >40%) and absence of criteria for vasovagal syncope or orthostatic hypotension	Echocardiogram+patient's history (item 22)
Non-cardiovascular causes	
(23) Acute haemorrhage	Hematocrit <30
(24) End-stage diseases (cancer, renal dialysis, etc.)	Patient's history
(25) Major physical injuries secondary to syncope	Physical examination
(26) Minor physical injuries *and* symptomatic orthostatic hypotension	Physical examination and orthostatic blood pressure measurement

ESC, European Society of Cardiology; ICD, implantable cardioverter–defibrillator; LBBB/RBBB, left/right bundle branch block; ARVD, arrhythmogenic right ventricular Dysplasia; WPW, Wolff–Parkinson–White; LVEF, left-ventricular ejection fraction.

we admit too many people for observation after syncope and that a serious cause is rarely found after an essentially normal history and physical examination and essentially normal electrocardiogram. Previous clinical decision rules include the San Francisco Syncope Rule, the Boston Syncope Rule, the EGSYS score, the OESIL risk score, the ROSE criteria, and others. Each decision rule appears to be great after the derivation set. The decision rules then appear to perform worse in internal validation studies, and then even worse in external validation studies.

This particular study was a retrospective analysis of patients with syncope at a single institution over a 6-month period. The primary outcome was any serious event that occurred during a 7-day period of the index presentation. They found

TABLE 4.—Comparison Between Clinical Practice and Faint-Algorithm Indications Among 254 Patients Referred to the ED

	Clinical Practice		Faint-Algorithm	
	Discharges	Admissions	Discharges	Admissions
Number (%)	136 (54%)	118 (46%)	197 (78%)	57 (22%)
Serious events within 7 days after the index visit (%)	5 (4%)	10 (8%)	6 (3%)	9 (16%)

ED, emergency department.

that of all the patients who were discharged, a "serious event" occurred in only 5 patients. This serious event in all 5 patients was a recurrence of syncope. So overall, the physicians did a good job in that there weren't really any discharged patients with what most physicians think of as a serious event, such as myocardial infarction, massive pulmonary embolus, intracranial hemorrhage, serious arrhythmia, new-onset heart failure, or death. Unfortunately, the prevalence of serious event was also low in the admitted group, as only 10 of 118 patients admitted had a serious event.

The authors used the Faint-Algorithm admission criteria (Table 1) to determine if, in using these 26 criteria in a web-based program, they could decrease the admission rate significantly and still have a very low rate of serious events in discharged patients. They concluded that the Faint-Algorithm would have had an excellent negative predictive value for discharged patients (Table 4). The admission rate would have been 52% lower and there would have only been 1 more serious event in the discharged group.

Obviously, given that this was a retrospective study, there are many limitations, and it can only be seen as hypothesis generating. A systemic prospective study using well-defined criteria is needed to actually determine if this approach is helpful. That said, I would certainly review the Faint-Algorithm criteria, as most physicians would agree that their list of reasons for admission make very good sense.

D. K. Mullin, MD

Safety and Resource Utilization

A Comparison of Cooling Techniques in Firefighters After a Live Burn Evolution

Colburn D, Suyama J, Reis SE, et al (Univ of Pittsburgh, PA)
Prehosp Emerg Care 15:226-232, 2011

Objective.—We compared the use of two active cooling devices with passive cooling in a moderate-temperature ($\approx 22°C$) environment on heart rate (HR) and core temperature (T_c) recovery when applied to firefighters following 20 minutes of fire suppression.

Methods.—Firefighters (23 men, two women) performed 20 minutes of fire suppression at a live-fire evolution. Immediately following the evolution, the subjects removed their thermal protective clothing and were randomized to receive forearm immersion (FI), ice water perfused cooling vest (CV), or passive (P) cooling in an air-conditioned medical trailer for 30 minutes. Heart rate and deep gastric temperature were monitored every 5 minutes during recovery.

Results.—A single 20-minute bout of fire suppression resulted in near-maximal mean ± standard deviation HR (175 ± 13 b·min^{-1}, P; 172 ± 20 b·min^{-1}, FI; 177 ± 12 b·min^{-1}, CV) when compared with baseline ($p < 0.001$), a rapid and substantial rise in T$_c$ (38.2° ± 0.7°, P; 38.3° ± 0.4°, FI; 38.3° ± 0.3°, CV) compared with baseline ($p < 0.001$), and body mass lost from sweating of nearly 1 kilogram. Cooling rates (°C·min) differed ($p = 0.036$) by device, with FI (0.05 ± 0.04) providing higher rates than P (0.03 ± 0.02) or CV (0.03 ± 0.04), although differences over 30 minutes were small and recovery of body temperature was incomplete in all groups.

Conclusions.—During 30 minutes of recovery following a 20-minute bout of fire suppression in a training academy setting, there is a slightly higher cooling rate for FI and no apparent benefit to CV when compared with P cooling in a moderate temperature environment.

▶ The human body functions at an optimal temperature, and if the body is exposed to thermal extremes, (ie, extreme heat or cold), bodily function becomes adversely affected. In this study, the focus is on the effect of heat on body function and what is the best, most efficient means of mitigating heat stress.

If the core body temperature increases and is not quickly corrected, severe physiologic consequences can occur (heat stress, heat exhaustion, heat stroke, severe dehydration, electrolyte imbalances leading to cardiac arrhythmias, cardiac ischemia, myocardial infarction, and even death).

Normal physiologic cellular metabolism emanates heat due to the thermodynamic inefficiency of the biochemical reactions that are taking place. The heat produced is distributed throughout the body via the circulatory system. Optimal chemical kinetics and physiologic functions of the integrated organ systems occur circa a core body temperature of (37°C/98.6°F). Thermal homeostasis is maintained by the modulation of sympathetic outflow from the autonomic nervous system (ANS). The ANS receives input from the hypothalamus in the central nervous system, which is sensitive to temperature and hence serves as a "thermo-regulator/thermostat" in the body. As body core temperature increases from an increase in metabolic demands secondary to muscle contraction, the nervous system responds by lowering the total peripheral resistance to blood flow in the cutaneous tissue, thus facilitating blood flow to the outer skin surface so that heat can be dissipated. Heart rate increases causing the increase in cardiac output needed to drive blood flow through the vasculature of the skin. In addition, the increase in sympathetic outflow to the skin initiates diaphoresis, which will further enhance heat dissipation from the skin via evaporation. When this system is overloaded by the actual heat, the normal means of dissipating heat are compromised. Yet this system must still mitigate the increase in temperature and it may become compromised. Providing assistance (active cooling) to this process by facilitating heat loss from the body may ameliorate/improve the actual outcome.

Heat is dissipated from or transferred from the body by radiation, convection, evaporation, and conduction. When the body is placed in a hot environment and metabolic demand increases due to increased activity, the efficiency of the work performed decreases, leaving the individual more prone to injury or an untoward outcome.

Firefighters are often called upon to work in a hot environment, which places a significant physiologic stress on these individuals Their duties often include performing many physical tasks such as fighting and extinguishing the fire, hauling and moving heavy equipment around, looking for and rescuing victims of the fire, setting up equipment to help dissipate the smoke that has been produced by the fire, and investigating the possible cause of the fire. Doing all of these things places an additional stress on the individual. This increase in activity increases metabolic demand, causing an elevation in heat production. During fire suppression, the firefighters wear thermal protective clothing (TPC) to protect them from burns, trauma, and injury subsequent to extreme heat exposure. The main threat is the heat from the flames. Another source of heat that can compound the problem is the high ambient temperature and humidity seen in the summer months. As a result of this heat exposure and heat generation, the body initiates physiologic processes to dissipate the heat being generated.

The hot environment impedes normal heat loss via radiation, conduction, and convection, and in fact, heat can be absorbed by the firefighter in this environment. TPC inhibits effective evaporation from the skin and also impedes radiation and convection, thus trapping heat close to the body. The solution to this is to remove the individual from the hot environment to a cooler environment, remove the thermal barrier and initiate cooling—active or passive.

To ensure the safety of these personnel and to maintain efficiency on their work/job performance, periods of rest or heat remediation are needed to re-establish homeostasis or "return to baseline" prestress conditions. In fact, this is mandated by the National Flight Paramedics Association Standard 1584. The safety of these personnel and the ability to maintain the workforce needed for completion of the job at hand often requires they be rotated and treated for heat exposure.

This article focuses on ways to mitigate heat stress. The authors attempt to compare several treatment modalities for dealing with heat stress. Specifically, they compare 2 active cooling techniques: (1) forearm immersion (FI) (ie, placing the forearm into cool water) or (2) placing an ice water perfused cooling vest (CV) onto the subject with passive cooling (P) in an air conditioned medical trailer (22°C). The source of the heat stress is a "live burn evolution" in which 23 men and 2 women perform fire suppression for 20 minutes immediately followed by 1 of 3 cooling interventions: FI, CV, or P. The parameters used to study the efficacy of these techniques are measurement of heart rate and deep gastric temperature (T_c) during the exposure and cool down.

Subjects for this study were voluntarily recruited from volunteer and career fire services. They were subjected to several pretests to ensure suitability for the study. The subjects were evaluated to rule out cardiac or respiratory problems and they were excluded if they were on medications that could affect or blunt heart rate response. Female participants were screened for pregnancy.

In this study, the data collected shows the following: an increase of heart rate to 172 to 177 beats per minute in the 3 groups and an increase in T_c to between 38.2°C and 38.3°C. Body mass decreased by nearly 1000 kg due to sweating. Subjects were randomly assigned to one of the 3 interventions, and the parameters specified were measured for 30 minutes.

The data showed little difference in the outcomes of cooling between the active and passive groups. Although cooling with FI may have increased the rate of cooling during the first 20 minutes of recovery, FI made no significant difference in the actual recovery of heart rate and T_c at 20 minutes. Measurements at the 30-minute interval showed virtually no significant differences in cooling rate, and the heart rate recovery was not yet complete.

When comparing these data with findings from a similar study performed in the laboratory environment in which they used 50 minutes of treadmill walking as the stressor, there appeared to be a discrepancy in the findings regarding FI cooling rate. The FI group in the laboratory did not appear to have a significant effect on the rate of cooling. This is thought to be because the laboratory cohort of subjects did not wear TPC in that study but had short sleeve cotton shirts versus the TPC in the live burn setting, causing an enhanced overall cooling rate ($°C.min^{-1}$) that did not differ with FI. This suggests that P in a cool low humidity environment with good skin exposure to facilitate the standard heat loss mechanisms may be the best way to restore the subjects to baseline physiologic function.

One potential confounder in this study was that this was a staged live burn, not an actual working structure fire in which the risks are greater and there are more unknown variables regarding the scene hazards. This alone may prompt a catecholamine surge and affect the cooling process due to the possibility of triggering vasoconstriction in the organ tissues, thus, affecting heat dissipation. Heart rate may also increase due to the presence of these adrenergic chemical stimuli in the blood. Therefore, removal to a low humidity, cool environment in which radiation, conduction, convection, and evaporation can appropriately take place seems to be the best intervention.

B. M. Minczak, MS, MD, PhD, PH-MD

A Descriptive Analysis of Occupational Health Exposures in an Urban Emergency Medical Services System: 2007–2009
Sayed ME, Kue R, McNeil C, et al (Boston Univ, MA; Boston EMS, MA)
Prehosp Emerg Care 15:506-510, 2011

Introduction.—Prehospital providers are exposed to various infectious disease hazards. Examining specific infectious exposures would be useful in describing their current trends as well as guidance with appropriate protective measures an emergency medical services (EMS) system should consider.

Objective.—To describe the types of infectious occupational health exposures and associated outcomes reported at an urban EMS system.

Methods.—A retrospective review of all reported exposures was performed for a three-year period from January 1, 2007, to December 31, 2009. Descriptive analysis was performed on data such as provider demographics, types of exposures reported, confirmation of exposure based on patient follow-up information, and outcomes.

Results.—Three hundred ninety-seven exposure reports were filed with the designated infection control officer (ICO), resulting in an overall exposure rate of 1.2 per 1,000 EMS incidents. The most common exposure was to possible meningitis ($n = 131$, 32.9%), followed by tuberculosis (TB) ($n = 68$, 17.1%), viral respiratory infections (VRIs) such as influenza or H1N1 ($n = 61$, 15.4%), and body fluid splashes to skin or mucous membranes ($n = 56$, 14.1%). Body fluid splashes involving the eyes accounted for 41 cases (10.3%). Only six cases (1.5%) of needlestick injuries were reported. Three hundred thirty-two of all cases (83.6%) were considered true exposures to an infectious hazard, of which 177 (53.3%) were actually confirmed. Half of all exposures required only follow-up with the ICO (52.6%). One hundred twenty-seven cases (31.9%) required follow-up at a designated occupational health services or emergency department. Of these, only 23 cases (18.1%) required treatment. There was a significant trend of increasing incidence of VRI exposures from 2008 to 2009 (6.3% vs. 26.8%, p < 0.001), while a significant decrease in TB exposures was experienced during the same year (22.9% vs. 8.2%, p = 0.002).

Conclusions.—Trends in our data suggest increasing exposures to viral respiratory illnesses, whereas exposures to needlestick injuries were relatively infrequent. Efforts should continue to focus on proper respiratory protection to include eye protection in order to mitigate these exposure risks.

▶ This study from Boston University and Boston emergency medical services (EMS) describes the epidemiology of occupational health exposures in a 2-tiered, urban, public EMS system that handles more than 100 000 calls annually. Most of the reports (84%) were "true exposures," although only a little over one-half were confirmed as exposures to an infectious hazard. The majority of the exposures (65%) were to respiratory-borne pathogens, that is, meningitis, tuberculosis, and viral respiratory infections. Splashes to either the skin or the mucous membranes of the nose and mouth and splashes to the eyes round out the top 5 types of exposures and account for 90% of the reports. Needlestick injuries accounted for only 6 reports over the 3 years of this study. Treatment was administered in 23 cases (18%), and the overwhelming majority (21/23) was for postexposure prophylaxis for meningococcal meningitis. Data such as these are useful for EMS directors to inform them where resources may be needed (ie, personal protective equipment) and what additional education and training is required (recognition of respiratory hazards).

E. A. Ramoska, MD, MPHE

A Descriptive Analysis of Occupational Health Exposures in an Urban Emergency Medical Services System: 2007–2009

Sayed ME, Kue R, McNeil C, et al (Boston Univ, MA; Boston EMS, MA)
Prehosp Emerg Care 15:506-510, 2011

Introduction.—Prehospital providers are exposed to various infectious disease hazards. Examining specific infectious exposures would be useful in describing their current trends as well as guidance with appropriate protective measures an emergency medical services (EMS) system should consider.

Objective.—To describe the types of infectious occupational health exposures and associated outcomes reported at an urban EMS system.

Methods.—A retrospective review of all reported exposures was performed for a three-year period from January 1, 2007, to December 31, 2009. Descriptive analysis was performed on data such as provider demographics, types of exposures reported, confirmation of exposure based on patient follow-up information, and outcomes.

Results.—Three hundred ninety-seven exposure reports were filed with the designated infection control officer (ICO), resulting in an overall exposure rate of 1.2 per 1,000 EMS incidents. The most common exposure was to possible meningitis ($n = 131$, 32.9%), followed by tuberculosis (TB) ($n = 68$, 17.1%), viral respiratory infections (VRIs) such as influenza or H1N1 ($n = 61$, 15.4%), and body fluid splashes to skin or mucous membranes ($n = 56$, 14.1%). Body fluid splashes involving the eyes accounted for 41 cases (10.3%). Only six cases (1.5%) of needlestick injuries were reported. Three hundred thirty-two of all cases (83.6%) were considered true exposures to an infectious hazard, of which 177 (53.3%) were actually confirmed. Half of all exposures required only follow-up with the ICO (52.6%). One hundred twenty-seven cases (31.9%) required follow-up at a designated occupational health services or emergency department. Of these, only 23 cases (18.1%) required treatment. There was a significant trend of increasing incidence of VRI exposures from 2008 to 2009 (6.3% vs. 26.8%, p < 0.001), while a significant decrease in TB exposures was experienced during the same year (22.9% vs. 8.2%, p = 0.002).

Conclusions.—Trends in our data suggest increasing exposures to viral respiratory illnesses, whereas exposures to needlestick injuries were relatively infrequent. Efforts should continue to focus on proper respiratory protection to include eye protection in order to mitigate these exposure risks.

▶ Prehospital emergency medical service (EMS) providers encounter various patients with a broad spectrum of pathology and trauma. Some patients have obvious injuries, such as fractures, lacerations, and extremity deformities. Yet other patients declare their chief complaint either verbally or manifesting some key "sign" or constellation of signs and symptoms that can be detected by the crew that may lead to a potential diagnosis. However, currently, EMS providers respond to various calls and provided many transports, both emergent and nonemergent, in which the nature of the call is vague, the source of the problem is obvious, the past medical history and the relevance of the history of present illness are not clearly linked to the present problem, or the data are simply not available. Subsequently, sometime after the transport when the patient's diagnosis is finally established, there are times when it is determined that there was a communicable, infectious source that caused the patient's illness and that the transporting crew has experienced an exposure to a potential pathogen that will require assessment, verification of actual exposure, confirmation of diagnosis if applicable, and follow-up treatment if indicated. Other times it is obvious that the person is "sick" and may have a communicable disease, but the crew may have already been exposed to the infectious agent at first contact, without taking any steps to protect themselves.

Despite education and awareness of Centers for Disease Control and Prevention guidelines on the use of universal precautions and Occupational Safety and Health Administration—mandated orientation and ongoing training on infectious diseases, universal precautions, and the application of prevention measures, occupational exposure to and potential spread of communicable diseases remains a major concern for EMS personnel and EMS administration. This problem can and does also impact the receiving facility that will admit and treat this patient without an initial awareness of the potential infection hazards. A former mentor of mine once stated: "the eyes cannot see what the mind does not know." This is certainly applicable in this scenario. To appropriately protect the prehospital providers, it must be known where and what the threats are. To this end, it would be beneficial to identify and examine the potential specific infectious exposures and determine their incidence, prevalence, and trends. Upon analysis of these data, EMS directors should modify current measures designed to provide protection and mitigation from initial exposure and subsequent dissemination of the infectious agent to the community.

The investigators in this study set out to describe the prevalent infectious occupational health exposures and to report on the associated outcomes of these exposures. They conducted a descriptive, epidemiologic, retrospective review of all reported exposures within the Boston EMS system over a 3-year period (January 1, 2007, to December 31, 2009). The data were in the form of electronic reports on file with the designated infection control officer for Boston EMS. They provided data describing what disease was reported, the relative incidence of these exposures, whether there was an actual exposure, and the subsequent outcome or treatment results, if treatment was indicated. The data were obtained via reports filed to the database. Limitations of this study include the fact that it was a retrospective study and that the data recorded may not represent all possible cases. Some data may not have been captured because of the lack of consistent documentation and reporting. Categories of exposures were created based on the existing exposures database. Much of the follow-up data were not captured. Data regarding reported exposures that were later determined not to be an actual exposure were also incomplete.

The data show that exposure to possible meningitis was the most common exposure followed by tuberculosis. The next highest reported cases were of viral respiratory infections (VRI), skin/mucous membrane splashes, eye splashes, various cutaneous rashes, mammalian bites, scratches, and finally needle stick injuries. The types of exposure rates reported suggest that air-borne pathogen exposure is a substantial infection hazard for EMS providers. These findings also emphasize the need for providing more attention to and use of personal protective equipment and respiratory droplet precautions when there is a suspicion for a potential respiratory pathogen. In addition, the finding that VRI exposure is on the increase stresses the need for the provision of proper annual influenza vaccination for prehospital providers to provide better defense for seasonal flu variants. In addition, better surveillance of possible meningitis is needed so that better prophylaxis can be made available to ward off the potential devastating consequences of this disease. Lastly, the frequency of exposures to needle sticks appears to have decreased. These data suggest better respiratory and eye protection, better surveillance for meningitis, and a continuation of practices regarding use of sharps in the prehospital arena.

B. M. Minczak, MS, MD, PhD, PH-MD

Air Medical Evacuations from a Developing World Conflict Zone
Low A, Vadera B (Med director for AMREF Flying Doctor Service in Nairobi, Kenya)
Air Med J 30:313-316, 2011

Somalia has been without effective government for close to two decades, with more than 1 million people internally displaced. The political unrest persists, with United Nations—backed African Union peacekeeping forces supporting the Transitional National government of Sharif Ahmed, struggling to maintain control of central Mogadishu from Islamist extremist groups, such as the reportedly Al-Qaeda—backed Al-Shabab. The African Union force of 5,000 troops is predominantly of Ugandan and Burundian origin, making up the African Mission in Somalia (AMISOM) effort. However, its mandate is limited to operations only in Mogadishu, and it is unauthorized to actively pursue insurgents. As with other ongoing high-profile conflicts, African Union troops face an enemy that blends into the civilian populace, fighting with a lethal mixture of improvised explosive devices and suicide bombers.

▶ Every emergency medical response has its potential hazards. No call, not even the most routine in nature, should be considered completely risk free. Emergency medical personnel are trained to look for hazards and have the concept of "scene safety" drilled into their psyche on a daily basis during their training. However, there are certain hazards that are not always foreseen, nor are some hazards even considered in most regions where established emergency medical services function on a day-to-day basis. This article describes the challenges and diversity of calls that the African Medical Research Foundation (AMREF) (a humanitarian, income generating service) personnel faced when providing air medical service, air ambulance repatriations, evacuation of injured patients, and medical escorts on commercial flights from a zone of conflict. The specific area was Somalia.

The article addresses the logistical considerations for these evacuations, the safety issues surrounding evacuations in areas where the government is unstable and where there is political unrest. In addition, there is a brief but comprehensive synopsis of an AMREF response on August 24, 2010, to a major incident in Mogadishu where there was an uprising. During this incident, trauma patients and medical cases were evacuated. The injuries consisted of blast injuries, (fragment and shrapnel injuries), gunshot wounds, long bone fractures, lumbar spine injuries, penetrating wounds of the thorax and abdomen, and a head injury. Due to the ongoing violent and potentially dangerous activities surrounding conflict, ground time was limited, thus hampering the provision of comprehensive medical interventions. Immediate treatment needs were identified and initiated followed by a prompt load-and- go evacuation with further treatment provided during the flight. Some of the treatments provided ranged from the delivery of supplemental oxygen, analgesia, intravenous fluid hydration, ketamine sedation, antiemetics, monitoring ventilation, splinting steroid administration, and even a few cases of blood transfusion.

Delivery of prehospital support and health care in a part of the world where the government is unstable or lacking altogether or there is anarchy, new issues arise that could precipitate a hazard and lead to dangerous and even fatal consequences for the rescue teams. This article delineates some of the issues in Somalia, such as the protection needed for aircraft to provide service and enter into Somali airspace and the need for interagency communication and cooperation so that both the services can be provided, mutual aid reciprocated, and that the safety of the responding air crews and prehospital medical personnel is ensured.

The information is useful as a guide for planning international support for disasters in politically unstable regions of the world. These issues demand special considerations, especially during civilian humanitarian responses to areas in need after earthquakes, floods, hurricanes, and tsunamis.

This article is descriptive in nature and brings to light pertinent issues.

B. M. Minczak, MS, MD, PhD, PH-MD

Assessing Air Medical Crew Real-Time Readiness to Perform Critical Tasks
Braude D, Goldsmith T, Weiss SJ (Univ of New Mexico, Albuquerque)
Prehosp Emerg Care 15:254-260, 2011

Background.—Air medical transport has had problems with its safety record, attributed in part to human error. Flight crew members (FCMs) must be able to focus on critical safety tasks in the context of a stressful environment. Flight crew members' cognitive readiness (CR) to perform their jobs may be affected by sleep deprivation, personal problems, high workload, and use of alcohol and drugs.

Objective.—The current study investigated the feasibility of using a computer-based cognitive task to assess FCMs' readiness to perform their job.

Methods.—The FCMs completed a short questionnaire to evaluate their physiologic and psychological state at the beginning and end of each shift.

The FCMs then performed 3 minutes of a computer-based cognitive task called synthetic work environment (SYNWIN test battery). Task performance was compared with the questionnaire variables using correlation and regression analysis. Differences between the beginning and end of each shift were matched and compared using a paired Students t test.

Results.—SYNWIN performance was significantly worse at the end of a shift compared with the beginning of the shift ($p = 0.028$) primarily because of decrement in the memory component. The SYNWIN composite scores were negatively correlated to degree of irritability felt by the participant, both before ($r = -0.25$) and after ($r = -0.34$) a shift and were significantly correlated with amount of sleep (0.22), rest (0.30), and life satisfaction (0.30).

Conclusions.—Performance by FCMs on a simple, rapid, computer-based psychological test correlates well with self-reported sleep, rest, life satisfaction, and irritability. Although further studies are warranted, these findings suggest that assessment of the performance of FCMs on a simple, rapid, computer-based, multitasking battery is feasible as an approach to determine their readiness to perform critical safety tasks through the SYNWIN task battery.

▶ Whether out in the field or in the hospital, emergency care providers can expect stressful circumstances to interfere with their work. Shift work, fatigue, and the need to respond rapidly to emergent problems are among the stressors.

It would be valuable to know how the members of any emergency care provider team are going to be able to function at any time. One of the challenges is to find meaningful tests of function and then find ways to intervene when deficits are found.

Consider the aspect of memory. How will memory be tested? If memory is tested by a task unrelated to those used by caregivers, such as by memorizing a string of numbers, how will the results of the test be related to the performance of memory tasks needed for taking care of patients? Imagine then the complexity of the problem if memory of strings of numbers is shown to be affected by lack of sleep; do we really know that lack of sleep affects the memory used to care for patients in the same way?

The authors chose the synthetic work environment (SYNWIN) system for testing readiness. This software provided a timed challenge of 4 competing tasks in different windows on a computer screen. It was the success at the memory task that was found to be significantly decreased after a shift when compared with the beginning of the shift.

How was memory tested? In this scheme, memory is tested by recognizing the presence of numbers that were presented in a set at the beginning of a test session. Is this type of memory related to that used in the delivery of patient care? This is an interesting result but does require that we spend time thinking about the meaning it and what to do about it.

N. B. Handly, MD, MSc, MS

Association Between Poor Sleep, Fatigue, and Safety Outcomes in Emergency Medical Services Providers

Patterson PD, Weaver MD, Frank RC, et al (Univ of Pittsburgh, PA; et al)
Prehosp Emerg Care 16:86-97, 2011

Objective.—To determine the association between poor sleep quality, fatigue, and self-reported safety outcomes among emergency medical services (EMS) workers.

Methods.—We used convenience sampling of EMS agencies and a cross-sectional survey design. We administered the 19-item Pittsburgh Sleep Quality Index (PSQI), 11-item Chalder Fatigue Questionnaire (CFQ), and 44-item EMS Safety Inventory (EMS-SI) to measure sleep quality, fatigue, and safety outcomes, respectively. We used a consensus process to develop the EMS-SI, which was designed to capture three composite measurements of EMS worker injury, medical errors and adverse events (AEs), and safety-compromising behaviors. We used hierarchical logistic regression to test the association between poor sleep quality, fatigue, and three composite measures of EMS worker safety outcomes.

Results.—We received 547 surveys from 30 EMS agencies (a 35.6% mean agency response rate). The mean PSQI score exceeded the benchmark for poor sleep (6.9, 95% confidence interval [CI] 6.6, 7.2). More than half of the respondents were classified as fatigued (55%, 95% CI 50.7, 59.3). Eighteen percent of the respondents reported an injury (17.8%, 95% CI 13.5, 22.1), 41% reported a medical error or AE (41.1%, 95% CI 36.8, 45.4), and 90% reported a safety-compromising behavior (89.6%, 95% CI 87, 92). After controlling for confounding, we identified 1.9 greater odds of injury (95% CI 1.1, 3.3), 2.2 greater odds of medical error or AE (95% CI 1.4, 3.3), and 3.6 greater odds of safety-compromising behavior (95% CI 1.5, 8.3) among fatigued respondents versus nonfatigued respondents.

Conclusions.—In this sample of EMS workers, poor sleep quality and fatigue are common. We provide preliminary evidence of an association between sleep quality, fatigue, and safety outcomes.

▶ Emergency medical services (EMS) providers work in an environment that is quite different from the in-hospital environment. The emergency medical technician (EMT) and paramedic often are initially working together and entering an environment that may be unsafe. Some of the potential hazards may be a potentially violent patient, aggressive bystanders, exposure to hazardous materials, fire, or an unstable vehicle that has just been involved in a motor vehicle crash. They may have to extricate an entrapped patient under hazardous conditions while initiating medical treatment to stabilize the patient. Decision making can be affected by the aforementioned issues causing significant distraction. If there are any complicated decisions that must be made or there are issues that require a deviation from standing protocols, input from medical command may be inaccessible or, at best, incomplete to the degree of communication that can be achieved from the emergency scene in the field. In the field, there is little "medical expertise back up." After the EMS providers stabilize the patient and initiate transport, usually the paramedic must work alone in the patient compartment, evaluating and treating the patient, communicating with the receiving facility, and if needed, managing the airway or administering medications. Hence, the ability to maintain situational awareness is of great importance and requires that the EMS providers be in top condition mentally and physically to prevent an adverse outcome for the patient or the medic. This article addresses issues relevant to patient and medic safety.

On first glance, this article appears to state the obvious—that sleep deprivation and chronic fatigue can lead to medical errors and injury to both the patient entrusted to the health care providers or the health care providers themselves. However, this publication provides an added significant modicum of detail regarding safety and the potential well being of EMS providers which is well worth review. In fact, I believe that managers who are responsible for work assignments, schedules, and determining shift lengths should read this article.

This team of investigators attempted to scientifically and methodically describe several parameters by surveying a convenience sample of EMS providers. To obtain the data, these authors utilized several survey tools: the Pittsburgh Sleep Quality Index and the Chalder Fatigue Questionnaire. They also used a consensus process to develop their own EMS Safety Inventory (EMS-SI). This was prepared to capture safety outcomes. The parameters of interest were perception of fatigue, sleep quality, and safety outcomes.

Some of the errors and injuries that can occur in the sleep-deprived, fatigued medic are failure to determine scene safety, deviation from protocol (warranted or unwarranted), failure to secure an airway due to multiple issues not found in the controlled hospital environment, dropping a stretcher and injuring the patient, or the medic sustaining a back injury while lifting the patient due to not following appropriate body mechanics needed to prevent spine injury during heavy lifting. Also, another big error is giving either the wrong medication or the wrong dosage. Needle sticks are also an occurrence that can be more likely to occur in the fatigued medic. As the patient is transported via ground or air, there is the risk of injury due to driver or pilot error.

The data collected show that many EMS personnel are tired, sleep deprived and thus more prone to make errors. Other issues that were briefly addressed but not measured were the effect of shift length, workload during a shift, frequencies of shifts, and actual number of shifts per week or month. This information should be incorporated in the scheduling process of EMS workers. Of note, several organizations such as the Accreditation Council for Graduate Medical Education, have modified resident work schedules; the Federal Aviation Administration has placed regulations on pilot flight hours. Maybe we should consider this when dealing with EMS staff issues.

Limitations of the study include the fact that this was a convenience sample, which relied on self-reporting. The subjective nature of the responses coupled with utilization of a new survey (EMS-SI) that may need validation may have biased or skewed the results. Nonetheless, this study brings to light that fatigue and sleep deprivation are indeed potentially qualifiable issues that need to be considered when scheduling and considering the safety of EMS providers and the patients.

B. M. Minczak, MS, MD, PhD, PH-MD

Factors at the Scene of Injury Associated with Air versus Ground Transport to Definitive Care in a State with a Large Rural Population
Stewart KE, Cowan LD, Thompson DM, et al (Oklahoma State Dept of Health; Univ of Oklahoma Health Sciences Ctr; et al)
Prehosp Emerg Care 15:193-202, 2011

Background.—Once emergency medical services (EMS) personnel decide to transport a trauma patient directly to definitive care, the next key decision at the scene of injury is whether to transport by air or ground.

Objective.—The aim of this study was to identify factors at the scene of injury that are associated with this decision.

Methods.—All trauma patients transported directly to a level I or level II trauma center by either air or ground EMS over a four-year period were selected from the Oklahoma State Trauma Registry. Initial scene vital signs, Glasgow Coma Scale score (GCS), injury mechanism, anatomic triage criteria, age, time of day, ground EMS service level, and scene location were collected. Scene location ZIP code centroids were geocoded and used to calculate distance to the trauma center. Following bivariate analyses, multivariable logistic regression models were developed within three strata defined by distance (>35, 16—35, and <16 miles).

Results.—More than 80% of the patients beyond 35 miles were transported by air, compared with 32% from 16—35 miles and only 4% from <16 miles. Regardless of distance, patients transported by helicopter tended to be younger, more often had abnormal vital signs, and more frequently came from areas served by a basic or intermediate ground EMS agency, as compared with patients transported by ground. Within each distance stratum, patients injured in severe motor vehicle crashes, motorcycle crashes, or pedestrian incidents were more likely to be transported by air. A GCS <14 was the only patient-related factor consistently associated with increased odds of air transport.

Conclusion.—Distance is the main factor in deciding whether to use air or ground EMS to transport a trauma patient from the scene of injury to a trauma center. With the exception of GCS <14, injury etiology was more strongly and consistently associated with the decision to transport by air than were patient related-factors. Identifying factors influencing the field transport decision will help develop transport guidelines that make efficient use of EMS resources.

▶ This study from the Oklahoma State Department of Health examined 10 248 patients transported by emergency medical services (EMS) directly from the scene of an injury to a level I or level II trauma center over a 4-year period. It gives us a picture of what is actually happening at the scene of a trauma when EMS personnel must decide on mode of transport. As might be expected, distance was the most influential factor associated with a decision to use helicopter emergency medical services (HEMS). Surprisingly, however, the time from EMS call to arrival at a trauma center was only 2 minutes shorter when HEMS was used, compared with ground EMS, in both the 35 miles or more and the 16- to 35-mile distance strata. In the miles or less distance stratum, HEMS averaged 10 minutes longer than ground transport.

Etiology of injury was also associated with mode of transport in all 3 distance strata: patients involved in severe motor vehicle collisions or those involving motorcycles or pedestrians were more likely to be transported by HEMS. Evidence of neurologic injury (Glasgow Coma Scale score < 14) was the only patient-related factor associated with the use of HEMS in all 3 distance strata. Other patient-related factors (abnormal heart rate and anatomic criteria) were associated with HEMS transport only in the middle-distance stratum (16-35 miles). It is unclear from the study why this was the case; however, it seems reasonable to speculate the EMS personnel feel more urgency when patients appear to have severe injuries and consequently have a lower threshold for using HEMS in this middle-distance strata because distance alone may not be a deciding factor.

Basic or intermediate ground EMS service level was also associated with a higher likelihood of using HEMS in all 3 distance strata. Although this is not an ideal proxy for expertise available at the scene, it may be that paramedics make more accurate assessments of a patient's status and thereby use HEMS less.

By considering what factors EMS personnel actually use in the field policy makers can develop useful guidelines for the use of HEMS.

E. A. Ramoska, MD, MPHE

Physical Stressors during Neonatal Transport: Helicopter Compared with Ground Ambulance
Bouchut J-C, Van Lancker E, Chritin V, et al (Hôpital Mère-Enfant, Bron, France; IAV Engineering, Tannay, Switzerland; et al)
Air Med J 30:134-139, 2011

Objectives.—This study was undertaken to assess concurrent mechanical stresses from shock, vibration, and noise to which a critically ill neonate is exposed during emergency transfer.

Methods.—For neonates transported by a French specialized emergency medical service, we measured and analyzed 27 physical parameters recorded during typical transport by ambulance and by helicopter. The noninvasive sensors were placed to allow better representation of the exposure of the newborn to the physical constraints.

Results.—Based on 10 hours of transport by ambulance and 2 hours by helicopter, noise, whole body vibration, rate of turn, acceleration, and pitch were extracted as the five most representative dynamic harshness indicators. A helicopter produces a higher-level but more stable (lower relative dispersion) whole body dynamic exposure than an ambulance, with a mean noise level of 86 ± 1 dBA versus 67 ± 3 dBA, mean whole body vibration of 1 ± 0.1 meter per second squared (m/s^2) versus 0.4 6 0.2 m/s^2, and acceleration of 1 6 0.05 m/s^2 versus 0.4 6 0.1 m/s^2. A ground ambulance has many more dynamic effects in terms of braking, shock, and impulsive noise than a helicopter (1 impulsive event per 2 minutes vs. 1 per 11 minutes).

Conclusions.—Our results show significant exposure of the sick neonate to both stationary and impulsive dynamic physical stressors during transportation, particularly in a ground ambulance. The study suggests opportunities to reduce physical stressors during neonatal transport.

▶ This study provides an in-depth discussion of the physics regarding forces imposed onto a neonate during 2 means of transport: ground ambulance and helicopter. Measurements of various force vectors were obtained by the strategic placement of a triaxial accelerometer and a temporal resolution inclinometer onto the incubator main frame. In addition, a microphone was placed in proximity to the neonate's ear, and a global positioning system antenna was placed on top of the vehicle.

The implication is that there are various vibrations and kinematic forces that may be adversely affecting an infant during transport. There are speculations that these physical forces may produce an adverse effect on the patient and should be controlled. To control the forces and mitigate their potential effects, the forces should be quantified. The quantification did not interfere with the care provided, because a trained engineer conducted the measurements.

A concise synopsis of the data suggests that forces during ground transport may be of greater concern than those imposed during flight. This venue of investigation is rather new and may initially prove useful to design engineers, emergency medical service (EMS) drivers, and helicopter pilots. Currently, the impact of these data on EMS operations is limited and has not directly caused any modification in protocols or operations.

B. M. Minczak, MS, MD, PhD, PH-MD

Prehospital Factors Associated with Mortality in Injured Air Medical Patients
Cudnik MT, Werman HA, White LJ, et al (The Ohio State Univ, Columbus; The Ohio State Univ Med Ctr, Columbus; et al)
Prehosp Emerg Care 16:121-127, 2011

Background.—Air medical transport provides rapid transport to definitive care. Overtriage and the expense and risk of transport may offset survival benefits.

Objective.—We assessed the ability of prehospital factors to predict resource need for helicopter-transported patients.

Methods.—We performed a prospective, observational cohort analysis of injured scene patients taken to one of two level I trauma centers from October 2009 to September 2010. Variables analyzed included patient

---

TABLE 1.—Prehospital Criteria for Helicopter Transport to a Trauma Center

---

Does the patient have two or more fractures of the humerus and/or femur?
Does the patient have second- or third-degree burns over >10% total body surface area?
Does the patient have abdominal tenderness or distention or a seat belt sign?
Does the patient have an amputation proximal to the wrist and/or ankle?
Does the patient have an arm and/or leg injury with neurovascular compromise?
Is this an automobile—vs.—pedestrian and/or bicycle collision that involved either being thrown, being run over, or a speed >20 mph?
Does the patient have one of the following comorbid conditions:
    Bleeding disorder or taking anticoagulants
    Diabetes
    End-stage renal disease and on hemodialysis
    Immunocompromised state
    Pregnancy
Does the patient have a crush injury of the head and/or neck and/or torso?
Does the patient have a crush injury of the arm and/or leg?
Is the patient failing to localize to pain?
Does the patient have a falling level of consciousness?
Did the patient have a fall >20 feet?
Does the patient have a flail chest?
Does the patient have a GCS ≤13?
Was the patient in a high-risk automobile crash, defined as:
    Death in the compartment
    Ejection
    Vehicle telemetry data show high risk of injury
Did the patient have a loss of consciousness >5 minutes?
Did this involve a motorcycle crash >20 mph?
Does the patient need endotracheal intubation?
Does the patient have evidence of a pelvic fracture?
Does the patient have a penetrating injury that is proximal to the knee and/or elbow with neurovascular compromise?
Does the patient have a penetrating injury to the head and/or neck and/or torso?
Does the patient have a pulse rate >120 bpm with signs of shock?
Does the patient have respirations <10 or >29/minute?
Does the patient have significant burns of the face and/or feet and/or hands and/or genitals and/or airway?
Does the patient have evidence of a spinal cord injury?
Does the patient have a systolic blood pressure <90 mmHg?
Does the patient have a tension pneumothorax?
Geriatric criteria (70 years of age and older)
    Was the patient in an MVC with one or more fractures of the humerus?
    And/or femur?
    Are there injuries of two or more body regions?
    Was the pedestrian struck by a vehicle or fall with traumatic brain injury?
    Does the patient have a systolic blood pressure <100 mmHg?

GCS = Glasgow Coma Scale score; MVC = motor vehicle crash.

---

demographics, diagnoses, and clinical outcomes (in-hospital mortality, emergent surgery within 24 hours, blood transfusion within 24 hours, and intensive care unit [ICU] admission ≥24 hours, as well as a combined outcome of all clinical outcomes). Prehospital variables were prospectively obtained from air medical providers at the time of transport and included past medical history, mechanism of injury, and clinical factors. We compared those variables with and without the outcomes of interest via χ^2 analysis and the Kruskal-Wallis test, where appropriate. Multivariate logistic regression identified factors associated with outcomes of interest with the intent of developing a clinical prediction tool.

TABLE 2.—Patient Demographics

	Population $N = 557$
Age—median [IQR], years	39 [24–52]
Gender—male	374 (67%)
Race—white	529 (95%)
Location—rural	321 (58%)
Distance—median [IQR], miles	39 [28–52]
Insurance	
Private	339 (60%)
Self-pay	92 (17%)
Medicare/Medicaid	109 (20%)
Workers' compensation	17 (3%)
Penetrating injury	19 (3%)
ED GCS <9	89 (16%)
ISS—median [IQR]	9 [5–17]
ISS >15	157 (28%)
EMS ETI	109 (20%)
ICU admission	182 (33%)
ICU stay >24 hours	179 (32%)
Blood transfusion within 24 hours*	59 (11%)
Emergent surgery within 24 hours	162 (29%)
ICU LOS—median [IQR], days	0 [0–2]
Hospital LOS—median [IQR], days	3 [1–7]
Mortality	20 (4%)
Early death, <24 hours	10 (2%)
DC alive <24 hours	6 (1%)
Hospital LOS 1 day†	93 (17%)

Data are expressed as *n* (%) unless otherwise specified.

DC = discharged; ED = emergency department; EMS = emergency medical services; ETI = endotracheal intubation; GCS = Glasgow Coma Scale score; ICU = intensive care unit; IQR = interquartile range; ISS = Injury Severity Score; LOS = length of stay.

*Two patients (<1%) had this outcome alone.

†Patients had none of the combined outcomes (death, ICU stay >24 hours, surgery within 24 hours, blood transfusion within 24 hours).

Results.—Five hundred fifty-seven patients were transported during the study period. The majority of the patients were male (67%) and white (95%) and had an injury that occurred in a rural location (58%). Most injuries were blunt (97%), and patients had a median Injury Severity Score (ISS) of 9. The overall mortality was 4%; 48% of the patients had one of the four outcomes. The most common reasons for requesting air transport were motor vehicle collision (MVC) with high-risk mechanism (18%), MVC at a speed greater than 20 mph (18%), Glasgow Coma Scale score (GCS) less than 14 (15%), and loss of consciousness (LOC) greater than 5 minutes (15%). Factors associated with mortality were age greater than 44 years, GCS less than 14, systolic blood pressure (SBP) less than 90 mmHg, and flail chest. This model had 100% sensitivity and 50% specificity and missed no deaths. The combined endpoint of all four outcomes (death, receipt of blood, surgery, ICU admission) included intubation by emergency medical services, two or more fractures of the humerus/femur, presence of a neurovascular injury, a crush injury to the head, failure to localize to pain on examination, GCS less than 14, or the presence of a penetrating head injury. This model had a sensitivity of 57% (53%–61%) and a specificity of 78% (75%–87%).

TABLE 3.—Prehospital Reasons for Helicopter Transport to a Trauma Center

Prehospital Criteria	Population $N = 557$
MVC with high-risk mechanism*	103 (18%)
MVC at speed >20 mph	102 (18%)
LOC >5 minutes	85 (15%)
GCS ≤13	82 (15%)
Abnormal vital signs (HR >120 bpm, SBP <90 mmHg, abnormal RR <10 or >29)	60 (11%)
Falling LOC	58 (10%)
Abdominal tenderness/distention/seat belt sign	52 (9%)
Crush head injury	37 (7%)
MVC with ejection	39 (7%)
Evidence of spinal cord injury	36 (6%)
Failure to localize to pain	36 (6%)
Fall >20 feet	31 (6%)
Penetrating head injury	36 (6%)
Evidence of pelvic injury	30 (5%)
Arm and/or leg injury with neurovascular compromise	23 (4%)
Crush injury of arm and/or leg	24 (4%)
≥2 Fractures of humerus and/or femur	22 (4%)
Automobile-vs.-pedestrian crash	15 (3%)
MVC with death of occupant	17 (3%)
Flail chest	6 (1%)
Second- or third-degree burns >10% BSA	4 (<1%)
Proximal amputation	3 (<1%)
Penetrating injury proximal to knee and/or elbow	2 (<1%)
Burns to face	5 (<1%)
Tension pneumothorax	1 (<1%)

Data are expressed as n (%).
Patients may have had more than one reason for transport by helicopter.
BSA = body surface area; GCS = Glasgow Coma Scale score; HR = heart rate; LOC = loss of consciousness; MVC = motor vehicle crash; RR = respiratory rate; SBP = systolic blood pressure.
*Death in compartment, ejection, or vehicle telemetry data show high risk of injury.

Conclusions.—Very few prehospital criteria were associated with clinically important outcomes in helicopter-transported patients. Evidence-based guidelines for the most appropriate utilization of air medical transport need to be further evaluated and developed for injured patients.

▶ When a patient appears to be seriously injured at the scene of an accident or if the presence of a mechanism that produced the injury suggests that there is a significant possibility that a complicated, undiscovered injury may be present, this precipitates the urgency for immediate, rapid transport of the victim to an appropriate facility. This decision is supported by significant evidence that timely evaluation, stabilization, and transport of a patient from an accident scene often produce much better outcomes. However, the mode of transport needed to achieve this can sometime create a dilemma. The question arises of when and who should be transported by ground versus by helicopter. Also, where should these patients go? Should they go to the nearest trauma center or to the highest level of care trauma center? What factors are useful in answering these questions?

The authors of this prospective project collected a vast compendium of variables from the helicopter emergency medical transport team regarding various issues at the scene and information pertinent to the level of injury to the patient. Data were also collected from the trauma centers regarding patient demographics, insurance status, and length of stay in the appropriate unit; injury severity scores; billing codes; and discharge diagnoses. For a more complete list of the variables, the reader is referred to Tables 1, 2, and 3 of the article. Outcomes data such as in-hospital mortality from any cause during the hospitalization were also scrutinized.

Upon compilation of the data from the patients transported, a compendium of descriptive statistics was used to scrutinize the data. The data suggest that a small number of patients had serious injures requiring transport to a level 1 trauma center. Furthermore, mechanism of injury was not identified as a good indicator of trauma mortality or the need for trauma center resource utilization. If overuse of helicopter emergency medical services subsequent to overtriage is to be attenuated, further evidence-based exploration of the variables is needed. Providing a solution to this dilemma may decrease overall costs, prevent unnecessary flights, and decrease injury to patients and helicopter crews. More meaning may be added to future data by comparing helicopter transports to ground transports.

B. M. Minczak, MS, MD, PhD, PH-MD

Termination of Resuscitation of Nontraumatic Cardiopulmonary Arrest: Resource Document for the National Association of EMS Physicians Position Statement

Millin MG, Khandker SR, Malki A (Johns Hopkins Univ School of Medicine, Baltimore, MD; Johns Hopkins Univ, Baltimore, MD)
Prehosp Emerg Care 15:547-554, 2011

In the development of an emergency medical services (EMS) system, medical directors should consider the implementation of protocols for the termination of resuscitation (TOR) of nontraumatic cardiopulmonary arrest. Such protocols have the potential to decrease unnecessary use of warning lights and sirens and save valuable public health resources. Termination-of-resuscitation protocols for nontraumatic cardiopulmonary arrest should be based on the determination that an EMS provider did not witness the arrest, there is no shockable rhythm identified, and there is no return of spontaneous circulation (ROSC) prior to EMS transport. Further research is needed to determine the need for direct medical oversight in TOR protocols and the duration of resuscitation prior to EMS providers' determining that ROSC will not be achieved. This paper is the resource document to the National Association of EMS Physicians position statement on the termination of resuscitation for nontraumatic cardiopulmonary arrest.

▶ Emergency medical personnel often are faced with the dilemma of whether to transport a patient to the hospital when the situation appears futile. An example of this situation is nontraumatic cardiopulmonary arrest. Patients found in asystole, with an unknown down time and who have not responded to on-scene resuscitative efforts, are often transported to the hospital by paramedics. Often this transport is done using lights and siren. The chances of an accident during transport or injury to the crew increase during such an endeavor. Furthermore, often upon arrival at the hospital, a futile and costly resuscitation is undertaken with little or no chance for the patient to survive with a favorable outcome. The cost for this entire endeavor can be a significant burden to the health care system if this scenario repeats itself many times over. There are potential mitigating circumstances: a pediatric patient, an adolescent, a patient who is hypothermic, a pregnant female, or the possibility of organ donation. To address what needs to be done in this circumstance and to provide guidelines for prehospital termination of resuscitation, the National Association of EMS Physicians has published a position paper on this issue. This paper provides a comprehensive discussion on the relevant issues.

B. M. Minczak, MS, MD, PhD, PH-MD

'Time critical' rapid amputation using fire service hydraulic cutting equipment
McNicholas MJ, Robinson SJ, Polyzois I, et al (North Cheshire Hosp NHS Trust, Warrington, UK; et al)
Injury 42:1333-1335, 2011

Introduction.—Entrapped trauma victims require extrication, which, on rare occasions, may involve amputation of a limb. Standard extrication techniques sometimes fail or may be impossible, leading to the death of the entrapped victim. We propose that the use of fire service hydraulic cutting equipment can be used effectively to urgently amputate a limb, where conventional techniques are unusable.

Method.—The study aims to determine: (i) the potential use of this equipment to achieve expeditious life-saving amputations and (ii) the effect the fire service hydraulic cutting equipment has on the bony and surrounding soft tissues. Initially a porcine limb was used followed by fresh-frozen cadaveric lower limbs. We recorded the time, number of cuts, proximal fracture propagation and quality of bone cut when performing amputations at five levels.

Results.—The experiment confirms that faster guillotine amputations in human cadaveric lower limb specimens can be achieved by using fire service hydraulic cutting equipment. Overall, the average time to complete an amputation in these ideal experimental circumstances at all five levels was quicker using the hydraulic cutting equipment. Either one or two cutting actions were required to achieve the amputation using fire service hydraulic cutting equipment. The degree and proximal extent of the comminution were greater using the fire service hydraulic cutting equipment.

Conclusion.—If circumstances and time constrains allow, a conventional amputation technique carried out by a trained medical practitioner would be preferable to the use of the fire service hydraulic cutting equipment. However, we feel that this technique could be used to perform emergent amputation under trained medical supervision, if it is felt that a standard amputation technique would take too long or the environment is too restrictive to perform a standard amputation safely.

▶ This limited, straightforward, yet provocative publication should be brought to the attention of state Emergency Medical Services (EMS) medical directors, trauma surgeons, and fire department leaders in the EMS community. The authors of this work set out to answer a simple question: "Can fire department heavy rescue equipment be used to amputate a limb when the situation calls for it?" Literature on this topic is limited. Protocols and policies regarding this procedure are sparse. I would like to see this study serve as a potential stimulus for the further exploration of field amputation procedures.

The amount of experienced trained personnel and the appropriate equipment for performing this procedure are lacking. Collaboration among active medical directors, experienced trauma surgeons, and EMS leaders should be initiated to explore this issue and make recommendations on a potential revision of this process.

Amputation of a limb in the prehospital arena is a rare occurrence. Usually amputation is considered as a last resort when a victim of a motor vehicle crash, building collapse, or flood is entrapped in a vehicle or structure and cannot be extricated by conventional means. As the event progresses, imminent danger of the victim perishing from a possible explosion, fire, fumes, hostile environmental conditions, or rising water may occur. Furthermore, the patient's condition may begin to deteriorate rapidly, precipitating the need to act quickly and definitively to release the victim from the wreckage. Hence, the situation turns into a "life over limb" scenario. When these situations occur and amputation is seriously contemplated, many decisions need to be made and appropriate action must be taken. All of this takes time and may cause additional delays in freeing the victim from the entrapment. As a result, the victim may suffer a fatal outcome. To this end, an expedient means of safely extricating the victim in a timely manner must be available and be promptly initiated.

Amputation of the limb by a surgeon experienced in prehospital amputation is the ideal option. However, for this to happen, an experienced surgeon with an appropriate team must be readily available. The equipment to perform this task must be on hand and ready for deployment, and the team should be based in relatively close proximity to the accident scene to decrease response times. Furthermore the team must be ready to respond immediately to the accident scene upon dispatch. After initiating the response, the team will need time to arrive at the scene, assess the situation, and develop an approach to the problem at hand. This will also add to scene time and possibly place the medical rescuers at some level of risk during the extrication. However, if fire department or rescue personnel already on scene and working to free this victim could simply use their specialized hydraulic heavy rescue equipment to expediently amputate the victim's limb without causing any further significant injury, why not just do that? The victim would be released from the wreckage in a more timely fashion, medical stabilization could progress, and afterwards, any further wound issues could be mitigated in the operating room. Although this is a very simplistic answer to this complex problem, many questions arise. The authors in this publication took the first step in attempting to answer these questions. Since designing a study to answer this question using human subjects presents many moral and ethical dilemmas, this group of professionals, the Anaesthetic Trauma and Critical Care organization in the United Kingdom, attempted to use a "bench science" approach and compare the appearance and quality of cuts made by the hydraulic rescue equipment with that of cuts made by an experienced surgeon. They started by performing several "cuts" in strategic locations on 4 lower hindquarters of a porcine model. After deeming this procedure successful and feasible on the porcine model, they were provided with the opportunity of performing strategic cuts on frozen, human cadaveric lower extremities and compared them with amputations done by the conventional amputation technique. To assess the amputation cuts, they used a description of the comminution of the bone fragments, proximal propagation of the fracture from the site of amputation, number of cuts needed to successfully make the amputation, and the total time needed to complete the amputation. They also assessed the appearance of the soft tissue. They used a grading system from grade 1, which was a "clean" cut, to a grade 4, which was considered a "ragged bone quality" cut. Due to the small sample size and limited design, the data were qualitative in nature, and the conclusions drawn were deductive inferences based on the findings reported.

In essence, performing an amputation with the hydraulic fire department equipment took less time than the standard technique. The degree of comminution of the bone was found to be less with the standard technique of surgical amputation. Also, the degree of proximal propagation of the fracture was observed to be less with the standard techniques versus the hydraulic cutting equipment amputation. However, as already mentioned, these issues can be appropriately mitigated in the operating room of the receiving medical facility.

One concern regarding the conclusions is that the specimens used in this study were previously fresh frozen, which may have altered tissue characteristics and affected the final appearance of the cuts made. Some of the parameters used in the study were not clearly defined; however, enough information was presented to provoke a further exploration into this issue.

The potential use of fire department heavy rescue equipment may decrease extrication/amputation time. Use of this equipment may also decrease unnecessary risks to the patient and to responding medical personnel without increasing the extent of the patient's injuries. More research needs to be done to elaborate on the possibilities.

B. M. Minczak, MS, MD, PHD, PH-MD

Who Has the Controls?
MacDonald E
Air Med J 30:236-280, 2011

Background.—The National Transportation Safety Board (NTSB) accident reports cite many pilots and crews who fly in conditions that Part 135 managers would never approve. Three major NTSB studies have indicated that more risk-mitigation tools are needed to reduce accident rates to as low as reasonably possible (ALARP) or 0. The Federal Aviation Administration (FAA) has issued advisory circulars and notices that suggest many valuable tools and processes, and many have been implemented. Although most notices have expired, the advice and guidance they provide remains valid and has resulted in the implementation of improved operational control systems and training programs in aviation decision making and situational awareness. However, confusion is still generated because of diverse interpretations of FAA guidelines and delay in implementation by region and between operators.

Analysis.—In 2006 the evaluation of the effectiveness of operational control and risk-management systems revealed several recurring questions, specifically, "What was the pilot and crew doing out under those conditions?," "What is the responsibility of the Part 135 operator in ensuring pilots have oversight?," and "What are the operational control responsibilities of the Part 135 operator?" The FAA defines operational control as the exercise of authority over beginning, conducting, or terminating a flight. Pilots today are usually well trained and aircraft and equipment are safer than in the past. Part 135 operators receive extensive training in situational awareness, air medical resource management, and aircrew decision making. Pilots and crew members also are aided by the availability of inadvertent instrumental meteorological conditions recovery, night training, and night vision devices, improving the risk mitigation processes. However, the implementation of operational control remains inconsistent. Most emergency medical services (EMS) operators have a system of operational control so they can determine whether the pilot is current and qualified, FAA medical is current, aircraft is airworthy, and flight-following systems are operational. These systems also monitor duty times to ensure they are not exceeded as well as other administrative details.

Improving Risk Management.—Changes in the operational control process are suggested. Included would be a risk-assessment matrix that assigns a certain value to each risk factor. The total point value would determine if the flight has a green (pilot decision only), yellow (pilot must seek higher approval), or red (no-go) status. The assigned point values would represent relative weighted risk, with certain factors given extra weight or an automatic yellow status. If the total point values reach a certain value or there is an automatic yellow risk factor, the flight is considered yellow and on hold until someone in the operational chain of command is called for approval to accept or continue the flight. Pilots would still be allowed to turn down a flight even if a certain numeric value or other criteria are not met. The pilot retains the final authority to accept the flight but any flight crewmember or higher operational control (op con) designee could turn it down. The op con designee becomes the fourth party in yellow conditions; four persons must agree when the risk matrix reaches a certain level and no pilot could launch in red status. Finally, the next level of operational control could not use this system to pressure or influence pilots to take flights with which they are uncomfortable.

Conclusions.—Having the suggested system would allow an experienced aviation decision maker to be involved in the process and provides a backup for the pilot if local pressure is being applied. EMS operators would benefit from having an experienced yet grounded or semi-retired EMS pilot to consult.

▶ The prehospital arena, where emergency medical service (EMS) providers perform their duties, routinely presents various risks and challenges to emergency medical technicians (EMTs) and paramedics. Incorporating the use of a helicopter into the provision of prehospital EMS (ie, helicopter emergency medical services [HEMS]) adds another layer of complexity to these issues. This article addresses the issue of safety and regulation in prehospital civilian aviation.

The author, who happens to be an HEMS pilot, expresses his concern for improving aviation safety. In the article, he discusses the importance of developing and complying with appropriate regulations pertaining to daily flight operations. He also stresses the need for better oversight of flight line operations. A brief overview of the development of a more effective operational control process that would potentially provide an action plan for risk mitigation is described. Various suggestions, such as the development of a risk assessment matrix that would assign point values to various issues relevant to making the decision to fly a medical mission, are proposed. A better way to decide on the acceptance or rejection of a flight is described. The process proposed also suggests the development of a decision-making scheme that involves seeking higher approval to launch an aircraft in questionable circumstances. The capability of the pilot or a single member of the crew to reject a flight is also noted. This article is informative and provides a means for potentially decreasing future aviation accidents while improving overall civilian aviation and HEMS safety.

B. M. Minczak, MS, MD, PhD, PH-MD

Treatment and Imaging

Medication Dosing Errors in Pediatric Patients Treated by Emergency Medical Services
Hoyle JD Jr, Davis AT, Putman KK, et al (Helen DeVos Children's Hosp/ Michigan State Univ College of Human Medicine, Grand Rapids; Grand Rapids Med Education and Res Ctr/Michigan State Univ; Michigan State Univ/Kalamazoo Ctr for Med Studies, Kalamazoo, Michigan; et al)
Prehosp Emerg Care 16:59-66, 2012

Background.—Medication dosing errors occur in up to 17.8% of hospitalized children. There are limited data to describe pediatric medication errors by emergency medical services (EMS) paramedics. It has been shown that paramedics have infrequent encounters with pediatric patients.

Objective.—To characterize medication dosing errors in children treated by EMS.

Methods.—We studied patients aged ≤11 years who were treated by paramedics from eight Michigan EMS agencies from January 2004 through March 2006. We defined a medication dosing error as ≥20% deviation from the weight-appropriate dose, as determined by the patient's reported weight in the prehospital medical record or by use of the Broselow-Luten tape (BLT). We studied errors in administering six EMS medications commonly given to children: albuterol, atropine, dextrose, diphenhydramine, epinephrine, and naloxone.

Results.—There were 5,547 children aged ≤11 years who were treated during the study period, of whom 230 (4.1%) received drugs and had a documented weight. These patients received a total of 360 medication administrations. Multiple drug administrations occurred in 73 cases. Medication dosing errors occurred in 125 of the 360 drug administrations (34.7%; 95% confidence interval [CI] 30.0, 39.8). Relative drug dosage errors (with 95% CI) were as follows: albuterol 23.3% (18.4, 29.1), atropine 48.8% (34.3, 63.5), diphenhydramine 53.8% (29.1, 76.8), and epinephrine 60.9% (49.9, 73.9). The mean error (± standard deviation) for intravenous/intraosseous 1:1000 epinephrine overdoses was 808% ± 428%. The mean error (± standard deviation) for intravenous/intraosseous 1:1000 epinephrine underdoses was 35.5% ± 27.4%.

Conclusions.—Medications delivered in the prehospital care of children were frequently administered outside of the proper dose range when compared with patient weights recorded in the prehospital medical record. EMS systems should develop strategies to reduce pediatric medication dosing errors.

▶ This retrospective analysis of data provided from an administrative emergency medical service (EMS) database provides insight into some of the obvious pitfalls confronting medics that can lead to medication errors.

Paramedics working in the prehospital arena are often challenged with treating a child during an emergency encounter without the benefit of detailed information regarding the patient. When a medication is indicated, they must determine allergy status, determine the correct dose, sometimes draw up the medication from a multidose vial, and then administer it to the patient. Second, the weight of the patient must be determined. Correct dosing usually involves doing a calculation based on the patient's weight. Medics do not usually carry a scale to determine how heavy the patient is. They rely on information from the parents or they may make an estimate of the patient's weight. They do have the Broselow-Luten tape (BLT), which provides a statistically based weight, based on the length of the patient. However, correct implementation of the tape in a stressful, prehospital encounter with a sick child can set the stage for a mistake to occur. Furthermore, if the medics lack significant experience with assessing and treating children, lack of familiarity with the use of the

BLT increases the possibility of making an error. Paramedic encounters with pediatric patients are infrequent, leading to the relative inexperience of medics in dealing with challenges in these situations. Furthermore, training to deal with pediatric patients is relatively limited so that when the medics encounter time-sensitive, urgent situations with minimal personnel available to provide for dose and drug verification, errors are more likely to occur.

Some proposed solutions suggested in this publication are to establish a set dosage for a particular treatment indication across a weight range to minimize calculations. Another option is to provide information cards that describe the number of milliliters of a drug to be administered from a standard medication vial to the patient. Then there is no need to ascertain the weight of the patient, and the need for a calculation to be performed under duress is alleviated.

Medical directors should revise the curriculum for paramedics with the intent of providing semiannual reviews and increasing training in how to deal with these types of encounters.

This study has its limitations. Lack of direct observation may have led to lost data pertinent to this study. Medics may have used the BLT or used some other means of determining the dosage needed and not documented it. The medics may have used an application on a handheld device to determine the dose. Self-reporting also introduces potential bias in the information.

Nonetheless, there is a lack of medication safety systems in the prehospital environment. Training needs to be modified to increase exposure of medics to simulated challenges with pediatric patients in the prehospital environment. Medication administration devices, vials, and dosage information cards should be reevaluated to increase patient safety, especially in the prehospital environment. Also, protocols should mandate some form of documented verification of medication dosing, such as the BLT, prior to administering the drug.

B. M. Minczak, MS, MD, PhD, PH-MD

Miscellaneous

Facing the Nuclear Threat: Thyroid Blocking Revisited
Hänscheid H, Reiners C, Goulko G, et al (Univ of Würzburg, Germany)
J Clin Endocrinol Metab 96:3511-3516, 2011

Context.—People being exposed to potentially harmful amounts of radioactive iodine need prophylaxis to prevent high radiation-absorbed doses to the thyroid.

Objective.—Parameters determining the individual protective effect of a pharmacological intervention were investigated.

Design and Participants.—Biokinetics of ^{123}I was evaluated in 27 healthy volunteers (aged 22–46 yr, median 25 yr, in total 48 assessments) twice in a baseline measurement of the undisturbed kinetics and in an intervention assessment 48 h later.

Interventions.—Seven regimens using single doses of potassium iodide (KI) or sodium perchlorate (SP) at different times relative to exposure were compared: 100 mg KI (−24, 2, 8, 24 h), 100 mg SP (2 h), or 1 g SP (2, 8 h).

Main Outcome Measures.—Different drugs and dosages and the influence of individual parameters of iodine kinetics should be tested.

Results.—Mean dose reductions for interventions at −24, 2, 8, and 24 h relative to the activity incorporation were 88.7, 59.7, 25.4, and 2.8%, respectively. One gram SP was equally effective as 100 mg KI; residual uptake was observed after 100 mg SP. The individual dose reduction decreased exponentially with the effective half-life of the activity in the blood. Kinetics in subjects older than 40 yr was as assumed in official guidelines for the prophylaxis after nuclear accidents but was faster in younger participants.

Conclusions.—Data on the efficacy of thyroid blocking used in the guidelines are adequate for older people but not for young individuals with their typically faster kinetics. SP may be used for thyroid blocking as alternative for individuals with iodine hypersensitivity.

▶ This is an important study for emergency department physicians who work near power plants. It provides an understanding of alternates to potassium iodide and also the need to adjust doses in the young. This is a good article to pull and discuss at your next Emergency Preparedness Meeting if you are responsible for pre- and postexposure prophylaxis in nuclear events.

R. J. Hamilton, MD

Active Cooling During Transport of Neonates with Hypoxic-Ischemic Encephalopathy

Hobson A, Sussman C, Knight J, et al (ShandsCair Flight Program, Gainesville, FL; Univ of Florida, Gainesville)
Air Med J 30:197-200, 2011

Background.—Morbidity or mortality can result from perinatal asphyxia causing hypoxic ischemic encephalopathy (HIE). Total body cooling is used to manage affected infants, with three multicenter trials showing that mild hypothermia improves the neurodevelopmental outcomes in infants at 36 weeks' gestation or greater who have experienced hypoxic-ischemic injury. Hypothermia must begin within 6 hours of birth, which presents a problem for infants born where this level of care is not available and needing transport to a neonatal intensive care unit (NICU) providing hypothermia therapy. Such infants are passively and/or actively cooled during transport, but neither method allows continuous monitoring of the temperature, so infants can be excessively or insufficiently cooled. The CritiCool temperature management unit uses a control algorithm that monitors skin and core temperature and adjusts circulating water temperature to maintain core temperate at 33.5°C. It is small enough for use on transports. The

CritCool was employed on a fixed-wing aircraft, a helicopter, and an ambulance transporting neonates to a NICU with hypothermia therapy facilities.

Case Reports.—Case 1: Boy, born at term, had fetal heart tones at 60 beats per minute (bpm) and was delivered by emergency Cesarean section. He was unresponsive, had a heart rate less than 60 bpm, and required intubation and endotracheal tube epinephrine administration. His Apgar scores were 1^1, 3^5, and 4^{10}. The NICU staff stabilized him and initiated passive cooling. A fixed-wing aircraft was dispatched. The transport vehicle arrived at the NICU to find the neonate's temperature was 31.5°C. Passive cooling was continued on the trip back to the plane, where the infant was placed on the CritiCool, beginning active temperature management with gradual rewarming. Once the aircraft landed, the neonate was transferred via ambulance to the hospital, with active cooling provided throughout the process. Passive cooling was used when the infant was transferred from the ambulance to the NICU, then active cooling therapy resumed. His admission temperature was 33.5°C, and he was classified as Sarnat stage III with a history of seizures and absent reflexes. Magnetic resonance imaging (MRI) revealed diminished brain volume and restricted diffusion in various areas of the brain, consistent with HIE. His health was stabilized but the diminished reflexes, seizures, and general low responsiveness persisted through his discharge on hospice care.

Case 2: Boy, a late preterm infant, was born via emergency Cesarean section after placental abruption and lack of fetal heart tones. His Apgar scores were 1^1, 2^5, 4^{10}, and 7^{15}. Initial arterial pH was 6.60 at 30 minutes; the base deficit was 26. Mechanical ventilation was begun to resuscitate the boy, with physicians classifying his condition as Sarnat stage II. He was passively cooled, achieving a rectal temperature of 31.8°C when the helicopter transport team assessed him. He was placed on the CritiCool device and transported for 50 minutes to the NICU facility, where his rectal temperature was 34.1°C. During 72 hours of systemic hypothermia the neonate's neurologic status continually improved. On day 4 MRI showed no evidence of neurologic injury.

Case 3: Girl, born at term via emergency Cesarean section, had initial Apgar scores of 1^1, 3^5, and 5^{10}. Her respiratory status was improving, but seizure activity prompted intubation and the administration of phenobarbital. Passive cooling was used during transport to the hospital, where physicians determined she required hypothermia therapy and had an ambulance sent for transport to the NICU. The ambulance team placed her on the CritiCool and actively cooled her during transport, achieving a temperature between 32.5° and 33.1°C. She was passively cooled when transferred from the ambulance to the hospital, then active cooling was reinitiated in the NICU. Her history of seizure activity and absent gag reflex led to her classification as Sarnat stage III, so active cooling was initiated for 72 hours. She improved with time, was eventually extubated, and had a normal MRI.

Practical Issues.—The CritiCool has no battery backup and weighs about 70 pounds when filled with water, so transport team members cannot easily move the device from the aircraft or helicopter once it is secured. During long transfers between the facility and fixed-wing aircraft, temperature fluctuations associated with passive cooling can occur unless there is an alternative way of monitoring the temperature. This prompted the use of a separate continuous rectal probe monitor and passive cooling for these transfers. If the neonate's temperature drops below 33.5°C, the incubator temperature should be raised to 0.5°C higher than the neonate's current temperature. On arrival at the transport vehicle, the rectal probe is replaced with the one for the CritiCool device.

Conclusions.—Overcooling an infant can increase the adverse effects of cooling, such as arrhythmias, electrocardiogram changes, electrolyte abnormalities, thrombocytopenia, and coagulopathies. The servo-controlled CritiCool offers a cooling device useful with multiple modes of transport that allows tight monitoring and adjustment of the neonate's temperature.

▶ Therapeutic hypothermia has become a key factor in the treatment of hypoxic ischemic encephalopathy (HIE) caused by perinatal asphyxia. Infants who manage to live through HIE without appropriate treatment often have developmental disabilities such as mental retardation, cerebral palsy, and seizures. If appropriately controlled hypothermia is promptly initiated within 6 hours of birth, studies have shown that infants born at 36 weeks' gestation have improved neurodevelopmental outcomes. If an infant is born in a facility that is capable of providing this treatment modality, starting the process within 6 hours can be easily achieved. However, if an infant is born at a facility without the means to initiate cooling, the neonate must be transported to a neonatal intensive care unit (NICU) that offers this therapy.

As soon as arrangements are made for transfer to the appropriate facility, cooling is initiated and maintained during transport. Both passive and active techniques are used to cool the infant. Passive cooling involves removing external heat sources. Active cooling involves using gel packs to achieve target temperatures between 32° and 35° C. Unfortunately, temperature monitoring is often suboptimal, with babies arriving at the receiving facility with temperatures actually below the recommended range. This resultant overcooling can lead to cardiac arrhythmias, electrocardiogram changed electrolyte abnormalities, thrombocytopenia, and coagulopathies. This problem can be avoided by having a device that incorporates feedback from the patients (ie, core and skin temperature) and makes temperature output adjustments as needed to keep the infant's body temperature in the appropriate range. In this article, the CritiCool, the microprocessor-controlled temperature management unit, manufactured by MTRE

(Southampton, PA), was studied. The publication describes the performance of this unit in ground, helicopter, and fixed-wing patient transports. The data reported suggest that this device can be used successfully during these various modes of transport. Limitations of the device, such as excessive weight and lack of a battery backup, are briefly described. The need for having alternative temperature measurements available during transport of the patients to airports for fixed wing transport are addressed to prevent significant temperature fluctuations during passive cooling. Lessons learned from this publication may be carried over to transports involving postcardiac arrest patients who are now currently undergoing neuroprotective hypothermia.

B. M. Minczak, MS, MD, PhD, PH-MD

EMS Provider Assessment of Vehicle Damage Compared with Assessment by a Professional Crash Reconstructionist
Lerner EB, Cushman JT, Blatt A, et al (Med College of Wisconsin, Milwaukee; Univ of Rochester, NY; CUBRC, Buffalo, NY; et al)
Prehosp Emerg Care 15:483-489, 2011

Objective.—To determine the accuracy of emergency medical services (EMS) provider assessments of motor vehicle damage when compared with measurements made by a professional crash reconstructionist.

Methods.—EMS providers caring for adult patients injured during a motor vehicle crash and transported to the regional trauma center in a midsized community were interviewed upon emergency department arrival. The interview collected provider estimates of crash mechanism of injury. For crashes that met a preset severity threshold, the vehicle's owner was asked to consent to having a crash reconstructionist assess the vehicle. The assessment included measuring intrusion and external automobile deformity. Vehicle damage was used to calculate change in velocity. Paired t-test, correlation, and kappa were used to compare EMS estimates and investigator-derived values.

Results.—Ninety-one vehicles were enrolled; of these, 58 were inspected and 33 were excluded because the vehicle was not accessible. Six vehicles had multiple patients. Therefore, a total of 68 EMS estimates were compared with the inspection findings. Patients were 46% male, 28% were admitted to hospital, and 1% died. The mean EMS-estimated deformity was 18 inches and the mean measured deformity was 14 inches. The mean EMS-estimated intrusion was 5 inches and the mean measured intrusion was 4 inches. The EMS providers and the reconstructionist had 68% agreement for determination of external automobile deformity (kappa 0.26) and 88% agreement for determination of intrusion (kappa 0.27) when the 1999 American College of Surgeons Field Triage Decision Scheme criteria were applied. The mean ($\pm$ standard deviation) EMS-estimated speed prior to the crash was 48 $\pm$ 13 mph and the mean reconstructionist-estimated change in velocity was 18 $\pm$ 12 mph (correlation -0.45). The EMS providers determined that 19 vehicles had rolled over, whereas the investigator identified 18 (kappa 0.96). In 55 cases, EMS and the investigator agreed on seat belt use; for the remaining 13 cases, there was disagreement (five) or the investigator was unable to make a determination (eight) (kappa 0.40).

Conclusions.—This study found that EMS providers are good at estimating rollover. Vehicle intrusion, deformity, and seat belt use appear to be more difficult for EMS to estimate, with only fair agreement with the crash reconstructionist. As expected, the EMS provider —estimated speed prior to the crash does not appear to be a reasonable proxy for change in velocity.

▶ This article attempts to describe whether the assessments of motor vehicle damage after a crash by emergency medical service (EMS) providers are accurate when compared with measurements and descriptions provided by a professional crash reconstructionist. The authors did a great job discussing the details of their study. They also provided a frank, detailed discussion of the limitations of this study. The data obtained from this investigation are certainly useful. However, there are many issues that make a valid comparison of the information provided by the EMS providers versus the accident reconstructionist difficult at best. When EMS providers arrive at the accident scene, they determine whether the scene is safe, approach the patients, assess them, and initiate treatment when appropriate. If extrication is required, they work with the rescue teams and maintain patient safety while providing whatever medical support is needed. Once the patient is stable, free from the wreckage, and ready for transport, they load the patient into the transport vehicle, ie, an ambulance or helicopter, and transport the patient to the appropriate receiving facility. Two major factors are considered in the decision as to where to take the patient: the severity of the patient's injuries and the mechanism of the injury. After a thorough patient assessment, components within The American College of Surgeons Field Triage Decision Scheme and other appropriate prehospital criteria are applied to determine the severity of the patient's condition. The mechanism is inferred from the visual information, and the cognitive estimates are made by the EMS crew while at the scene. The amount of scene time dedicated to assessing how much damage was done to the vehicle is limited and rightfully so, since the issue of patient care takes priority. However, there is a quick "Rorschach impression" or mental picture that the medics can and do obtain. As the EMS team initiates transport, they usually notify the receiving hospital of the patient's condition, and they provide a generalization of the mechanism. Upon arrival at the receiving facility, they usually provide a more detailed hand-off report to the trauma team. The information they provide regarding the degree of vehicular damage provides information relevant to the medical decision making. The team can then reset their index of suspicion regarding the patient's condition and determine what testing and imaging are indicated. Now a question arises: how accurate is the medic's report when compared with actual measurements by a trained accident reconstructionist?

Based on the data collected by these investigators, they correctly state that the EMS personnel are reasonably accurate when it comes to determining whether the vehicle rolled over or not. However, there is only fair agreement regarding the data of the EMS provider versus the expert when it comes to comparing the degree of vehicular deformity and intrusion. There is also disagreement regarding the use of seat belts. Some of the reasons why this is the case are addressed below.

The accident reconstructionist, an individual trained in analyzing the damage done to a vehicle from a crash, was not at the scene nor did he/she see the condition of the vehicle immediately after the crash. Most likely, the first contact with the vehicle was at the destination to which the vehicle was towed—body shop or junkyard. There is a potential confounder here in that the appearance of the vehicle may have been altered during the towing/wrecking process. Also, potential repairs may have already begun. Furthermore, the trained investigator can take his/her time-making measurements without the stress of working a live accident scene and taking care of a patient. The EMS personnel are not specifically trained in accident reconstruction. They received a limited amount of training in their EMT/paramedic training and are not considered experts.

Again, this study is very useful in illustrating that the information gathered from the accident scene by medics is very important, but the intrinsic issues that affect the accuracy of the information are inextricable from the situation. Nonetheless, getting a rough idea about what the accident scene looked like and appropriately factoring the suspected potential mechanism into the medical decision making can only benefit the patient. The health care team must be aware that the information provided about the mechanism of injury has its limitations. The potential for some overtriage will be inevitable. Hopefully, undertriage will not override the clinician's index of suspicion regarding the extent of patient's potential injuries and will not precipitate a missed diagnosis.

One possible future solution could be to take appropriate images of the scene via a digital camera or the equivalent and bring this information to the treating facility.

B. M. Minczak, MS, MD, PhD, PH-MD

Helicopters and the Civilian Trauma System: National Utilization Patterns Demonstrate Improved Outcomes After Traumatic Injury

Brown JB, Stassen NA, Bankey PE, et al (Univ of Rochester School of Medicine, NY)
J Trauma 69:1030-1036, 2010

Background.—The role of helicopter transport (HT) in civilian trauma care remains controversial. The objective of this study was to compare patient outcomes after transport from the scene of injury by HT and ground transport using a national patient sample.

Methods.—Patients transported from the scene of injury by HT or ground transport in 2007 were identified using the National Trauma Databank version 8. Injury severity, utilization of hospital resources, and outcomes were compared. Stepwise logistic regression was used to determine whether transport modality was a predictor of survival or discharge to home after adjusting for covariates.

Results.—There were 258,387 patients transported by helicopter (16%) or ground (84%). Mean Injury Severity Score was higher in HT patients (15.9 ± 12.3 vs. 10.2 ± 9.5, $p < 0.01$), as was the percentage of patients with Injury Severity Score >15 (42.6% vs. 20.8%; odds ratio [OR], 2.83; 95% confidence interval [CI], 2.76—2.89). HT patients had higher rates of intensive care unit admission (43.5% vs. 22.9%; OR, 2.58; 95% CI, 2.53—2.64) and mechanical ventilation (20.8% vs. 7.4%; OR, 3.30; 95% CI, 3.21—3.40). HT was a predictor of survival (OR, 1.22; 95% CI, 1.17—1.27) and discharge to home (OR, 1.05; 95% CI, 1.02—1.07) after adjustment for covariates.

Conclusions.—Trauma patients transported by helicopter were more severely injured, had longer transport times, and required more hospital resources than those transported by ground. Despite this, HT patients were more likely to survive and were more likely to be discharged home after treatment when compared with those transported by ground. Despite concerns regarding helicopter utilization in the civilian setting, this study shows that HT has merit and impacts outcome.

▶ The decision to "launch the bird" to transport a patient to a tertiary care center should not be taken lightly. Medical transport helicopter pilots and crew are conditioned and probably self-selected to minimize risk for the betterment of the patient. Given that this is one of the most dangerous modes of transportation, the benefits of transporting this patient to the next level of care must clearly outweigh the risks of weather, night operations, electrical wires, and other unforeseen hazards. The authors of this article dredged the National Trauma Databank to assess outcomes in patients transported via helicopters and ground ambulances. Although the overall mortality was higher in the aeromedical evaluation patients, they did report improved survival to hospital discharge. Unfortunately, comparisons between helicopter and ambulance transport will remain flawed. Until patients are randomized to air or ground transport, too many variables contribute to the ultimate outcomes. Generally, scene medical personnel decide who is too sick to drive, more remote hospitals recommend that the sicker patients "go downtown" because of resource availability, and administrators encourage the flying commercial to be out over the catchment area. These factors all blur the research question.

E. C. Bruno, MD

Management of ingested foreign bodies and food impactions
Ikenberry SO, Jue TL, Anderson MA, et al
Gastrointest Endosc 73:1085-1091, 2011

This is one of a series of statements discussing the use of GI endoscopy in common clinical situations. The Standards of Practice Committee of the American Society for Gastrointestinal Endoscopy (ASGE) prepared this text. In preparing this guideline, a search of the medical literature was performed by using PubMed. Studies or reports that described fewer than 10 patients were excluded from analysis if multiple series with more than 10 patients addressing the same issue were available. Additional references were obtained from the bibliographies of the identified articles and from recommendations of expert consultants. Guidelines for appropriate use of endoscopy are based on a critical review of the available data and expert consensus at the time that the guidelines are drafted. Further controlled clinical studies may be needed to clarify aspects of this guideline. This guideline may be revised as necessary to account for changes in technology, new data, or other aspects of clinical practice. The original guideline was published in 1995 and last updated in 2002. The recommendations are based on reviewed studies and are graded on the strength of the supporting evidence. The strength of individual recommendations is based both on the aggregate evidence quality and an assessment of the anticipated benefits and harms. Weaker recommendations are indicated by phrases such as "we suggest," whereas stronger recommendations are typically stated as "we recommend."

This guideline is intended to be an educational device to provide information that may assist endoscopists in providing care to patients. This guideline is not a rule and should not be construed as establishing a legal standard of care or as encouraging, advocating, requiring, or discouraging any particular treatment. Clinical decisions in any particular case involve a complex analysis of the patient's condition and available courses of action. Therefore, clinical considerations may lead an endoscopist to take a course of action that varies from these guidelines (Table 2).

▶ This is a great position paper by the American Society for Gastrointestinal Endoscopy on the management of ingested foreign bodies and food impactions. It is a must-read for emergency physicians. See Table 2 for the major recommendations in terms of timing of endoscopy for ingested foreign bodies. The other major recommendations made in the article include the following: (1) Avoid contrast radiographic examinations before removal of foreign bodies

---

TABLE 2.—Timing of Endoscopy for Ingested Foreign Bodies

Emergent endoscopy
    Patients with esophageal obstruction (ie, unable to manage secretions)
    Disk batteries in the esophagus
    Sharp-pointed objects in the esophagus
Urgent endoscopy
    Esophageal foreign objects that are not sharp-pointed
    Esophageal food impaction in patients without complete obstruction
    Sharp-pointed objects in the stomach or duodenum
    Objects >6 cm in length at or above the proximal duodenum
    Magnets within endoscopic reach
Nonurgent endoscopy
    Coins in the esophagus may be observed for 12-24 hours before endoscopic removal in an asymptomatic patient
    Objects in the stomach with diameter >2.5 cm
    Disk batteries and cylindrical batteries that are in the stomach of patients without signs of GI injury may be observed for as long as 48 hours. Batteries remaining in the stomach longer than 48 hours should be removed.

because of risk of aspiration and because it makes removal more difficult. (2) Get an ear-nose-throat consultation for foreign bodies at or above the level of the cricopharyngeus. (3) Glucagon 1 mg (intravenous) can be given in the setting of an impacted esophageal food bolus to induce the relaxation of the distal esophagus, but generally it does not work and it should not delay definitive endoscopic removal. (4) Coins within the esophagus may be observed in asymptomatic patients but should be removed endoscopically within 24 hours if spontaneous passage into the stomach does not occur. (5) Drug-containing packets should not be removed endoscopically because of the dangerous risk of bag rupture. These generally are treated with whole bowel irrigation with a polyethylene glycol solution. (6) In general, more than 80% of foreign objects will likely pass through the entire gastrointestinal tract without the need for intervention as long as physicians and patients are patient.

D. K. Mullin, MD

Mother's Little Helper: The Problem of Narcotic Diversion
Clark J R
Air Med J 30:294-296, 2011

Background.—Prescription drug diversion is removing prescription drugs from their medical sources and transferring them into the illegal market. The US Drug Enforcement Administration (DEA) investigates situations that involve diversion in medical settings. The current status of this problem and suggestions to improve oversight were explained.

Diversion Facts.—The three most commonly abused classes of prescription drugs are opioids, central nervous system depressants, and stimulants. These drugs are not always diverted for personal use, but also represent a lucrative business, with the street value of pharmaceutical-grade drugs up to 10 times their retail value. Diversion is especially prevalent in areas of autonomous practice, such as emergency medical services (EMS) and helicopter EMS. Practitioners in these settings have ready access to a supply of controlled substances and fewer watchdogs than in institutional settings.

Prevention.—All programs involving controlled substances have a system-level strategy to prevent and detect the diversion of these agents. However, lapses occur. Access is the common denominator in diversion cases and is created when shortcuts are taken for convenience or familiarity with the controls permits rigging or tampering with the system. Typically nurses obtain drugs by asking a physician to write a prescription for them, by forging a prescription, by administering a partial dose to a patient and keeping the rest, by fraudulently documenting a narcotics record about waste, or by obtaining as-needed medications for patients who have refused or not requested them.

Leaders should be aware of warning signs that an employee or co-worker is at risk. They are responsible for ensuring the systems in place will prevent diversion. If an addiction is identified, the individual should be directed toward help to overcome it. Because drug addiction is not treated the same as other physical and mental impairments under the Americans with Disabilities Act and the Rehabilitation Act of 1973, persons currently diverting drugs for personal use may be discharged or denied employment. However, drug addicts not currently using drugs or rehabilitated, those who have a history of drug addiction only, and those in a rehabilitation program must not be discriminated against.

Results of Diversion.—Diverting drugs compromises patient safety, destroys goodwill and the public image of the program or hospital, and exposes persons and institutions to criminal and civil liability. When a theft or significant loss of any controlled substance is discovered, the DEA registrant must notify the local DEA Field Division Office immediately and complete an online form regarding the loss or theft. Penalties for diversion are significant, depending on the drug involved, its schedule, the quantity, the number of previous offenses, any harm caused, and the number of persons involved. Failure to report a diversion incident can incur a fine of up to $10,000 per occurrence.

Conclusions.—Enforcement and consistency are important when dealing with maintaining the effectiveness of safety nets such as drug diversion prevention programs. Strong procedures are needed to track distribution and monitor compliance with narcotic use policies. Continuous quality improvement programs that validate medication use, regular audits of security systems and logs, and routine continuing education of all staff are important components of an effective drug diversion prevention program.

▶ Substance abuse is prevalent across all levels of society. From the stereotypical street drug addict, the college professor, the local government official, the religious leader to the health care provider, people have their idiosyncrasies, areas of weakness, and vulnerabilities. In addition, different people have very dissimilar coping mechanisms when dealing with the stressors in their lives. Some cope and compensate well, whereas others turn to pharmacology for help—the old sarcastic adage of "better living through chemistry." This article brings to light the issue of substance abuse and diversion among health care providers, specifically those working in an autonomous practice arena such as emergency medical services (EMS) or helicopter EMS (HEMS). These providers have been noted as particularly problematic. Nurses and physicians, working together, also have the opportunity to help each other out by doing things that facilitate access and diversion of drugs. What makes things even easier for this to occur is the lack of active vigilance/surveillance and control. Nurses are reported to have a prevalence of substance abuse that parallels the general population. It is estimated that 6% to 8% of nurses are practicing while impaired.

This publication serves to provide a concise presentation on the scope of the problem of substance abuse. Within this article diversion is defined, some facts regarding motive for diversion are addressed, and readers are provided with some clues of what to look for in their immediate work environment so that they can more easily detect whether a coworker may be involved in diversion or abuse of prescription drugs. The information provided is not for the purpose of instigating conflict among colleagues but can serve as a tool for dealing with substance abuse and diversion in the workplace.

Diversion is defined by Title 21 of the United States Code (USC) Controlled Substances Act as "the use of prescription drugs for recreational purposes." The Drug Enforcement Administration (DEA) is tasked with investigating circumstances where diversion is suspect. The Office of National Drug Control Policy reports that the most commonly abused substances are opioids, central nervous system depressants, and stimulants. The motivation for diversion is not always for self-administration and recreation; some parties who divert make significant financial gains diverting and distributing drugs on the street. This activity destroys trust in individual professionals, damages the reputation of the health care providers guilty of and involved in this activity, and affects the overall impression of a given hospital or health care facility.

The common issue in almost all cases of diversion is access and lack of adequate accountability and surveillance. Some of the tricks of the trade for obtaining the substances are searching through waste containers for analgesic patches, asking a physician for a prescription because the person "ran out of their meds" and can't get to their doctor in the next few days, forging a prescription or medication record, unsupervised "wasting" of unused medication, and fraudulently appropriating or outright stealing narcotic medications that were unexpectedly discontinued for a given patient. Some nurses have been observed taking some of the patient's as-needed narcotics and logging that the medication was given to the patient. Other clues are found in documentation aberrancies: a physician documents more medications than others; the "count" is often off when this person is working; there is no documentation provided regarding the patient's response to the analgesic given; or a health care provider mistakenly draws up too much medication for a patient which then has to be "thrown away." Some health care providers administer medications when the drug drawer is being restocked and manage to sneak out an extra dose from the supply cart. Other health care workers joke or state that they inadvertently took home medication in their pocket and "wasted" it at home.

The article finishes with a presentation of the facts regarding implications of diversion, that is, the mandate and need for reporting diversion to the appropriate authorities, as well as the potential financial penalties, licensure consequences, and incarceration guidelines.

The take-home message is that health care leadership must provide and enforce policies that will curb the opportunity for diversion and provide help and rehabilitation with an avenue for rehabilitation of the potential addict or dealer. I recommend that all health care providers who serve in some form of leadership role, and even those that do not, become familiar with this publication.

B. M. Minczak, MS, MD, PhD, PH-MD

Semiautomatic Intraosseous Devices in Pediatric Prehospital Care

Myers LA, Russi CS, Arteaga GM (Mayo Clinic, Rochester, MN)
Prehosp Emerg Care 15:473-476, 2011

Background.—Intraosseous (IO) access is attempted when intravenous access cannot be established during an emergency. The U.S. Food and Drug Administration—cleared semiautomatic IO access device (EZ-IO; Vidacare Corp., Shavano Park, TX) has been shown to be safe and effective.

Objective.—To examine the characteristics of pediatric patients receiving IO infusions, primary clinical impressions of emergency medical services providers, success rates, and subsequent treatment after use of a manual IO device or the semiautomatic IO device.

Methods.—A midwestern, 12-site, statewide ambulance service began using the semiautomatic device instead of a manual IO device in 2007. Retrospective review included analysis of device placement rates and subsequent treatment of children (younger than 18 years) who underwent an IO access procedure with either the manual device (January 2003 through February 2007) or the semiautomatic device (March 2007 through May 2009).

Results.—First-attempt success was achieved in 80.6% of patients (25 of 31) in the manual device group and in 83.9% of patients (52 of 62) in the semiautomatic device group (p = 0.98). In the manual device group, there were 37 attempts for 25 successful device placements (67.6% success), and in the semiautomatic group, there were 72 attempts for 58 successful placements (80.6% success) (p = 0.52). Intravenous attempts were made before IO attempts in 35.5% of patients (11 of 31) in the manual group and in 1.7% of patients (1 of 60) in the semiautomatic group (p < 0.001). Treatment (medication use, excluding lidocaine for local anesthetic purposes and intravenous crystalloid) was administered IO in 84.0% of the patients (21 of 25) in the manual device group and in 73.2% of the patients (41 of 56) in the semiautomatic device group.

Conclusions.—For the pediatric cohort, use of a semiautomatic IO access device in place of a manual device offered no statistically significant difference in first-attempt success (3.3%) or in success per attempt (13.0%). However, the rate at which IO access was used by emergency medical services providers more than tripled with use of the semiautomatic device.

▶ Intravenous access is often attempted in the prehospital arena to administer fluids or medication. However, obtaining this access in compromised patients who have lost blood, are dehydrated, or have other mitigating circumstances that can compromise the ease of placing the line is often a challenge. Furthermore, this challenge becomes even greater when access is needed in a child less than 6 years old.

When an attempt to start an intravenous (IV) line on a child in an emergency fails, usually intraosseous (IO) access is attempted. Several manual devices are available, but now the semiautomatic IO access device (EZ-IO; Vidacare Corp,

Shavano Park, Texas) is available. These authors set out to examine and describe if any changes in practices occur when this device was available to medics.

The study found that there were no significant changes in first-attempt success with the semiautomatic device versus manual means. However, the rate of semiautomatic IO use increased. Medics used the EZ-IO more than the manual IO. In fact, medics made more attempts to start an IV before turning to the manual IO device.

From this study, we can infer that the medics appear to be more comfortable using the EZ-IO than the manual IO in pediatric patients. Limitations inherent in the study design may have affected the final outcome demonstrated by the data. The data failed to show a difference in first-success attempts between the techniques. This may possibly be attributed to the sample size. In addition, the data were obtained from self-generated patient care reports from the medics. No outcome measurements were provided regarding the subsequent clinical treatment and disposition of the patients.

Having used the EZ-IO myself, this device does facilitate placement of the line, and the technique appears less brutal during the actual procedure of placing the IO. Having the semiautomatic device makes IO line placement easier and more likely when IV access fails.

B. M. Minczak, MS, MD, PhD, PH-MD

Sensitivity of erythrocyte sedimentation rate and C-reactive protein for the exclusion of septic arthritis in emergency department patients

Hariharan P, Kabrhel C (Boston Univ Med Ctr, MA; Massachusetts General Hosp, Boston)
J Emerg Med 40:428-431, 2011

Background.—Previous studies in post-operative orthopedic and pediatric patients suggest that erythrocyte sedimentation rate (ESR) and C-reactive protein (CRP) testing may be helpful in ruling out septic arthritis. However, these tests have not been evaluated in a population of adult Emergency Department (ED) patients.

Study Objective.—Determine the sensitivity of ESR and CRP in patients with septic arthritis.

Methods.—Retrospective analysis of ED patients with septic arthritis from 2003 to 2008. Eligible patients had an International Classification of Diseases-Ninth Revision diagnosis of pyogenic arthritis (711.0x) plus: positive synovial fluid culture, positive synovial Gram stain, or operative irrigation. Patients were excluded if no ESR or CRP was performed within 24 h. Sensitivity of ESR and CRP at various cutoffs was calculated with 95% confidence intervals (CI).

Results.—We identified 167 patients with septic arthritis. We included 143 (86%) who had ESR (n = 140, 84%) or CRP (n = 96, 57%) performed. Mean age was 49 (±22) years, and 85 (59%) were male. Race was: 125 (87%) white, 4 (3%) black, and 12 (8%) Hispanic. Thirty-five

(24%) had infection of prosthetic joints. Synovial cultures were positive in 102 (71%). Sensitivity of ESR was: 98% (95% CI 94–100%) using a cutoff of ≥10 mm/h (n = 134) and 94% (95% CI 88–97%) using a cutoff of ≥15 mm/h (n = 131). The sensitivity of CRP was 92% (95% CI 84–96%) using a cutoff of ≥20 mg/L (n = 88).

Conclusion.—ESR and CRP have sensitivities of > 90% for septic arthritis, but only when low thresholds are used. Further study is required to determine the clinical usefulness of ESR and CRP testing.

▶ Patients presenting with a hot swollen joint represent a diagnostic challenge. Questions abound regarding the cause of the warmth, erythema, and possible effusion. Furthermore, arthrocentesis, a procedure designed to obtain the synovial fluid for cell count, Gram stain, and culture, is not a benign procedure and may cause an inflammatory condition to convert to an infectious one. The procedure also may be technically difficult, depending on the joint(s) affected. The ability to exclude septic arthritis as the reason for the joint complaints without arthrocentesis is an enviable option.

This retrospective study sought to determine if use of erythrocyte sedimentation rate (ESR) and C-reactive protein (CRP) predicted infectious arthritis. Retrospectively looking at patients with confirmed septic arthritis, they determined that ESR of < 10 mm/h and CRP of < 15 mg/L may be adequate to exclude septic arthritis, with a sensitivity of > 90%. Unfortunately, the diagnostic test results necessary to the achieve requisite sensitivities are so low that the clinical use is limited. A 2010 *Lancet* article further clouds the evaluation of patients with suspected septic arthritis, refuting the use of cell count, Gram stain, culture, and concurrent arthritis (gout, pseudogout, etc).[1]

E. C. Bruno, MD

Reference

1. Mathews CJ, Weston VC, Jones A, Field M, Coakley G. Bacterial septic arthritis in adults. *Lancet*. 2010;375:846-855.

The Use of Epinephrine for Out-of-Hospital Treatment of Anaphylaxis: Resource Document for the National Association of EMS Physicians Position Statement
Jacobsen RC, Millin MG (Univ of Missouri—Kansas City School of Medicine; Johns Hopkins Univ School of Medicine, Baltimore, MD)
Prehosp Emerg Care 15:570-576, 2011

Anaphylaxis is a potentially life-threatening condition that requires both prompt recognition and treatment with epinephrine. All levels of emergency medical services (EMS) providers, with appropriate physician oversight, should be able to carry and properly administer epinephrine safely when caring for patients with anaphylaxis. EMS systems and EMS medical directors should develop a mechanism to review the charts of patients who received epinephrine and were not in cardiac arrest. This will help to ensure the safe and appropriate use of epinephrine in order to provide continued quality improvement. Despite the safety of epinephrine, EMS systems that carry epinephrine autoinjectors should establish protocols to deal with patients or emergency responders who have an unintentional injection of epinephrine into the hand or digit. Continued research is needed to better define the role that EMS plays in the management of anaphylaxis. This paper serves as a resource document to the National Association of EMS Physician position on the use of epinephrine for the out-of-hospital treatment of anaphylaxis.

▶ Anaphylaxis occurs with a frequency ranging from 30 to 2000 episodes per 100 000 persons, with a prevalence of 2% over a lifetime. This condition has many triggers, such as food allergies and bee stings, and can develop as a result of treatment with a new medication. Some patients experience this condition without ever determining what the exact trigger of the event was.

Anaphylaxis is an acute-onset, rapidly developing, systemic allergic reaction that is potentially life threatening. When anaphylaxis occurs, capillaries start to leak, blood pressure decreases, and the airway and pulmonary system become compromised secondary to swelling, edema, and bronchospasm. The patient may manifest changes in the skin and experience hypoxia, wheezing, cardiovascular collapse, and ultimately death. Prompt recognition and treatment of this condition can effectively reverse these signs and symptoms and stabilize the allergic reaction, preventing death. The most effective universal standard treatment for anaphylaxis is the prompt administration of epinephrine.

Emergency medical service (EMS) personnel (ie, paramedics) have protocols for the administration of epinephrine for cardiac arrest. When it comes to treating anaphylaxis, guidelines are not as clear. Many EMS units with emergency medical technicians (EMTs) currently do not have protocols for carrying and treating patients with anaphylaxis. However, many patients who suffer from this condition and have no medical training carry "epi-pens"or epinephrine autoinjectors. Furthermore, many regions and states throughout the country are now considering protocols and means to allow EMTs and even camp counselors, scout leaders, tour guides, and teachers to administer epinephrine to patients suffering from anaphylaxis.

The National Association of EMS Physicians has now provided a statement to support that all levels of EMS providers, with appropriate physician oversight, should be able to carry and properly administer epinephrine safely when caring for patients with anaphylaxis. The data from many publications show that epinephrine is a safe drug to administer for anaphylaxis. Bad outcomes occur in older patients who have comorbidities. This drug should be administered promptly to patients who are experiencing anaphylaxis.

Another point of this publication is that administration of epinephrine should be intramuscular. Data from a study to determine blood levels of epinephrine after administration of the drug into the lateral thigh of healthy pediatric patients appears to achieve better, quicker blood levels. This route of administration has gained acceptance for the treatment of anaphylaxis.

B. M. Minczak, MS, MD, PhD, PH-MD

9 Emergency Center Activities

Clinical Skills

Tibial subacute osteomyelitis with intraosseous abscess: an unusual complication of intraosseous infusion
Henson NL, Payan JM, Terk MR (Emory Univ School of Medicine, Atlanta, GA; Veterans Affairs Med Ctr and Emory Univ School of Medicine, Decatur, GA)
Skeletal Radiol 40:239-242, 2011

Intravenous (IV) access is a critical step in patient care, especially in the emergency and/or trauma setting. Recently, intraosseous (IO) infusion has re-emerged as a recommended alternative to central venous access in both the pediatric and the adult patient. We present the case of an older adult male patient several months after emergency tibial IO infusion, now with left shin pain, and the MRI and culture findings diagnostic of subacute osteomyelitis with IO abscess, an unusual complication of IO infusion.

▶ With the advent of battery-powered intraosseous (IO) devices (making IO insertion easier and faster) and the updated recommendations of the American Heart Association and the International Liaison Committee on Resuscitation (suggesting IO infusion as an alternative to central venous access), the use of IO infusion is becoming more commonplace. This case report serves to remind us of the complications that may be encountered with this increased use of IO access in both pediatric and adult patients.

The most common complication of IO infusion is infiltration, occurring in up to 12% of patients in 1 study. Other complications are rare; these include osteomyelitis (as in this case report), compartment syndrome, air embolism, fat embolism, growth plate injuries, and fractures. Emergency physicians should keep intraosseous access in mind as a possible etiology when considering any of the aforementioned events.

E. A. Ramoska, MD, MPHE

Emergency Medicine and Society

"Family Plan"—Multiple-Patient Visits From the Same Family to an Inner-City Pediatric Emergency Department

Kannikeswaran N, Sethuraman U, Rao S, et al (Wayne State Univ, Detroit, MI; West Virginia Univ Children's Hosp, Morgantown)
Pediatr Emerg Care 27:390-393, 2011

Objectives.—The issue of multiple family members presenting to the emergency department (ED) for care during a single visit is unique to pediatric EDs (PEDs). The epidemiology of such multiple-patient visits (MPVs) has not been well characterized. The aims of this study were to describe patient characteristics, Emergency Severity Index (ESI) triage categories, length of stay, ED disposition, and payer characteristics of such MPV and to compare these characteristics to that of the overall ED visits (OEVs).

Methods.—We conducted a retrospective chart review of MPVs to an inner-city PED from June to December 2006. We collected patient demographics, ESI triage categories, ED disposition, length of stay, and payer characteristics. Descriptive methods and comparative methods were used to summarize the sample characteristics and compare group differences, respectively.

Results.—Multiple-patient visit constituted 2.2% (1166/52,491) of the total ED visits with a total of 2511 patients. The majority (88%; 1025/1166) of such visits were with 2 patients in a family. Ninety-one percent (2285/2511) of patients presented for medical complaints. Compared with the OEV, MPV belonged significantly more to ESI triage category 5 (51.2% vs 28.6%) and less to ESI triage category 3 (10.0% vs 24.6%; $\chi^2 = 775.4$; $P < 0.01$). A significantly higher percentage of MPV patients belonged to Medicaid Health Maintenance Organization compared with the OEV patients (72.4% vs 47.6%; $P < 0.01$). Only 3.3% of MPV patients required hospital admission.

Conclusions.—In our inner-city PED, most of the MPVs are for medical complaints, belong to a lower acuity, and have a low hospital admission rate.

▶ Is there any characteristic of patients who come in to the emergency department as family members that is distinct from other patients? Answering this question is the goal of the authors of this article. The first part of the study was to determine whether patterns of acuity and length of stay are different for these family presentations.

Take a moment to think about your own emergency department. Family members might come as victims of an automobile accident, perhaps all exposed to carbon monoxide, or suffering from the same viral infection. In some cases, multiple family members will come at once because there is no adequate child care for the children to be left at home or even in the waiting room. I think we can appreciate the situations when all the family members are suffering from common illnesses. By the way, is it likely that more than one person in the family will suffer from sepsis at the same time?

The authors found that the length of stay for patients of the family visit were generally unlikely to have longer lengths of stay than those of single-patient visits. A small but significant increase in length of stay was noted for lowest acuity patient—these are the patients getting doctor and nurse contacts without any use of resources. This is not so surprising because the first child will have his or her workup completed while the other children wait, then the next child is examined and so forth. The more children, the longer the stay for the last child interviewed. However, in the setting of higher-acuity patients, it is less surprising that children are all waiting for some resource provision, such as a radiograph which would equalize the duration of stay for all the children. I do wonder, however, if there is a difference in time consumed for charting and other postcare workload for these patients.

Once we have an idea of what is going on with multiple family members, it is possible to make plans for how to care for them. This study gives us some idea that there is not a lot of difference for these types of presentations compared with what we do already.

N. B. Handly, MD, MSc, MS

"Sign Right Here and You're Good to Go": A Content Analysis of Audiotaped Emergency Department Discharge Instructions
Vashi A, Rhodes KV (Mount Sinai School of Medicine, NY; Univ of Pennsylvania School of Medicine, Philadelphia)
Ann Emerg Med 57:315-322, 2011

Study Objective.—The goal of this study is to quantitatively and qualitatively assess the quality and content of verbal discharge instructions at 2 emergency departments (EDs).

Methods.—This was a secondary data analysis of 844 ED audiotapes collected during a study of patient–emergency provider communication at 1 urban and 1 suburban ED. ED visits of nonemergency adult female patients were recorded with a digital audiotape. Of 844 recorded ED visits, 477 (57%) audiotapes captured audible discharge instructions suitable for analysis. Audiotapes were double coded for the following discharge content: (1) explanation of illness, (2) expected course, (3) self-care, (4) medication instructions, (5) symptoms prompting return to the ED, (6) time-specified for follow-up visit, (7) follow-up care instructions, (8) opportunities for questions, and (9) patient confirmation of understanding. Analysis included descriptive statistics, χ^2 tests, 2-sample t tests, and logistic regression models.

Results.—Four hundred seventy-seven of 871 (55%) patient tapes contained audible discharge instructions. The majority of discharges were conducted by the primary provider (emergency physician or nurse practitioner). Ninety-one percent of discharges included some opportunity to ask questions, although most of these were minimal. Only 22% of providers confirmed patients' understanding of instructions.

Conclusion.—Verbal ED discharge instructions are often incomplete, and most patients are given only minimal opportunities to ask questions or confirm understanding.

▶ Surely you have seen situations like this: a patient comes in to your emergency department (ED) complaining that, despite being seen at another ED, the patient did not understand what to expect about the course of the illness or injury and wants a chance to talk to a doctor again. This reencounter includes waiting-room time, triage, conversations with nurses and doctors, and possible repeated or additional tests before discharge. If only the patient had a better understanding of the discharge information the first time.

To even begin talking about making improvements, it is important to find ways to measure the quality and quantity of the discharge process. The next step would be to identify a baseline activity and design interventions. The authors do provide a useful introduction to the types of studies done, including some concepts and measures of provider-patient communication.

It is not enough to think about the problem of an inadequate discharge instruction process as a cause of lost time and energy; it should be considered that patient satisfaction would also depend on the quality of interaction throughout the ED visit, including at the time of discharge.

The authors have a data set of audio recordings of ED visits repurposed to analyze the discharge instruction process. Studies like this are time consuming; the discharge process must be identified by listening to many hours of tape, which then must be transformed to coded events such as "time of discharge information session" or "quality of provider's encouragement to ask questions."

The results are not very surprising: there are many gaps in providing information at discharge. It is not clear whether the constraints of working in the ED setting can be easily overcome, but there is likely to be a cultural process through which our residents are learning to minimize the effort while attendings and nurses often continue to fail delivering good discharge encounters.

N. B. Handly, MD, MSc, MS

"Sign Right Here and You're Good to Go": A Content Analysis of Audiotaped Emergency Department Discharge Instructions
Vashi A, Rhodes KV (Mount Sinai School of Medicine, NY; Univ of Pennsylvania School of Medicine, Philadelphia)
Ann Emerg Med 57:315-322, 2011

Study Objective.—The goal of this study is to quantitatively and qualitatively assess the quality and content of verbal discharge instructions at 2 emergency departments (EDs).

Methods.—This was a secondary data analysis of 844 ED audiotapes collected during a study of patient-emergency provider communication at

1 urban and 1 suburban ED. ED visits of nonemergency adult female patients were recorded with a digital audiotape. Of 844 recorded ED visits, 477 (57%) audiotapes captured audible discharge instructions suitable for analysis. Audiotapes were double coded for the following discharge content: (1) explanation of illness, (2) expected course, (3) self-care, (4) medication instructions, (5) symptoms prompting return to the ED, (6) time-specified for follow-up visit, (7) follow-up care instructions, (8) opportunities for questions, and (9) patient confirmation of understanding. Analysis included descriptive statistics, χ^2 tests, 2-sample t tests, and logistic regression models.

Results.—Four hundred seventy-seven of 871 (55%) patient tapes contained audible discharge instructions. The majority of discharges were conducted by the primary provider (emergency physician or nurse practitioner). Ninety-one percent of discharges included some opportunity to ask questions, although most of these were minimal. Only 22% of providers confirmed patients' understanding of instructions.

Conclusion.—Verbal ED discharge instructions are often incomplete, and most patients are given only minimal opportunities to ask questions or confirm understanding.

▶ This interesting study scrutinized actual audiotapes of emergency department (ED) personnel giving patients their discharge instructions. The primary provider, either a physician or a nurse practitioner, gave about 53% of the instructions. Communication during the discharge process lasted an average of 4 minutes. Most patients were given instructions to follow up in a clinic or with their primary care physician (73%), an explanation of their illness (76%), and instructions about medication use (80%). Approximately one half of the patients were provided with information about the expected course of their illness. Only about two-fifths of the patients were specifically told when to follow up; and only about one-third were given specific signs that should prompt a return visit to the ED. Roughly one-fifth of providers confirmed that their patient understood the discharge instructions, and in the vast majority of cases (90%), this interaction was of a minimal quality (eg, the provider simply asked, "OK?").

Communication is 1 of the 6 core competencies that are taught during emergency medicine residency training. This study suggests that, in general, we could do a better job of communicating with our patients, especially during the discharge process. Previous research has shown that the quality of discharge instructions is related to overall patient satisfaction, and patient satisfaction is related to malpractice risk. We all should examine how we provide discharge instructions to patients, strive to be more complete, and most important, ensure that our patients have understood our instructions.

E. A. Ramoska, MD, MPHE

A Content Analysis of Parents' Written Communication of Needs and Expectations for Emergency Care of Their Children

Hoppa EC, Porter SC (Cohen Children's Med Ctr of New York/Long Island Jewish Med Ctr, New Hyde Park; Univ of Toronto, Ontario, Canada)
Pediatr Emerg Care 27:507-513, 2011

Objective.—We investigated the potential value of information shared by parents on a written form designed to capture needs and expectations for care to an emergency department (ED) system that values patient-centeredness.

Methods.—We conducted a retrospective content analysis of parent-completed written forms collected during an improvement project focused on parent-provider communication in a pediatric ED. The primary outcome was potential value of the completed forms to a patient-centered ED system, defined as a form that was legible, included observations that mapped to medical problems, and included reasonable parental requests. We analyzed variation in potential value and other form attributes across a priori–defined visit type and acuity. Visit type was validated by a separate, blinded medical record review.

Results.—A random stratified sample of 1008 forms was established from 6937 parent-completed forms collected during the 6-month improvement project; 995 of 1008 forms had matching medical records; 922 (92.7%) of 995 forms demonstrated potential value; 990 (99.5%) of 995 forms were legible; 948 (95.3%) of 995 forms included observations that mapped to a medical problem, and 599 (93.3%) of 642 forms contained reasonable parental requests. There was good agreement between the form and medical record for visit type ($\kappa = 0.62$). The potential value of forms did not vary significantly across visit type (88.2%–92.8%) or acuity (88.9%–93.4%).

Conclusions.—Information shared by parents on written forms designed to capture needs and expectations provides potential value to a patient-centered ED system. The high level of informational value is consistent across patient type and acuity level.

▶ Can we get value from a questionnaire completed by parents in a pediatric emergency department (ED) encounter before beginning the interview? How might the information from this effort contribute to improved patient care and doctor-patient/-parent relationship? ED encounters are often rushed, and there may not be an opportunity for parents to express their concerns before the encounter is over. It may be that if we provide an uninterrupted opportunity for parents to describe their concerns, then a greater satisfaction with care will result.

The authors reviewed the content of responses to questionnaires provided to parents in the ED and compared these responses to the medical chart. For those parents who did complete at least some of the surveys, greater than 90% could have provided some guidance for care delivery. However, this written form of communication may not have been a preferred or comfortable way for parents to express their questions and requests because less than a third of surveys were completed by parents. Are there other ways to bring parents satisfactorily into the care episode?

Previously, the authors had found parents were more satisfied when offered a chance to complete this type of questionnaire. Subjects of this study did not rate their satisfaction, and it was not possible to determine if physicians found the information on the questionnaires useful during the actual patient encounter.

There is likely to be a balance point between gathering more data from patients and their families and the need to see more patients. Studies in this area should continue.

N. B. Handly, MD, MSc, MS

A Hierarchical Communication Model of the Antecedents of Health Care Professionals' Support for Donations after Cardiac Death
Peltier JW, D'Alessandro AM, Hsu M, et al (Univ of Wisconsin-Whitewater, McFarland; UW Organ Procurement Organization, Madison; et al)
Am J Transplant 11:591-598, 2011

Using structural equation modeling, the direct and indirect impact of five variables on the support of donation after cardiac death from the perspective of health care professionals were investigated: knowledge, trust in the transplant team, whether patients are in a state of irreversibility, whether health care professionals participate in a patient's death, and perceptions about the brain death versus cardiac death donation process. In total, 10/15 relationships posited in the model had significant pathways. The results provide insight into sequential communication strategies for generating support for donations after cardiac death.

▶ It is difficult to keep up with the types of methods used in studies both to have some sense of what the authors have done and to consider your use of the same tools.

Structural equation modeling (SEM) tools are being used more frequently as they are becoming less expensive. Graphical models are often built first to help identify linked factors, and then some kind of mathematical relationship is suspected or a relationship is fitted to the data available. Behind the scenes, the model is treated as a system of simultaneous equations so that all variables are considered at the same time. This is a significant difference from regression models in which each variable is considered while holding all the other variables constant (such as at their mean values).

The authors apply the SEM approach to the problem of how to increase support among health care practitioners for cardiac death organ donation. However, there was a lot of work to develop the questions for the survey used so that there could be a clear idea of how the responses to questions described the subject's attitude according to the model concepts.

It is one thing to apply SEM to a problem and demonstrate that some of the hypothesized relationships were significant. It is another task to transform that understanding of how health care practitioners think to then create an intervention to increase organ donations as the authors were able to show in this study.

Besides all the methodological work, it should be remembered that the subject of this study is part of our world. The emergency department is a place where conversations about organ donation is going to happen.

N. B. Handly, MD, MSc, MS

Antithrombotic effect of grape seed proanthocyanidins extract in a rat model of deep vein thrombosis

Zhang Y, Shi H, Wang W, et al (First Affiliated Hosp of Sun Yat-sen Univ, Guangzhou, China; et al)
J Vasc Surg 53:743-753, 2011

Objective.—Proanthocyanidins are abundantly found in grape seeds and have been suggested to inhibit the pathogenesis of systemic diseases. We investigated the antithrombotic effects of proanthocyanidins in a rat model of deep vein thrombosis (DVT) and examined the underlying mechanisms.

Methods.—DVT was induced in rat model by inferior vena cava (IVC) ligation. Grape seed proanthocyanidins extract (GSPE, 400 mg/kg/d) dissolved in saline (2 mL) was orally administered to the experimental rats. Control rats were administrated saline (2 mL) only. The thrombi were harvested and weighed. The IVC was analyzed histologically and by transmission electron microscopy. The cytokines interleukin (IL)-6, IL-8, and tumor necrosis factor-α (TNF-α) were detected by enzyme-linked immunosorbent assay. Expression of cellular adhesion molecules (CAMs) in thrombi was examined by Western blot.

Results.—GSPE significantly reduced thrombus length and weight ($P < .01$) and protected the integrity of the endothelium. GSPE inhibited thrombogenesis-promoting factors P-selectin, von Willebrand factor, and CAMs, and promoted thrombogenesis- demoting factors CD34, vascular endothelial growth factor receptor-2, and ADAMTS13 (a disintegrin and metalloproteinase with a thrombospondin type one motif, member 13). Compared with the control, GSPE significantly lowered the cytokines IL-6 (74.19 ± 13.86 vs 189.54 ± 43.76 pg/mL; $P < .01$), IL-8 (80.71 ± 21.42 vs 164.56 ± 39.54 pg/mL; $P < .01$), and TNF-α (43.11 ± 17.58 vs 231.84 ± 84.11 pg/mL; $P < .01$).

Conclusions.—GSPE significantly inhibited the propagation of thrombus induced by IVC ligation in a rat model. The antithrombotic properties of proanthocyanidins are likely to be directly associated with endothelial protection and regeneration, platelet aggregation, and inhibition of inflammatory cell and thrombus adhesion. Thus, proanthocyanidins may have a clinical application in DVT treatment.

▶ We read and hear about the beneficial effects of red wine drinking—whether as part of a "Mediterranean diet" or more specifically about the anti-inflammatory factors in peels or seeds. In this study, the authors created a thrombotic model by ligating the inferior vena cava and then assessed clot formation and status of the vessel endothelium in rats treated with either saline (control) or with grape seed proanthocyanidins extract (GSPE).

They found a significant decrease in the amount of clot formed when the rat was treated with GSPE (compared with saline-treated animals) and were able to show that many of the expected inflammatory mediators were also reduced in the clot and vessel wall biopsies.

Their work further extended to the observation of decreased injury to endothelia among animals treated with GSPE. This fits with a concern that our treatments of deep vein thrombosis only manage one part of the disease—the clot itself but not the inflammatory storm that persists and perhaps may increase the risk of future clot formation.

More work is needed, but this work certainly suggests that GSPE might be a valuable prevention and treatment for deep vein thrombi. How about other inflammatory disorders? Can I pour you a glass?

N. B. Handly, MD, MSc, MS

Association between waiting times and short term mortality and hospital admission after departure from emergency department: population based cohort study from Ontario, Canada
Guttmann A, Schull MJ, Vermeulen MJ, et al (Inst for Clinical Evaluative Sciences, Toronto, Ontario, Canada)
BMJ 342:d2983, 2011

Objective.—To determine whether patients who are not admitted to hospital after attending an emergency department during shifts with long waiting times are at risk for adverse events.

Design.—Population based retrospective cohort study using health administrative databases.

Setting.—High volume emergency departments in Ontario, Canada, fiscal years 2003-7.

Participants.—All emergency department patients who were not admitted (seen and discharged; left without being seen).

Outcome Measures.—Risk of adverse events (admission to hospital or death within seven days) adjusted for important characteristics of patients, shift, and hospital.

Results.—13 934 542 patients were seen and discharged and 617 011 left without being seen. The risk of adverse events increased with the mean length of stay of similar patients in the same shift in the emergency department. For mean length of stay ≥ 6 v <1 hour the adjusted odds ratio (95% confidence interval) was 1.79 (1.24 to 2.59) for death and 1.95 (1.79 to 2.13) for admission in high acuity patients and 1.71 (1.25 to 2.35) for death and 1.66 (1.56 to 1.76) for admission in low acuity patients). Leaving without being seen was not associated with an increase in adverse events at the level of the patient or by annual rates of the hospital.

Conclusions.—Presenting to an emergency department during shifts with longer waiting times, reflected in longer mean length of stay, is associated with a greater risk in the short term of death and admission to hospital in patients who are well enough to leave the department. Patients who leave without being seen are not at higher risk of short term adverse events.

▶ What happens to clinical suspicion or the type of workup performed when the line of patients grows longer and total ED visit times increase? Could it be that the rush to empty the place affects our thinking or our performance in some way? The work of these authors is important enough to review here.

The authors reviewed the short-term (within 7 days after the index visit) outcomes of patients seen at emergency departments and not admitted. This group included those individuals who were seen and discharged or those who left without being seen (LWBS). The outcomes chosen were death or admission to hospital. Patients were assigned a length-of-stay value based on the average length of stay of all patients arriving in the same shift with the same triage acuity score, whether patients from the same acuity group were admitted or not. Thus, patients waiting for inpatient beds were included in the mean length of stay if they had the same triage acuity level.

Average times of stay were broken into categorical groups by number of hours of total stay (< 1 hour was the reference for group comparison), and patients whose average length of stay value was more than 6 hours were grouped together.

The 2 outcomes for patients who LWBS were not related to average length of stay. The authors noted that these patients were typically of lower acuity and younger. Whether these LBWS patients took advantage of other health resources to prevent need for admission or death was unknown. One thing is certain: these patients were not subject to any care process involving physicians the ED.

For those patients who were seen and discharged, a different and concerning pattern was observed. Patients whose average length of stay was greater than 6 hours were nearly twice as likely to die or be admitted as those whose average length of stay was less than 1 hour.

This result is based on the average length of stay for patients with the same triage acuity level. It may be that patients with the same triage acuity level are not really the same clinically; however, the fact that patients grouped together did not just have a spread of lower and higher risk makes it seem less likely that acuity values are not appropriate measures of clinical similarity.

This is a retrospective study, and thus what we know is that there is an association, not a cause, between average length of stay and either admission or death within 7 days of the visit. Is there a way to determine what a physician might do with these patients uncoupled from the stress of the ED? The challenge is to understand the care process better to avoid these "errors of disposition."

N. B. Handly, MD, MSc, MS

Availability and Potential Effect of Rural Rotations in Emergency Medicine Residency Programs

Talley BE, Moore SA, Camargo CA Jr, et al (Denver Health Med Ctr, CO; Univ of Colorado Denver School of Medicine, Aurora; Massachusetts General Hosp, Boston; et al)
Acad Emerg Med 18:297-300, 2011

Objectives.—Increased exposure of emergency medicine (EM) residents to rural rotations may enhance recruitment to rural areas. This study sought to characterize the availability and types of rural rotations in EM residency programs and to correlate rotation type with rural practice after graduation.

Methods.—Program directors from all 126 Accreditation Council for Graduate Medical Education (AC-GME)-accredited EM residency programs with at least 2 years of graduates were surveyed. Directors were asked about availability of rural rotations, categorized as: 1) required, 2) elective (with or without predesignated sites), or 3) not available. Completion of rotations and initial practice location after graduation by rotation type were compared.

Results.—The 111 (88%) directors reported 2,380 graduates over the past 2 years. Rural rotations were required by six (5%) programs, elective at 92 (83%), and not available at 13 (12%). Overall, 197 (8%) residents completed a rural rotation during residency, and 160 (7%) selected their initial job in a rural area. More residents completed an elective rural rotation in programs with versus without a predesignated site (7% vs. 4%, respectively). EM residency graduates were more likely to select a rural job when rural rotations were required (22%), compared to other options: predesignated (7%) or no predesignated (6%) elective or not available (7%; $p < 0.001$).

Conclusions.—Elective rural rotations at predesignated sites increase resident exposure to rural areas compared to programs without predesignated sites, but neither approach was associated with rural practice after graduation. EM residency programs that required a rural rotation had increased resident selection of rural jobs, but only 5% of programs had this requirement.

▶ I think there might be a problem with association and cause when trying to understand what is involved with increasing emergency medicine residents seeking rural positions. The authors found that residency programs with required rural rotation have a higher fraction of residents seeking rural jobs.

While it is easier to contact a program director to find out the summary information about the program and graduates, it misses (and maybe to a great extent) the possibility that the residents who were amenable to choosing rural jobs made the choice to match to those specific residencies precisely because they had a required rural rotation.

The authors acknowledge that sampling attitudes from individual residents would be important to understanding what factors influence choices to practice in rural areas. I think this is absolutely correct. If a resident has personal experience in rural life, or if the family (especially partner) has expectations of life after residency, these factors will greatly affect the decision-making process. I spoke to a nurse manager just last week from a 9000-patient-per-year emergency department who told me that partners have little to do in her town, so it is hard to recruit physicians to her hospital. What about salary or the chance the partner can find opportunities for work?

I think we will find that the program experience has less to do with the choice to work in rural environments than personal attitudes. However, there is no doubt that learning to practice in a more austere environment is a good experience, whether it happens due to local resources or regulations to control costs.

N. B. Handly, MD, MSc, MS

Can we identify women at risk of pregnancy despite using emergency contraception? Data from randomized trials of ulipristal acetate and levonorgestrel

Glasier A, Cameron ST, Blithe D, et al (Univ of Edinburgh, Scotland, UK; Natl Inst of Child Health and Human Development, Bethesda, MD; et al)
Contraception 84:363-367, 2011

Background.—Emergency contraception (EC) does not always work. Clinicians should be aware of potential risk factors for EC failure.

Study Design.—Data from a meta-analysis of two randomized controlled trials comparing the efficacy of ulipristal acetate (UPA) with levonorgestrel were analyzed to identify factors associated with EC failure.

Results.—The risk of pregnancy was more than threefold greater for obese women compared with women with normal body mass index (odds ratio (OR), 3.60; 95% confidence interval (CI), 1.96−6.53; p<.0001), whichever EC was taken. However, for obese women, the risk was greater for those taking levonorgestrel (OR, 4.41; 95% CI, 2.05−9.44, p=.0002) than for UPA users (OR, 2.62; 95% CI, 0.89−7.00; ns). For both ECs, pregnancy risk was related to the cycle day of intercourse. Women who had intercourse the day before estimated day of ovulation had a fourfold increased risk of pregnancy (OR, 4.42; 95% CI, 2.33−8.20; p<.0001) compared with women having sex outside the fertile window. For both methods, women who had unprotected intercourse after using EC were more likely to get pregnant than those who did not (OR, 4.64; 95% CI, 2.22−8.96; p=.0002).

Conclusions.—Women who have intercourse around ovulation should ideally be offered a copper intrauterine device. Women with body mass index >25 kg/m^2 should be offered an intrauterine device or UPA. All women should be advised to start effective contraception immediately after EC.

▶ Notwithstanding issues of conscience about the use of contraception, it remains an appropriate concern about whether use of emergency contraception is actually efficacious. Emergency contraception may be a problem for the emergency physician, especially after a rape.

The authors combined data from 2 studies to explore patterns of failure of use of emergency contraception with 2 common agents, levonorgestrel and ulipristal acetate. The former has a track record of about 50% effectiveness, over a period of 72 hours after intercourse and the latter more effective as a contraceptive for up to 120 days after intercourse. The lengths of action suggest that there may be a window for use of these medications that may extend beyond the emergency encounter, and thus emergency physicians might think they can put off conversations about and prescriptions for these medications. However, in times of high emotion (such in the settings of confusion or fear) it may be critical to provide a complete "package" of care that includes the discussion of what these medications can provide. This article provides a significant assist in doing just that.

It does seem odd that the authors chose to include post—emergency contraception unprotected intercourse as a possible risk factor for failure for the use of the medications. Sure, we can include discussion of the need for further protection from pregnancy, but this behavior is not, surprisingly, going to raise the risk of pregnancy after treatment. However, it is hard to think of this as a cause of failure of the emergency contraceptive action. More appropriate is the finding that body mass index (BMI; or weight) and temporal proximity to ovulation were significant factors influencing success of contraception. It was already known that the time of intercourse around the time of ovulation does influence the chance of pregnancy. New in this study, however, was that the risk of failure increased with increased BMI. The reason for this is not yet known but may be a result of inadequate concentration of medication because all the patients were given the same mass of medication.

N. B. Handly, MD, MSc, MS

Catheter-directed ultrasound-accelerated thrombolysis for the treatment of acute pulmonary embolism

Engelhardt TC, Taylor AJ, Simprini LA, et al (Louisiana Heart, Lung and Vascular Inst, Metairie; Washington Hosp Ctr, DC; et al)
Thromb Res 128:149-154, 2011

Background.—Systemic thrombolysis rapidly improves right ventricular (RV) dysfunction in patients with acute pulmonary embolism (PE) but is associated with major bleeding complications in up to 20%. The efficacy of low-dose, catheter-directed ultrasound-accelerated thrombolysis (USAT) on the reversal of RV dysfunction is unknown.

Materials and Methods.—We performed a retrospective analysis of 24 PE patients (60 ± 16 years) at intermediate (n = 19) or high risk (n = 5) from the East Jefferson General Hospital who were treated with USAT (mean rt-PA dose 33.5 ± 15.5 mg over 19.7 hours) and received multiplanar contrast-enhanced chest computed tomography (CT) scans at baseline and after USAT at 38 ± 14 hours. All CT measurements were performed by an independent core laboratory.

Results.—The right-to-left ventricular dimension ratio (RV/LV ratio) from reconstructed CT four-chamber views at baseline of 1.33 ± 0.24 was significantly reduced to 1.00 ± 0.13 at follow-up by repeated-measures analysis of variance (p<0.001). The CT-angiographic pulmonary clot burden as assessed by the modified Miller score was significantly reduced from 17.8 ± 5.3 to 8.7 ± 5.1 (p<0.001). All patients were discharged alive, and there were no systemic bleeding complications but four major access site bleeding complications requiring transfusion and one suspected recurrent massive PE event.

Conclusions.—In patients with intermediate and high risk PE, low-dose USAT rapidly reverses right ventricular dilatation and pulmonary clot burden.

▶ Have you done anything new with your ultrasound equipment lately? Well, this study suggests a different use than normal for your ultrasound machine.

Some years back there were some reports that ultrasound at the right energy level could assist thrombolysis, and the effect was not related to the local heating of the sample from the ultrasound wave.

The authors present their experience using a combination of drug delivering and ultrasound broadcasting catheter in patients with significant pulmonary embolism (those that cause changes to the right ventricle to left ventricle diameter ratios).

Thrombolysis has been a useful agent to recover right ventricular function, but its use has risks of bleeding. The goal of the combination of thrombolysis and ultrasound is that it would be possible to use lower doses of thrombolytics to minimize the risks while obtaining the benefits of therapy to preserve right ventricular function.

The general goals appear to be met in this pilot study. A prospective study with longer follow-up would be in order.

N. B. Handly, MD, MSc, MS

Changes in Barriers to Primary Care and Emergency Department Utilization
Cheung PT, Wiler JL, Ginde AA (Univ of Colorado School of Medicine, Aurora)
Arch Intern Med 171:1397-1399, 2011

Background.—The aims of the 2010 Patient Protection and Affordable Care Act (ACA) include expanding health insurance coverage, improving access to medical care, and controlling health care costs. By improving access to and use of primary care services, it was hoped that the use of higher-cost emergency care would be minimized. Barriers to timely primary care and emergency department (ED) utilization rates were evaluated in Massachusetts, where legislation similar to the ACA has been in effect since 2006. However, ED visits remained high even with over 98% of working adults having health care coverage. Changes in national barriers to timely primary care access between 1999 and 2009 were evaluated, along with their relationship to ED utilization.

Methods.—Data came from the National Household Interview Survey and covered 317,497 adults. Five barriers to timely primary care were studied: (1) couldn't reach via telephone, (2) couldn't get an appointment soon enough, (3) once there, had to wait too long to see the doctor, (4) office was not open when needed, and (5) no transportation. Barriers were used to predict self-reported ED visits over the previous 12 months. Analyses were adjusted for demographic, socioeconomic, health status, and access-to-care variables.

Results.—Per year, 9.7% of adults reported one barrier and 20.1% reported at least one ED visit. More barriers were associated with the greater likelihood of an ED visit. Overall, barriers to timely primary care were associated with an increased use of ED facilities. The prevalence of barriers increased from 6.3% for a single barrier to 12.5%. Among adults with at least one ED visit, the prevalence of having at least one barrier increased from 12.0% to 18.9%.

Conclusions.—Limited access to primary care services has become increasingly important as a contributor to the rising use rates for ED services. The primary care provider shortage will likely accelerate this trend and result in even higher patient ED utilization. Optimal health care delivery and attempts to limit ED use will probably require solutions beyond expanding insurance coverage, likely including increasing the supply and availability of primary care providers.

▶ What are the alternatives for reducing the use of the emergency department (ED)? Either some other care site must be available, or there must be a way to refuse care to some number of people who come to the ED.

This study was based on analyses of multiple years of the National Health Interview Survey (NHIS). However, reasons why patients delay care and not why they end up in the ED as opposed to their primary care office were questions posed to subjects. It is not clear that delays in care meant the same thing as using the ED instead of the primary care practitioner for care, and thus the conclusions of this work have to be viewed with some suspicion.

It does seem likely that the availability of care via the ED does matter, but this dataset cannot be used to prove this. In fact, it did seem so likely to me that I did not even question the authors' interpretation, and it was only because I wanted to know more about the NHIS for my own understanding that I reviewed the questions (available online[1,2]).

Availability should matter—lack of transportation (does this mean that these patients were using ambulances to get to the ED instead of the primary care office?) or the fact that the office would be open, contribute to patients choosing to go to the ED. But what is it that makes a patient decided that if the doctor's office is not available the patient would seek any care until some later time? It is interesting that some complaints about the primary care visit included wait times before being seen by the doctor; this, however, does not sound like the ED has an advantage here.

If insurance reform is expected to increase patient visits for care and as long as primary care offices are unlikely to deliver the care that patients want, these patients will come to the ED. The other aspect to be determined is if the patients actually need this care.

N. B. Handly, MD, MSc, MS

References

1. Centers for Disease Control and Prevention. National Health Interview Survey. http://www.cdc.gov/nchs/nhis/quest_data_related_1997_forward.htm. Updated September 20, 2011. Accessed November 3, 2011.
2. 2007 NHIS questionnaire - sample adult survey: adult identification. http://ftp.cdc.gov/pub/health_statistics/nchs/Survey_Questionnaires/NHIS/2007/English/qadult.pdf. Published May 27, 2008. Accessed November 3, 2011.

Charlson Comorbidity Index Adjustment in Intracerebral Hemorrhage
Bar B, Hemphill JC III (Univ of California, San Francisco)
Stroke 42:2944-2946, 2011

Background and Purpose.—Previous studies of intracerebral hemorrhage (ICH) outcome prediction models have not systematically included adjustment for comorbid conditions. The purpose of this study was to assess whether the Charlson Comorbidity Index (CCI) was associated with early mortality and long-term functional outcome in patients with intracerebral hemorrhage.

Methods.—We performed a retrospective analysis on a prospective observational cohort of patients with ICH admitted to 2 University of California San Francisco hospitals from June 1, 2001 to May 31, 2004. Components of the ICH score and use of early care limitations were recorded. Outcome was assessed using the modified Rankin Scale to 12 months. The CCI was derived using hospital discharge International Classification of Diseases, revision 9 codes and patient history obtained from standardized case report forms.

Results.—In this cohort of 243 ICH patients, comorbid conditions were common, with CCI scores ranging from 0 to 12. Only 29% of patients with high CCI scores (≥ 3) achieved a 12-month modified Rankin Scale score of ≥ 3 compared with 48% of patients with CCI scores of 0 ($P=0.02$). CCI score was independently predictive of 12-month functional outcome, with higher CCI having a greater impact (CCI=2: odds ratio, 2.3; $P=0.06$; CCI=≥ 3: odds ratio, 3.5; $P=0.001$).

Conclusions.—Comorbid medical conditions as measured by the CCI independently influence outcome after ICH. Future ICH outcome studies should account for the impact of comorbidities on patient outcome.

▶ The Charlson Comorbidity Index (CCI) is a tool to stratify patients according to the burden of diseases already present when outcome of disease or treatment is being analyzed. This can be important if the preexisting diseases are alone likely to lead to poor outcomes that need to be distinguished from the disease or treatment of consideration.

The authors were able to compare values of the CCI at admission of patients suffering from nontraumatic intracerebral hemorrhage (and in some cases, modified values were available if the patient returned to the hospital before 12 months after the index event) with 30-day mortality and functional outcome at 12 months.

In each outcome analysis, increasing CCI did independently predict worsening outcome. No attempt was made to identify particular elements of the CCI (prior diseases such as connective tissue disease or congestive heart failure) with the functional outcome, however. It may be that certain comorbidities play a greater role in combination with the post—intracerebral hemorrhage outcome. This will have to be determined in future studies.

In the meantime, knowing the CCI for patients when they arrive in the emergency department, we can begin to have conversations with our patients and families about what to expect in the future.

N. B. Handly, MD, MSc, MS

Combination warfarin-ASA therapy: Which patients should receive it, which patients should not, and why?
Douketis JD (McMaster Univ and St Joseph's Healthcare, Hamilton, Ontario, Canada)
Thromb Res 127:513-517, 2011

Combination warfarin-ASA therapy is currently used in approximately 800,000 patients in North America as long-term treatment for the primary and secondary prevention of atherothrombotic and thromboembolic diseases. Despite a potentially complementary action of anticoagulant and antiplatelet drugs, the use of combination warfarin-ASA therapy is not based on compelling evidence of a net therapeutic benefit, with the exception of patients with a mechanical heart valve. On the other hand, there is more compelling and consistent evidence that combination warfarin-ASA therapy confers a 1.5- to 2.0-fold increased risk for serious bleeding compared with use of warfarin alone. In everyday practice, clinicians should combine the best available evidence with clinical judgment, considering that in most clinical scenarios, clinical practice guideline may not provide clear recommendations for patients who should, and should not, receive combination warfarin-ASA therapy. The objectives of this review are to describe which patients are receiving combined warfarin-aspirin therapy, to summarize the evidence for the therapeutic benefit and harm of combined warfarin-ASA therapy, and to suggest practical guidelines as to which patients should, and should not, receive such treatment.

▶ Think about the concept of "if some is good then more is better."
You see a patient with chronic atrial fibrillation on Coumadin presenting with acute coronary syndrome. Among the steps to follow, you start aspirin therapy.

It seems only natural, and you do not think much about it. But what is the risk-benefit picture for using Coumadin and aspirin?

This review seeks to address just this issue. It does turn out that there may be few reasons for using both medications long term (although in the setting of patients with mechanical valves or those individuals receiving drug eluting stents, there is good reason for long-term use of both medications). However, the risk of significant bleeding may otherwise outweigh combined use of Coumadin and aspirin.

As emergency physicians, we are not going to be making the decisions about starting patients on long-term combination therapy. But it will be useful when talking with our consultants and primary physicians to remain abreast of this review and its recommendations. Of course, on the horizon we can expect to be challenged with medication reconciliation tasks involving these medications.

N. B. Handly, MD, MSc, MS

Comparing National Institutes of Health Funding of Emergency Medicine to Four Medical Specialties
Bessman SC, Agada NO, Ding R, et al (Johns Hopkins Univ School of Medicine, Baltimore, MD; et al)
Acad Emerg Med 18:1001-1004, 2011

Objectives.—The purpose of this study was to compare National Institutes of Health (NIH) funding received in 2008 by emergency medicine (EM) to the specialties of internal medicine, pediatrics, anesthesiology, and family medicine. The hypothesis was that EM would receive fewer NIH awards and less funding dollars per active physician and per medical school faculty member compared to the other four specialties.

Methods.—Research Portfolio Online Reporting Tools (RePORT) were used to identify NIH-funded grants to 125 of the 133 U.S. allopathic medical schools for fiscal year 2008 (the most recent year with all grant funding information). Eight medical schools were excluded because six were not open in 2008, one did not have a website, and one did not have funding data available by medical specialty. From RePORT, all grants awarded to EM, internal medicine, family medicine, anesthesiology, and pediatric departments of each medical school were identified for fiscal year 2008. The authors extracted the project number, project title, dollars awarded, and name of the principal investigator for each grant. Funds awarded to faculty in divisions of EM were accounted for by identifying the department of the EM division and searching for all grants awarded to EM faculty within those departments using the name of the principal investigator. The total number of active physicians per medical specialty was acquired from the Association of American Medical Colleges' 2008 Physician Specialty report. The total number of faculty per medical specialty was collected by two research assistants who independently counted the faculty listed on each medical school website. The authors compared the total number of NIH awards and total funding per 1,000 active physicians and per 1,000 faculty members by medical specialty.

Results.—Of the 125 medical schools included in the study, 84 had departments of EM (67%). In 2008, NIH awarded over 9,000 grants and approximately $4 billion to the five medical specialties of interest. Less than 1% of the grants and funds were awarded to EM. EM had the second-lowest number of awards and funding per active physician, and the lowest number of awards and funding per faculty member. A higher percentage of grants awarded to EM were career development awards (26%, vs. a range of 11% to 19% for the other specialties) and cooperative agreements (26%, vs. 2% to 10%). In 2008, EM was the only specialty of the five not to have a fellowship or T32 training grant. EM had the lowest proportion of research project awards (42%, vs. 58% to 73%).

Conclusions.—Compared to internal medicine, pediatrics, anesthesiology, and family medicine, EM received the least amount of NIH support per active faculty member and ranked next to last for NIH support by active physician. Given the many benefits of research both for the specialty and for society, EM needs to continue to develop and support an adequate cohort of independent investigators.

▶ The authors present the numbers of grants and amounts of awards in the National Institutes of Health (NIH) funds for the specialties of emergency medicine, internal medicine, pediatrics, and anesthesiology in this article. It is certainly interesting to be aware of the differences because now it is a reasonable step to understand why the differences exist.

We know that it may be hard to compare the interests of emergency physicians with organ-based specialties, such as orthopedics or nephrology. It may be a great problem trying to find appropriate comparable specialties for this kind of study, however. Internal medicine may be too broad a group of interests, including organ-based specialties and general care. Similarly, pediatrics would also have both organ-based and general research interests. The authors suggested that emergency medicine might have resuscitation and operations as key research topics. If so, then it would be a better comparison for how well emergency physicians do at receiving grants in the resuscitation area (and be compared with cardiac and trauma resuscitation efforts among other specialties). The operations aspect of emergency care is likely to fall far outside the kind of funding that the NIH would provide and might better be supported by the National Science Foundation.

The differences found for numbers and values of grants received per faculty (or total practicing emergency physician) may say quite a lot about expectations from residents and faculty and the experience they have toward performing research. Perhaps shift work does not provide the same kind of routine focus on research as part of the practice of emergency medicine even at academic training sites.

Success in grantsmanship will increasingly depend on institutional support (medical schools, hospitals, and residencies). Do emergency physicians get the same kind of support in the process as members of other specialties? This article starts the thinking process.

N. B. Handly, MD, MSc, MS

Constructing a Composite Quality Score for the Care of Acute Myocardial Infarction Patients at Discharge: Impact on Hospital Ranking

Couralet M, Guérin S, Le Vaillant M, et al (Institut Gustave Roussy, Villejuif, France)
Med Care 49:569-576, 2011

Objective.—To determine the impact on hospital ranking of different aggregation methods when creating a composite score from a set of quality indicators relating to a single clinical condition.

Design.—The analysis was based on 14966 medical records taken from all French hospitals that treated over 30 patients with acute myocardial infarction in 2008 (n = 275). Five quality indicators measuring the quality of care delivered to patients with acute myocardial infarction at hospital discharge were aggregated by 5 methods issued from a variety of activity sectors (indicator average, all-or-none, budget allocation process, benefit of the doubt, and unobserved component model).

Main Outcome Measures.—Each aggregation method was used to rank hospitals into 3 categories depending on the position of the 95% confidence interval of the composite score relative to the overall mean. Variations in rank according to method were estimated using weighted κ coefficients.

Results.—Agreement between methods ranged from poor (κ = 0.20) to almost perfect (κ = 0.84). A change of method led to a change in rank for 71% (196 of 275) of hospitals. Only 14 of 121 hospitals which were ranked top and 20 of 118 which were ranked bottom, by at least 1 of the 5 methods, held their rank on a switch to the 4 other methods.

Conclusion.—Hospital ranking varied widely according to 5 aggregation methods. If one method has to be chosen, for instance for reporting to governments, regulatory agencies, payers, health care professionals, and the public, it is necessary to provide its rationale and characteristics, and information on score uncertainty.

▶ Do you receive a patient satisfaction score? Medicare and Medicaid will be paying based on satisfaction scores soon. Scores are all around us, and this article offers an interesting look at how scores may be combined and what are the implications of that.

You and your hospital have agreed that there is a cluster of 8 meaningful actions that should be completed before discharge after acute myocardial infarction (AMI). It is now time to read the report of how well you are managing these patients by how well you have successfully met the 8 actions (this is what the authors have done).

You read with surprise that for more than half of your patients this past month, there is no data found for actions 1 and 2. Can you just leave out patients for whom some data are missing? Imputing, the process of filling in missing data, might be in order, but if you know little about how your hospital has been practicing, it might be hard to know at first whether these missing values should be successes or failures. Perhaps you institute better data recording procedures after the first month.

After the second month, you see that you have improved your data recording and collection skills and can provide results for 98% of your discharged AMI patients. At this point, you feel that the numbers actually mean something about your practices. You find that step 1 is accomplished about 20% of the time, whereas all the other actions are accomplished more than 90% of the time. Because you have results for the individual actions, you can make up a plan to improve the successes of step 1.

At the same time as your hospital has made these data available to the public, so have 2 other hospitals in your community. Each site makes efforts to improve their success rates to above 90% at the start (maybe even going for Six Sigma?). Now, how should prospective patients look at these data? The public might recognize that low frequencies of success of various steps mean that something is not right. But if each hospital has a different profile of successes and failures, how will an individual decide which hospital is truly better?

That is the point of this study. The authors looked at different ways of combining scores from different processes into a single number, the idea being that it would be easier for the public to understand a single number when deciding which hospital is best. It does matter how the final result is obtained—hospitals were grouped differently on the basis of these methods.

It matters when communicating results to patients, and likewise it matters when trying to create a single patient satisfaction score. You may not want to get into the math, but you better be ready to ask how someone is calculating the score.

N. B. Handly, MD, MSc, MS

Diagnostic Blood Loss From Phlebotomy and Hospital-Acquired Anemia During Acute Myocardial Infarction
Salisbury AC, Reid KJ, Alexander KP, et al (Saint Luke's Mid America Heart and Vascular Inst, Kansas City, MO; Duke Clinical Res Inst, Durham, NC; et al)
Arch Intern Med 171:1646-1653, 2011

Background.—Hospital-acquired anemia (HAA) during acute myocardial infarction (AMI) is associated with higher mortality and worse health status and often develops in the absence of recognized bleeding. The extent to which diagnostic phlebotomy, a modifiable process of care, contributes to HAA is unknown.

Methods.—We studied 17 676 patients with AMI from 57 US hospitals included in a contemporary AMI database from January 1, 2000, through December 31, 2008, who were not anemic at admission but developed moderate to severe HAA (in which the hemoglobin level declined from normal to <11 g/dL), a degree of HAA that has been shown to be prognostically important. Patients' total diagnostic blood loss was calculated by multiplying the number and types of blood tubes drawn by the standard volume for each tube type. Hierarchical modified Poisson regression was used to test the association between phlebotomy and moderate to severe HAA, after adjusting for site and potential confounders.

Results.—Moderate to severe HAA developed in 3551 patients (20%). The mean (SD) phlebotomy volume was higher in patients with HAA (173.8 [139.3] mL) vs those without HAA (83.5 [52.0 mL]; $P < .001$). There was significant variation in the mean diagnostic blood loss across hospitals (moderate to severe HAA: range, 119.1-246.0 mL; mild HAA or no HAA: 53.0-110.1 mL). For every 50 mL of blood drawn, the risk of moderate to severe HAA increased by 18% (relative risk [RR], 1.18; 95% confidence interval [CI], 1.13-1.22), which was only modestly attenuated after multivariable adjustment (RR, 1.15; 95% CI, 1.12-1.18).

Conclusions.—Blood loss from greater use of phlebotomy is independently associated with the development of HAA. These findings suggest that HAA may be preventable by implementing strategies to limit blood loss from laboratory testing.

▶ We all have seen unnecessary blood draws, but what about blood draws that contribute to worsening anemia? The authors chose to follow the hospital courses for patients with normal hemoglobin levels on arrival who were admitted for acute myocardial infarction.

The data did not contain specific values of volume of blood drawn at specific times; however, blood volumes were estimated based on the tests completed and amount of blood needed for that test. This likely would be a lower bound on total blood collected.

Among patients reaching a state of significant anemia while in the hospital, there was a pattern of larger total volume of blood drawn. This does not prove that the blood loss that was the basis of the diagnosis of in-hospital anemia was due to the blood draws alone, however. Consider that the patient developed bleeding problems (after anticoagulation), and more blood draws were done to manage this in-hospital bleeding.

Reducing the amount of blood drawn is one corrective action to apply (if lab equipment can accommodate smaller tubes). Also, a more judicious use of blood tests would be in order.

N. B. Handly, MD, MSc, MS

Effects of Benefits and Harms on Older Persons' Willingness to Take Medication for Primary Cardiovascular Prevention

Fried TR, Tinetti ME, Towle V, et al (Yale Univ School of Medicine, New Haven, CT)
Arch Intern Med 171:923-928, 2011

Background.—Quality-assurance initiatives encourage adherence to evidenced-based guidelines based on a consideration of treatment benefit. We examined older persons' willingness to take medication for primary cardiovascular disease prevention according to benefits and harms.

Methods.—In-person interviews were performed with 356 community-living older persons. Participants were asked about their willingness to take medication for primary prevention of myocardial infarction (MI) with varying benefits in terms of absolute 5-year risk reduction and varying harms in terms of type and severity of adverse effects.

Results.—Most (88%) would take medication, providing an absolute benefit of 6 fewer persons with MI out of 100, approximating the average risk reduction of currently available medications. Of participants who would not take it, 17% changed their preference if the absolute benefit was increased to 10 fewer persons with MI, and, of participants who would take it, 82% remained willing if the absolute benefit was decreased to 3 fewer persons with MI. In contrast, large proportions (48%-69%) were unwilling or uncertain about taking medication with average benefit causing mild fatigue, nausea, or fuzzy thinking, and only 3% would take medication with adverse effects severe enough to affect functioning.

Conclusions.—Older persons' willingness to take medication for primary cardiovascular disease prevention is relatively insensitive to its benefit but highly sensitive to its adverse effects. These results suggest that clinical guidelines and decisions about prescribing these medications to older persons need to place emphasis on both benefits and harms.

▶ The human brain has a hard time working out the balance of benefit and risks when making decisions. So are these rational decisions? Not likely, but they are informed in some way.

As emergency physicians, we are not often going to be prescribing primary prevention medications such as statins. However, we will have the opportunity to start new medications even if for short periods. Thus it would be worth becoming aware of how our patients think about medications and how they consider benefits and risks of using them.

The authors surveyed older individuals at senior centers about a theoretical new medicine and whether these individuals would take this medicine. First, a series of benefit scenarios (no side effects were assumed for these scenarios) were posed, and patients were asked if they would take the medicine. The greater the relative and absolute benefit, the greater the number of respondents who agreed they would take the medication.

A subsequent set of scenarios included not just the variation in benefit but a variety of side effects and of different levels of severity. Even slight side effects changed respondents' willingness to use a medication.

I am sure there is a similar process going through most of our patients' heads when we prescribe new medications. They want to know the side effects, how severe these effects are, and how likely they are to occur. We may also run into this kind of problem as we participate more in medication reconciliation. Sure it is easy to just ask, "What are you taking now?" But it makes sense that we should also ask, "Which ones have you chosen to stop and why?"

N. B. Handly, MD, MSc, MS

Emergency Department Utilization After the Implementation of Massachusetts Health Reform

Smulowitz PB, Lipton R, Wharam JF, et al (Beth Israel Deaconess Med Ctr, Boston, MA; Harvard Med School and Harvard Pilgrim Health Care Inst, Boston, MA)
Ann Emerg Med 58:225-234, 2011

Study Objective.—Health care reform in Massachusetts improved access to health insurance, but the extent to which reform affected utilization of the emergency department (ED) for conditions potentially amenable to primary care is unclear. Our objective is to determine the relationship between health reform and ED use for low-severity conditions.

Methods.—We studied ED visits, using a convenience sample of 11 Massachusetts hospitals for identical 9-month periods before and after health care reform legislation was implemented in 2006. Individuals most affected by the health reform law (the uninsured and low-income populations covered by the publicly subsidized insurance products) were compared with individuals unlikely to be affected by the legislation (those with Medicare or private insurance). Our main outcome measure was the rate of overall and low-severity ED visits for the study population and the comparison population during the period before and after health reform implementation.

Results.—Total visits increased from 424,878 in 2006 to 442,102 in 2008. Low-severity visits among publicly subsidized or uninsured patients decreased from 43.8% to 41.2% of total visits for that group (difference=2.6%; 95% confidence interval [CI] 2.25% to 2.85%), whereas low-severity visits for privately insured and Medicare patients decreased from 35.7% to 34.9% of total visits for that group (difference=0.8%; 95% CI 0.62% to 0.98%), for a difference in differences of 1.8% (95% CI 1.7% to 1.9%).

Conclusion.—Although overall ED volume continues to increase, Massachusetts health reform was associated with a small but statistically significant decrease in the rate of low-severity visits for those populations most affected by health reform compared with a comparison population of individuals less likely to be affected by the reform. Our findings suggest that access to health insurance is only one of a multitude of factors affecting utilization of the ED (Fig 4).

▶ Whether you agree with the merits of the Patient Protection and Affordable Care Act (PPACA or Obamacare), it is likely here to stay. In general, the best predictor of the future comes from studying the past. The Massachusetts Health Reform was, in all practical purposes, the precursor to the PPACA. Studying its effects on the medical system is important to understanding what may occur in the future and may allow the rest of the nation to be prepared.

This study was conducted to examine the effects of the health care reform legislation on emergency department use in the state of Massachusetts. This was done by using a convenience sample of 11 hospitals and comparing 3

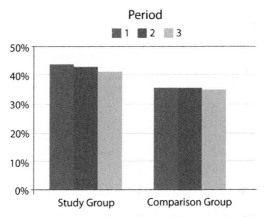

Period

FIGURE 4.—Low severity ED visit volume. (Reprinted from Annals of Emergency Medicine, Smulowitz PB, Lipton R, Wharam JF, et al. Emergency department utilization after the implementation of Massachusetts health reform. *Ann Emerg Med.* 2011;58:225-234. Copyright 2011, with permission from the American College of Emergency Physicians.)

periods of time: before reform, during the enrollment period, and after health reform. Overall emergency department visits increased by 4.1% from 2006 to 2008. Using a previously validated algorithm that helped classify patients as having low-, indeterminate-, high-severity, or unclassified visits, the authors were able to determine that low-severity visits in the study group decreased by 2.6% (see Fig 4). Interestingly, the percentage of low-severity emergency department visits did not decrease to the level of the comparison group (those unaffected by the law, such as Medicare patients).

So why did health reform have such a limited effect on emergency department utilization? First, although access to health care should be improved when insurance is acquired, limitations in the availability of primary care may have limited the effect. This, despite the fact that Massachusetts has the most primary care physicians per capita in the United States, should concern the rest of the nation. In addition, even with adequate coverage, it might take time and effort to alter care-seeking patterns that have become ingrained in some communities. Many previously uninsured patients have never had insurance before, so they may be used to relying on the emergency department instead of other care settings. This behavior may take years to unlearn. Because most of the newly insured patients are of low income, they had low or nonexistent co-pays for emergency department visits. Unfortunately, it appears that even people who may previously have had good insurance, such as Medicare or other private health insurances, still have a high rate of low-severity emergency department visits, approximately 35%. This will likely not change for several reasons, including lack of primary care physicians. Additionally, many Americans find emergency departments convenient because of the hours of operation, the ability to obtain a comprehensive evaluation and testing at 1 time, patient perceptions about the severity of their illness, and some financial factors. This study is a good start, and I am sure many more will roll out as different parts of the PPACA become effective.

D. K. Mullin, MD

National Survey of Preventive Health Services in US Emergency Departments

Delgado MK, Acosta CD, Ginde AA, et al (Stanford Univ School of Medicine, Palo Alto, CA; Univ of Colorado Denver School of Medicine, Aurora; et al)
Ann Emerg Med 57:104-108, 2011

Study Objective.—We describe the availability of preventive health services in US emergency departments (EDs), as well as ED directors' preferred service and perceptions of barriers to offering preventive services.

Methods.—Using the 2007 National Emergency Department Inventory (NEDI)—USA, we randomly sampled 350 (7%) of 4,874 EDs. We surveyed directors of these EDs to determine the availability of (1) screening and referral programs for alcohol, tobacco, geriatric falls, intimate partner violence, HIV, diabetes, and hypertension; (2) vaccination programs for influenza and pneumococcus; and (3) linkage programs to primary care and health insurance. ED directors were asked to select the service they would most like to implement and to rate 5 potential barriers to offering preventive services.

Results.—Two hundred seventy-seven EDs (80%) responded across 46 states. Availability of services ranged from 66% for intimate partner violence screening to 19% for HIV screening. ED directors wanted to implement primary care linkage most (17%) and HIV screening least (2%). ED directors "agreed/strongly agreed" that the following are barriers to ED preventive care: cost (74%), increased patient length of stay (64%), lack of follow-up (60%), resource shifting leading to worse patient outcomes (53%), and philosophical opposition (27%).

Conclusion.—Most US EDs offer preventive services, but availability and ED director preference for type of service vary greatly. The majority of EDs do not routinely offer Centers for Disease Control and Prevention—recommended HIV screening. Most ED directors are not philosophically opposed to offering preventive services but are concerned with added costs, effects on ED operations, and potential lack of follow-up.

▶ This study provides a snapshot of the availability of preventive health services in US emergency departments (EDs) and what services ED medical directors would prefer to implement. It also catalogs what barriers to offering preventive health services the directors perceived. The study was conducted from September 2008 through April 2009. The median number of services offered was 4 (interquartile range 2-5). Ten percent of the EDs claimed to offer no preventive health services.

Intimate partner violence screening was the most common service offered, being available in 66% of the EDs surveyed. This means that one-third of the EDs are either not compliant with a Joint Commission mandate or their medical directors are unaware of the screening actually being conducted in their EDs. More than one half of the EDs offered reliable primary care clinic linkage (54%) and hypertension screening/referral (51%). Only about one-fifth of the

EDs have implemented the Centers for Disease Control 2006 guideline calling for human immunodeficiency virus screening and referral.

Of the services they did not already offer, ED medical directors most wanted to offer a reliable linkage of patients without a usual source of care to primary care (17%). The second most desired service was smoking cessation counseling/referral (14%).

Almost three-quarters of ED directors were concerned that offering preventive health services would lead to unreimbursed costs. More than one-quarter (27%) thought that preventive services should not be offered in the ED.

E. A. Ramoska, MD, MPHE

Outcomes in Patients Visiting Hospital Emergency Departments in the United States Because of Periodontal Conditions

Elangovan S, Nalliah R, Allareddy V, et al (Harvard Univ, Boston, MA; The Univ of Iowa)
J Periodontol 82:809-819, 2011

Background.—The chances of presenting to hospital emergency departments (EDs) are significantly higher in individuals who ignore regular dental care and in those with medical conditions. Little is known about nationwide estimates of hospital-based ED visits caused by periodontal conditions in the United States. The objective of this study is to determine the incidence of ED visits caused by periodontal conditions that occurred in a 2006 nationwide sample and to identify the risk factors for hospitalization during the ED visits.

Methods.—The Nationwide Emergency Department Sample (NEDS) for 2006 was used for this study. Patients who visited the ED with a primary diagnosis of acute gingivitis, chronic gingivitis, gingival recession, aggressive or acute periodontitis, chronic periodontitis, periodontosis, accretions, other specified periodontal disease, or unspecified gingival and periodontal disease were selected for this study. Estimates were projected to the national levels using the discharge weights. The association between patient characteristics and the odds of being hospitalized was examined using a multivariable logistic regression analysis.

Results.—A total of 85,039 visits to hospital-based EDs with a mean charge per visit of $456.31 and total charges close to $33.3 million were primarily attributed to gingival and periodontal conditions in the United States. Close to 36% and 33% of all visits occurred among the lowest income group and uninsured population, respectively. The total ED charges for those covered by Medicare, Medicaid, private insurance, and other insurance plans were close to $4.95 million, $9.14 million, $8.01 million, and $0.92 million, respectively. The uninsured were charged a total of $10.06 million. Inpatient admission to the same hospital was required for 1,167 visits. The total hospitalization charge for this group was $17.51 million. Patients with comorbid conditions (congestive heart failure, valvular disease, hypertension, paralysis, neurologic disorders, chronic pulmonary disease, hypothyroidism, liver disease, AIDS, coagulopathy, deficiency anemia, obesity, alcohol abuse, or drug abuse) were associated with higher odds for hospitalization during an ED visit for periodontal conditions compared to those without comorbid conditions ($P<0.05$). Patients who had a primary diagnosis of acute or aggressive periodontitis were associated with significantly higher odds of being hospitalized during ED visits.

Conclusions.—Estimates from the NEDS suggest that a total of 85,039 hospital-based ED visits had a primary diagnosis for periodontal conditions. Close to \$33.3 million was charged by hospitals for treating these conditions on an emergency basis. ED visits with a primary diagnosis for acute and aggressive periodontitis, covered by Medicare insurance, and comorbid conditions were more likely to result in hospitalization based on the analysis of the NEDS. However, when interpreting these conclusions, one should keep the limitations inherent to hospital discharge datasets in perspective.

▶ During 2006, a little more than 85 000 people visited emergency departments (EDs) for periodontal conditions. This was 0.07% of all ED visits for that year. The vast majority were treated and released, with only approximately 1.5% being admitted to the hospital. As might be expected, a slightly disproportionate share of the visits occurred during the weekend. Furthermore, one-third of the visits occurred among the uninsured, and almost 36% of all visits occurred among the lowest income group (< \$38 000/y). This study provides a snapshot of one type of dental condition seen in the ED and confirms what we probably all instinctively thought: most dental complaints are benign, more present on the weekend, and the patients are commonly uninsured and/or poor.

E. A. Ramoska, MD, MPHE

The Effect of Triage Diagnostic Standing Orders on Emergency Department Treatment Time

Retezar R, Bessman E, Ding R, et al (Johns Hopkins Univ School of Medicine, Baltimore, MD; et al)
Ann Emerg Med 57:89-99, 2011

Study Objective.—Triage standing orders are used in emergency departments (EDs) to initiate evaluation when there is no bed available. This study evaluates the effect of diagnostic triage standing orders on ED treatment time of adult patients who presented with a chief complaint for which triage standing orders had been developed.

Methods.—We conducted a retrospective nested cohort study of patients treated in one academic ED between January 2007 and August 2009. In this ED, triage nurses can initiate full or partial triage standing orders for patients with chest pain, shortness of breath, abdominal pain, or genitourinary complaints. We matched patients who received triage standing orders to those who received room orders with respect to clinical and temporal factors, using a propensity score. We compared the median treatment time of patients with triage standing orders (partial or full) to those with room orders, using multivariate linear regression.

Results.—Of the 15,188 eligible patients, 25% received full triage standing orders, 56% partial triage standing orders, and 19% room orders. The unadjusted median ED treatment time for patients who did not receive triage standing orders was 282 minutes versus 230 minutes for those who received a partial triage standing order or full triage standing orders (18% decrease). Controlling for other factors, triage standing orders were associated with a 16% reduction (95% confidence interval −18% to −13%) in the median treatment time, regardless of chief complaint.

Conclusion.—Diagnostic testing at triage was associated with a substantial reduction in ED treatment time for 4 common chief complaints. This intervention warrants further evaluation in other EDs and with different clinical conditions and tests.

▶ This study from Johns Hopkins University School of Medicine was conducted at a community teaching hospital emergency department (ED) that was staffed with emergency medicine residents and midlevel providers, under the supervision of 1 to 2 attending physicians per shift. Of the 132 589 patients who presented to the ED during the 32-month study period, 38 719 patients (29%) were eligible for inclusion (ie, these patients had 1 of the 4 chief complaints for which triage standing orders were developed: chest pain, shortness of breath, abdominal pain, or genitourinary complaints). Ultimately, 12 323 patients (32% of the eligible patients and 9.3% of the census) had either partial or full triage standing orders implemented. Overall, the unadjusted median ED treatment time, for patients who received either partial or full triage standing orders, declined 52 minutes (18%) when compared with patients who received diagnostic orders only after being placed in a room. After adjusting for patient, clinical, and temporal factors, the reduction was 16%.

Treatment times varied substantially by chief complaint. There were decreases in treatment time for each of the chief complaint categories for patients who received either full or partial triage standing orders when compared with patients receiving only room orders. Interestingly, this generalization breaks down when the authors examined the implementation of partial triage standing orders versus full triage standing orders. In this comparison the adjusted change in treatment time was decreased for shortness of breath (−14%) but increased for abdominal pain (+ 13%). The other 2 categories (chest pain and genitourinary) as well as the 4 categories combined did not show a statistically significant difference in treatment time.

This study appears to demonstrate that triage standing orders implemented by the nurse can decrease treatment time compared with waiting for the patient to be placed in a room. What remains to be defined is which particular chief complaints and specific diagnostic studies will lead to a reduction in treatment time.

E. A. Ramoska, MD, MPHE

Miscellaneous

A pragmatic randomised trial of stretching before and after physical activity to prevent injury and soreness

Jamtvedt G, Herbert RD, Flottorp S, et al (Norwegian Knowledge Centre for the Health Services, Oslo, Norway; The George Inst for International Health, Sydney, Australia; et al)
Br J Sports Med 44:1002-1009, 2010

Objective.—To determine the effects of stretching before and after physical activity on risks of injury and soreness in a community population.

Design.—Internet-based pragmatic randomised trial conducted between January 2008 and January 2009.

Setting.—International.

Participants.—A total of 2377 adults who regularly participated in physical activity.

Interventions.—Participants in the stretch group were asked to perform 30 s static stretches of seven lower limb and trunk muscle groups before and after physical activity for 12 weeks. Participants in the control group were asked not to stretch.

Main Outcome Measurements.—Participants provided weekly on-line reports of outcomes over 12 weeks. Primary outcomes were any injury to the lower limb or back, and bothersome soreness of the legs, buttocks or back. Injury to muscles, ligaments and tendons was a secondary outcome.

Results.—Stretching did not produce clinically important or statistically significant reductions in all-injury risk (HR=0.97, 95% CI 0.84 to 1.13), but did reduce the risk of experiencing bothersome soreness (mean risk of bothersome soreness in a week was 24.6% in the stretch group and 32.3% in the control group; OR=0.69, 95% CI 0.59 to 0.82). Stretching reduced the risk of injuries to muscles, ligaments and tendons (incidence rate of 0.66 injuries per person-year in the stretch group and 0.88 injuries per person-year in the control group; HR=0.75, 95% CI 0.59 to 0.96).

Conclusion.—Stretching before and after physical activity does not appreciably reduce all-injury risk but probably reduces the risk of some injuries, and does reduce the risk of bothersome soreness.

Trial Registration.—anzctr.org.au 12608000044325.

▶ There are 2 important points to this report. One is the result of the study, and the other is the way it was done.

It is easy to picture the situation when either preparing to exercise ourselves or when talking to our patients about exercise that the issue of stretching comes up. So what is the evidence for stretching as a means to prevent injuries or reduce soreness? The authors find that there are not many studies that apply well to the typical setting of amateur athletes we would encounter. The authors devised a setting for those who exercise on a regular basis to participate randomly to either a no-stretch or active-stretch group and measure outcomes at the beginning of the study and for each week for 12 weeks.

The results showed statistically insignificant results for most outcomes and perhaps clinically insignificant results overall. What should be a meaningful difference on a 0 to 10 scale for soreness or looseness? Some interesting patterns appear, however: as one ages, the effect of stretching may turn from helpful to harmful, and not surprisingly, if one believes that stretching should help, there is greater likelihood of self-reported better outcomes with stretching.

The other important aspect to this study is how it was designed. This was an Internet study in which the subjects participated through e-mail and Web responses. Randomization was driven by computers without human interaction, and recruitment occurred only by traditional radio or TV media. Of course one could wonder about the validity of results obtained. (Were the subjects lying in their responses? Could subjects bias the study by enrolling multiple times?) These kinds of problems occur in most survey studies. As long as there are safeguards built into the studies, using the Internet will likely prove to be a valuable medium for studies.

N. B. Handly, MD, MSc, MS

Assessment of a Training Curriculum for Emergency Ultrasound for Pediatric Soft Tissue Infections

Marin JR, Alpern ER, Panebianco NL, et al (Univ of Pittsburgh School of Medicine, PA; Univ of Pennsylvania School of Medicine, Philadelphia)
Acad Emerg Med 18:174-182, 2011

Objectives.—The objective was to evaluate a training protocol for pediatric emergency physicians (EPs) learning emergency ultrasound (EUS) for the evaluation of skin and soft tissue infections (SSTIs) by assessing technical ability and interrater reliability.

Methods.—Pediatric emergency medicine (EM) fellows and attending physicians completed a 1-day training course taught by an expert emergency sonologist. After the course, EPs performed proctored examinations on patients with SSTIs until they reached predefined performance criteria, after which they performed independent EUS examinations. All EUS examinations were recorded using still images and video clips that were reviewed and rated by the expert sonologist on four technical measures and combined into a composite score. The expert's opinion regarding the presence or absence of an abscess was also compared to the study sonologist's opinion and analyzed for interrater reliability.

Results.—Seven EPs performed 107 EUS examinations. The mean ($\pm$ SD) composite score for the evaluation of technical ability for the first EUS was 3.3 $\pm$ 0.14 (on a 4-point scale), indicating a high level of quality following the training course. There was a small amount of improvement in the quality score (0.015, 95% confidence interval [CI] = 0.0003 to 0.03) with each consecutive EUS examination. The interrater reliability between the sonologist and the expert for the presence of an abscess as measured by the kappa statistic was 0.80 (95% CI = 0.63 to 0.97), indicating substantial agreement.

Conclusions.—After a brief training program, pediatric EPs can perform technically successful emergency EUS examination of SSTIs, with excellent agreement with an expert sonologist.

▶ Emergency ultrasound (EUS) is rapidly becoming an adjunctive tool for bedside clinical evaluation, much like the stethoscope, otoscope, or ophthalmoscope. The Accreditation Council for Graduate Medical Education has made EUS a mandatory core competency in emergency medicine (EM) residency training. All EM residents, for at least the past decade, have had EUS training as part of their curriculum. This study shows that after a brief training program and a short period of supervised exams, novice physicians can be taught how to competently use EUS in the evaluation of skin and soft-tissue infections. Moreover, they retained the skill for up to 14 months after the initial training.

Older physicians who have not been trained in the use of EUS should not be put off by this newfangled technology. The skills are easily obtained after brief educational sessions and a few proctored exams. The use of EUS at the bedside can be valuable in select patients and will increase diagnostic acumen.

E. A. Ramoska, MD, MPHE

ED handoffs: observed practices and communication errors
Maughan BC, Lei L, Cydulka RK (Rhode Island Hosp & Warren Alpert School of Medicine of Brown Univ, Providence; Univ of Rochester Med Ctr, NY; MetroHealth Med Ctr and Case Western Reserve Univ, Cleveland, OH)
Am J Emerg Med 29:502-511, 2011

Objective.—The study objectives were to identify emergency department (ED) handoff practices and describe handoff communication errors among emergency physicians.

Methods.—Two investigators observed patient handoffs among emergency physicians in a major metropolitan teaching hospital for 8 weeks. A data collection form was designed to assess handoff characteristics including duration, location, interruptions, and topics including examination, laboratory examinations, diagnosis, and disposition. Handoff errors were defined as clinically significant examination or laboratory findings in physician documentation that were reported significantly differently during or omitted from verbal handoff. Multivariate negative binomial regression models assessed variables associated with these errors. The study was approved by the institutional review board.

Results.—One hundred ten handoff sessions encompassing 992 patients were observed. Examination handoff errors and omissions were noted in 130 (13.1%) and 447 (45.1%) handoffs, respectively. More examination errors were associated with longer handoff time per patient, whereas fewer examination omissions were associated with use of written or electronic support materials. Laboratory handoff errors and omissions were noted in 37 (3.7%) and 290 (29.2%) handoffs, respectively. Fewer laboratory errors were associated with use of electronic support tools, whereas more laboratory handoff omissions were associated with longer ED lengths of stay.

Conclusions.—Clinically pertinent findings reported in ED physician handoff often differ from findings reported in physician documentation. These errors and omissions are associated with handoff time per patient, ED length of stay, and use of support materials. Future research should focus on ED handoff standardization protocols, handoff error reduction techniques, and the impact of handoff on patient outcomes.

▶ Emergency department handoffs have always plagued emergency physicians. They now are affecting all fields thanks to what seems to be stricter intern and resident work hours being enforced each year. Poor communication is recognized as a major factor contributing to the estimated 44 000 to 195 000 patient deaths that occur each year because of medical errors. A recent survey of surgical and medical residents found that 59% reported one or more of their patients harmed as a result of inadequate handoffs.

This was a fairly well-done study. There were 2 major take-home points. One was that the longer a patient stayed in the emergency department, the more likely it was that the handoff was going to be associated with omissions of both examination and laboratory results. Second, if handoffs were done via typed, handwritten, or electronic medical record notes, omissions of examination and laboratory results were less likely.

This study will hopefully be used as a starting point for future ones to determine the best ways to handoff between physicians. As of now, almost 90% of emergency medicine residencies have no existing uniform handoff policy. This obviously needs to change, but we first need to understand what the problems are and then attempt to fix them.

D. K. Mullin, MD

ED handoffs: observed practices and communication errors
Maughan BC, Lei L, Cydulka RK (Rhode Island Hosp & Warren Alpert School of Medicine of Brown Univ, Providence; Univ of Rochester Med Ctr, NY; MetroHealth Med Ctr and Case Western Reserve Univ, Cleveland, OH)
Am J Emerg Med 29:502-511, 2011

Objective.—The study objectives were to identify emergency department (ED) handoff practices and describe handoff communication errors among emergency physicians.

Methods.—Two investigators observed patient handoffs among emergency physicians in a major metropolitan teaching hospital for 8 weeks. A data collection form was designed to assess handoff characteristics including duration, location, interruptions, and topics including examination, laboratory examinations, diagnosis, and disposition. Handoff errors were defined as clinically significant examination or laboratory findings in physician documentation that were reported significantly differently during or omitted from verbal handoff. Multivariate negative binomial regression models assessed variables associated with these errors. The study was approved by the institutional review board.

Results.—One hundred ten handoff sessions encompassing 992 patients were observed. Examination handoff errors and omissions were noted in 130 (13.1%) and 447 (45.1%) handoffs, respectively. More examination errors were associated with longer handoff time per patient, whereas fewer examination omissions were associated with use of written or electronic support materials. Laboratory handoff errors and omissions were noted in 37 (3.7%) and 290 (29.2%) handoffs, respectively. Fewer laboratory errors were associated with use of electronic support tools, whereas more laboratory handoff omissions were associated with longer ED lengths of stay.

Conclusions.—Clinically pertinent findings reported in ED physician handoff often differ from findings reported in physician documentation. These errors and omissions are associated with handoff time per patient, ED length of stay, and use of support materials. Future research should focus on ED handoff standardization protocols, handoff error reduction techniques, and the impact of handoff on patient outcomes.

▶ Consistency is surely a critical component for error-free hand-offs. But it is hard to imagine how to do this without a different view of how information is used in patient care. In this report, the authors identified variability during sign out—by itself, this characteristic of hand-off practice is useful—and several other patterns when errors or omissions occur. (Because they did not study outcomes, it was not possible to show if these were clinically significant.) Much of what they found is similar to that seen in other hand-off studies in the emergency department although some changes may be a result of the local practice environment and culture.

One way to be consistent is to tell all, but this would be like reading the entire clinical chart (historical, physical examination, and test values) and make room for time to present clinical suspicions and differential diagnoses (probably the most important and difficult to describe in a medical record). Somewhere in this discussion needs to be time to present a task list of what else there is to be done. This is a large menu and would not likely be practical in terms of time and energy. The hand-off needs to be an edited or abridged version of this story. In fact, the content of hand-offs might be akin to translation, and we are seeking the right idioms in this translation that communicate the story well enough to our colleagues in very brief moments.

I do not know if computers or forms are the answer; perhaps a short course in journalism would help us get our thoughts clearer for communication?

N. B. Handly, MD, MSc, MS

Evaluation of the Effectiveness of Systematized Training of Advanced Trauma Life Support Protocol in the Interpretation of Cervical Spine and Chest Radiographs in Three Different Emergency Services
Job PM Jr, Von Bahten LC, de Oliveira N Jr (Hospital Universitario Cajuru and Pontificia Universidade Católica do Paraná, Brazil)
J Trauma 70:E122-E124, 2011

Introduction.—Most Brazilian hospitals have no medical radiologists for emergencies. The radiologic evaluation is provided by doctors with heterogeneous generalist training. The objective is to demonstrate the need for systematization in the care of trauma in the interpretation of cervical spine and chest radiographs. Is it possible that, through a continuing education program, generalist doctors could be trained in the evaluation of these radiographs?

Materials and Methods.—Twenty-five doctors of various specialties were evaluated in the mid region of Santa Catarina Stage, in three stages. Initially, the doctors evaluated seven cervical spine radiographs and seven chest radiographs (stage I). After this evaluation (without knowing the results of the examinations), the doctors received advanced trauma life support protocol training for the interpretation of cervical spine and chest radiographs, through an exhibition class (stage II). Three weeks later, the same doctors were evaluated again, interpreting the same radiographs.

Results.—The mean percentage of correct answers was 60.73% in the first interpretation of cervical radiographs and 65.25% for the chest radiographs. None of the participants had reached 100%. In stage III, the average success rates in cervical spine and chest radiographs were 86.95% and 87.53%, respectively, an improvement of 21.72% and 26.18% ($p < 0.001$). During evaluation in the stage III, seven doctors obtained 100% success in the evaluation of cervical spine radiographs and two doctors achieved 100% success in the evaluation of chest radiographs.

Conclusion.—The systematized training, through the advanced trauma life support protocol, significantly increased the success rate of the evaluation of cervical spine and chest radiographs.

▶ This Brazilian study may not seem to have much to do with emergency medicine (EM) in the United States; however, remember that there are still many smaller hospitals in rural areas of the United States that are staffed with non-EM-trained physicians and with midlevel practitioners. Until we reach a time when board-certified emergency physicians staff all of our emergency departments, these hospitals and their practitioners would benefit from a standardized approach to the care of trauma patients, such as is offered by courses like advanced trauma life support (ATLS). In hospitals where the practitioners are not residency-trained EM physicians, it is paramount to ensure that they have the basic knowledge required to adequately assess and treat any and all patients. Merit-badge courses, such as Advanced Cardiac Life Support, Pediatric Advanced Life Support, Advanced Paediatric Life Support, and Advanced Trauma Life

Support, are essential for non-EM physicians and midlevel practitioners to ensure that a basic level of clinical competence is attained.

E. A. Ramoska, MD, MPHE

Hot water irrigation as treatment for intractable posterior epistaxis in an out-patient setting
Novoa E, Schlegel-Wagner C (Kantonsspital Luzern, Switzerland)
J Laryngol Otol 126:58-60, 2012

The management of intractable posterior epistaxis is challenging for any physician. Nasal packing, often combined with use of an endonasal balloon system, is painful for the patient, and torturous to maintain for two to three days. If conservative treatment fails, the most commonly used treatment options are currently invasive procedures such as endoscopic coagulation of bleeding arteries, external ligation and, rarely, embolisation. This paper describes a simple, non-invasive technique of treating posterior epistaxis with hot water irrigation. Technical information is presented, and the benefits of the method are discussed.

▶ Epistaxis management in the emergency department can make even the most seasoned physician cringe. Stubborn anterior bleeding and posterior bleeding generally results in balloon tamponade, which is uncomfortable and may require admission. Although more of an informational article, the authors present an alternative method of epistaxis control—hot water irrigation. First used in the 19th century, the hot water irrigation technique faded away with the advent of nasal packing and vascular surgical procedures, despite being more effective (55% vs 45%) than nasal packing for the management of posterior epistaxis. The authors present a description of the method itself (with an included video) and practical advice to enhance success. The technique uses 500 mL simple tap water heated to a temperature of 50°C and is infused continuously via a balloon catheter over 3 minutes to induce nasal edema and enhancement of the coagulation pathway. The authors use dedicated heater/irrigation device, but a clever emergency physician could devise a similar method with the equipment available in any emergency department.

E. C. Bruno, MD

10 Respiratory Distress

Accuracy of a transcutaneous carbon dioxide pressure monitoring device in emergency room patients with acute respiratory failure

Gancel P-E, Roupie E, Guittet L, et al (Département d'Accueil et de Traitement des Urgences, Caen, France; Evaluations et Recherches en épidémiologie, Caen, France; et al)
Intensive Care Med 37:348-351, 2011

Purpose.—Transcutaneous CO_2 monitors are widely used in neonatal ICUs. Until recently, these devices performed poorly in adults. Recent technical modifications have produced transcutaneous CO_2 monitors that have performed well in adults with chronic illnesses. We evaluated the accuracy of one of these devices, the TOSCA® 500, in adults admitted to an emergency department for acute respiratory failure.

Methods.—We prospectively collected 29 pairs of simultaneous transcutaneous arterial CO_2 ($PtcCO_2$) and arterial CO_2 ($PaCO_2$) values in 21 consecutive adults with acute respiratory failure (acute heart failure, $n = 6$; COPD exacerbation, $n = 8$; acute pneumonia, $n = 6$; and pulmonary embolism, $n = 1$). Agreement between $PaCO_2$ and $PtcCO_2$ was evaluated using the Bland-Altman method.

Results.—Mean arterial oxygen saturation was 90%, arterial oxygen tension ranged from 32 to 215 mmHg, and $PaCO_2$ ranged from 23 to 84 mmHg. The mean difference between $PaCO_2$ and $PtcCO_2$ was 0.1 mmHg, and the Bland-Altman limits of agreement (bias ± 1.96 SD) ranged from −6 to 6.2 mmHg. None of the patients experienced adverse effects from heating of the device clipped to the earlobe.

Conclusion.—$PtcCO_2$ showed good agreement with $PaCO_2$ in adults with acute respiratory failure.

▶ As the authors point out, frequent use of invasive arterial sticks for blood gas sampling is a painful and impractical way to monitor patients with complex respiratory problems. Sure, one of the problems is the arterial stick or indwelling arterial catheter. Another is that readings are actually spot checked, and there is a physical disconnect between the sampling and the blood gas machine; the blood has to be carried to the machine, and there is a dwell time to get the reading from the machine.

So how about a continuous reading device for carbon dioxide that is noninvasive? These devices exist and are coming into more use in adults after years of service in pediatric and neonatal settings.

What makes any device practical is for it to be easy to apply, work in a broad set of disease states, and give reliable results. This is the study that answers reliability (accuracy) and ease of application. There is still some concern about how it might operate in low flow and shock states when there would be decreased perfusion, but that is another experiment.

N. B. Handly, MD, MSc, MS

Nebulized Budesonide Added to Standard Pediatric Emergency Department Treatment of Acute Asthma: A Randomized, Double-Blind Trial
Upham BD, Mollen CJ, Scarfone RJ, et al (Univ of New Mexico, Albuquerque; The Children's Hosp of Philadelphia, PA)
Acad Emerg Med 18:665-673, 2011

Objectives.—The goal was to determine if adding inhaled budesonide to standard asthma therapy improves outcomes of pediatric patients presenting to the emergency department (ED) with acute asthma.

Methods.—The authors conducted a randomized, double-blind, placebo-controlled trial in a tertiary care, urban pediatric ED. Patients 2 to 18 years of age with moderate to severe acute asthma were randomized to receive either a single 2-mg dose of budesonide inhalation suspension (BUD) or normal sterile saline (NSS) placebo, added to albuterol, ipratropium bromide (IB), and systemic corticosteroids (SCS). The primary outcome was the difference in median asthma scores between treatment groups at 2 hours. Secondary outcomes included differences in vital signs and hospitalization rates.

Results.—A total of 180 patients were enrolled. Treatment groups had similar baseline demographics, asthma scores, and vital signs. A total of 169 patients (88 BUD, 81 NSS) were assessed for the primary outcome. No significant difference was found between groups in the change in median asthma score at 2 hours (BUD −3, NSS −3, p = 0.64). Vital signs at 2 hours were also similar between groups. Fifty-six children (62%) were admitted to the hospital in the BUD group and 55 (62%) in the NSS group (difference 0%, 95% confidence interval [CI] = −14% to 14%). Neither multivariate adjustment nor planned subgroup analysis by inhaled corticosteroids (ICS) use prior to the ED significantly altered the results.

Conclusions.—For children 2 to 18 years of age treated in the ED for acute asthma, a single 2-mg dose of budesonide added to standard therapy did not improve asthma severity scores or other short-term ED-based outcomes.

▶ Pediatric patients presenting with moderate to severe asthma exacerbations generally receive inhaled bronchodilators (with or without ipratroprium bromide) and systemic corticosteroids. Addition of nebulized budesonide is considered to be a viable intervention that may hasten clinical improvement. The authors of this randomized, double-blind, placebo-controlled trial compared the nebulized budesonide to control when added to conventional asthma management. They assessed clinical improvement at the 2-hour mark and were unable to identify any clinical difference between the intervention or control groups. Asthma severity scores were similar in both groups. Secondary end points of need for hospital admission and the need for readmission also did not differ between the groups. Without demonstrated clinical improvement, addition of budesonide is not necessary in the emergency management of moderate to severe asthma. Patients with severe asthma may continue to receive nebulized budesonide when the patient is not improving and the treating physician's plan is proceeding toward admission.

E. C. Bruno, MD

Two Days of Dexamethasone Versus 5 Days of Prednisone in the Treatment of Acute Asthma: A Randomized Controlled Trial
Kravitz J, Dominici P, Ufberg J, et al (St Barnabas Health System, Toms River, NJ; Albert Einstein Med Ctr, Philadelphia, PA; Temple Univ, Philadelphia, PA; et al)
Ann Emerg Med 58:200-204, 2011

Study Objective.—Dexamethasone has a longer half-life than prednisone and is well tolerated orally. We compare the time needed to return to normal activity and the frequency of relapse after acute exacerbation in adults receiving either 5 days of prednisone or 2 days of dexamethasone.

Methods.—We randomized adult emergency department patients (aged 18 to 45 years) with acute exacerbations of asthma (peak expiratory flow rate less than 80% of ideal) to receive either 50 mg of daily oral prednisone for 5 days or 16 mg of daily oral dexamethasone for 2 days. Outcomes were assessed by telephone follow-up.

Results.—Ninety-six prednisone and 104 dexamethasone subjects completed the study regimen and follow-up. More patients in the dexamethasone group reported a return to normal activities within 3 days compared with the prednisone group (90% versus 80%; difference 10%; 95% confidence interval 0% to 20%; $P=.049$). Relapse was similar between groups (13% versus 11%; difference 2%; 95% confidence interval $-7%$ to 11%, $P=.67$).

Conclusion.—In acute exacerbations of asthma in adults, 2 days of oral dexamethasone is at least as effective as 5 days of oral prednisone in returning patients to their normal level of activity and preventing relapse.

▶ Corticosteroids, in conjunction with bronchodilators, are the mainstay of treatment in acute asthma exacerbations. In adults, oral prednisone in burst or taper form are generally prescribed for outpatient management. The authors of this prospective, randomized, double-blind study assessed the effectiveness of a 2-day course of dexamethasone compared with a 5-day course of prednisone. They were able to demonstrate that 10% more patients in the dexamethasone group returned to normal activities than in the prednisone group, suggesting that dexamethasone is superior to prednisone. The authors found no difference between the groups in terms of bronchodilator use. The overall results of the study were similar to pediatric studies referenced in the article as well. Although clinical improvement is important in the patient's overall health, patient compliance with prescriptions is a contributing factor. Shorter courses of medications will likely lead to improved patient compliance, which may decrease rebound events.

E. C. Bruno, MD

Comparison of Succinylcholine and Rocuronium for First-attempt Intubation Success in the Emergency Department
Patanwala AE, Stahle SA, Sakles JC, et al (Univ of Arizona, Tucson)
Acad Emerg Med 18:11-14, 2011

Objectives.—The objective was to determine the effect of paralytic type and dose on first-attempt rapid sequence intubation (RSI) success in the emergency department (ED).

Methods.—This was a retrospective evaluation of information collected prospectively in a quality improvement database between July 1, 2007, and October 31, 2008. Information regarding all intubations performed in a tertiary care ED was recorded in this database. All RSI performed using succinylcholine or rocuronium were included. Logistic regression was used to analyze the effect of paralytic type and dosing, as well as age, sex, body mass index, physician experience, device type, and presence of difficult airway predictors on first attempt RSI success.

Results.—A total of 327 RSI were included in the final analyses. All patients received etomidate as the induction sedative and were successfully intubated. Of these, 113 and 214 intubations were performed using succinylcholine and rocuronium, respectively. The rate of first-attempt intubation success was similar between the succinylcholine and rocuronium groups (72.6% vs. 72.9%, p = 0.95). Median doses used for succinylcholine and rocuronium were 1.65 mg/kg (interquartile range [IQR] = 1.26–1.95 mg/kg) and 1.19 mg/kg (IQR = 1–1.45 mg/kg), respectively. In the univariate logistic regression analyses, variables predictive of first-attempt intubation success were laryngeal view (more success if Grade 1 or 2 compared to Grade 3 or 4 of the Cormack-Lehane classification, odds ratio [OR] = 55.18, 95% confidence interval [CI] = 18.87 to 161.39), intubation device (less success if direct laryngoscopy, OR = 0.57, 95% CI = 0.34 to 0.96), and presence of a difficult airway predictor (OR = 0.55, 95% CI = 0.31 to 0.99). In the multivariate analysis, the only variable predictive of first-attempt intubation success was laryngeal view.

Conclusions.—Succinylcholine and rocuronium are equivalent with regard to first-attempt intubation success in the ED when dosed according to the ranges used in this study.

▶ Rapid sequence induction and subsequent intubation is a critical procedure in emergency medicine. The choice of paralytic hinges on the balance of speed, familiarity, and adverse effects. The authors of this retrospective review compared the first-pass effectiveness of succinylcholine and rocuronium. Although the researchers' results demonstrate similar rates of success, some questions remain. First, the authors define airway success by placement of the endotracheal intubation, but there is no mention of method or adjunct, eg, intubating laryngeal mask airway, Bougie, etc. Second, rocuronium was used disproportionately more often (2:1) than succinylcholine. With the retrospective nature of the data, more competent airway managers may choose 1 agent over the other more often, skewing the results in favor of their preference paralytic.

Succinylcholine will remain in the armamentarium of the airway manager but has inherent risks related to contraindications. Food and Drug Administration approval of sugammadex, the rocuronium reversal agent, would likely result in greatly expanded use of rocuronium, based on improved side-effect profile without duration of action concerns.

E. C. Bruno, MD

Out-of-Hospital Lingual Dystonia Resulting in Airway Obstruction
Jacobsen RC (Truman Med Ctr, Kansas City, MO)
Prehosp Emerg Care 15:537-540, 2011

This article discusses a case of antipsychotic-induced, focal lingual dystonia causing airway obstruction that was managed completely in the out-of-hospital environment by emergency medical services (EMS) providers. With the ever-increasing use of antipsychotic medications by the general population, it is important for EMS providers and emergency medicine physicians to be aware of rare presentations of dystonic reactions that can sometimes be life-threatening when they involve the lingual, pharyngeal, or laryngeal musculature. This article identifies the medications most likely to induce dystonic reactions, risk factors that predispose individuals to the development of dystonia, and the pathophysiology behind these adverse reactions. It also discusses differential diagnoses to consider, and emergent treatment options.

▶ Treating a patient with an unfamiliar condition can be a challenge even for the experienced health care practitioner. The urgency of the situation especially increases when the condition involves an inevitable compromise of the airway.

This document describes a condition in which the musculature of the tongue is involved in an antipsychotic medication—induced dystonia, which affects the airway. The use of antipsychotic medication is increasing. As a result so are

---

TABLE 1.—Manifestations of Acute Dystonia

Oculogyric crisis	Spasm of the extraorbital muscles, causing upwards and outwards deviation of the eyes. Blepharospasm.
Torticollis	Head held turned to one side.
Opisthotonos	Painful forced extension of the neck. When severe, the back is involved and the patient arches off the bed.
Macroglossia	The tongue does not swell, but it protrudes and feels swollen.
Buccolingual crisis	May be accompanied by trismus, risus sardonicus, dysarthria, and grimacing.
Laryngospasm	Uncommon, but frightening.
Spasticity	Trunk muscles and less commonly limbs can be affected.

Table from: Campbell D. The management of acute dystonic reactions. Aust Prescriber. 2001;24:19-20. Reprinted with permission from *Australian Prescriber.*

---

presentations of patients with dystonic reactions. Signs and symptoms of dystonia include oculogyric crisis, torticollis, opisthotonus, macroglossia, buccolingual crisis, laryngospasm, and spasticity. For more detail the reader is referred to Table 1 of the publication. Treatment of this condition, even if the health care provider is not sure of the diagnosis, is diphenhydramine, 25—50 mg intravenously (IV) or intramuscularly (IM), and for pediatric patients, 1—2 mg/kg, or, alternatively, 1—2 mg IV or IM of benztropine and for pediatric patients 0.02—0.05 mg/kg IV or IM not to exceed 2 mg/d. A small dose of benzodiazepines may prove helpful in some situations for alleviating anxiety and providing muscle relaxation.

B. M. Minczak, MS, MD, PhD, PH-MD

11 Pulmonary

Critical Issues in the Evaluation and Management of Adult Patients Presenting to the Emergency Department With Suspected Pulmonary Embolism
American College of Emergency Physicians Clinical Policies Subcommittee (Writing Committee) on Critical Issues in the Evaluation and Management of Adult Patients Presenting to the Emergency Department With Suspected Pulmonary Embolism
Ann Emerg Med 57:628-652, 2011

This clinical policy from the American College of Emergency Physicians is the revision of a 2003 clinical policy on the evaluation and management of adult patients presenting with suspected pulmonary embolism (PE). A writing subcommittee reviewed the literature to derive evidence-based recommendations to help clinicians answer the following critical questions: (1) Do objective criteria provide improved risk stratification over gestalt clinical assessment in the evaluation of patients with possible PE? (2) What is the utility of the Pulmonary Embolism Rule-out Criteria (PERC) in the evaluation of patients with suspected PE? (3) What is the role of quantitative D-dimer testing in the exclusion of PE? (4) What is the role of computed tomography pulmonary angiogram of the chest as the sole diagnostic test in the exclusion of PE? (5) What is the role of venous imaging in the evaluation of patients with suspected PE? (6) What are the indications for thrombolytic therapy in patients with PE? Evidence was graded and recommendations were given based on the strength of the available data in the medical literature.

▶ Responsible for approximately 200 000 deaths annually, pulmonary embolism (PE) remains an evasive diagnostic entity for all physicians. The American College of Emergency Physicians (ACEP) have revised and updated the 2003 clinical policy addressing PEs. This version included only 1 level A recommendation for the diagnosis and management of PE. During the initial evaluation of the patient with suspected PE, the authors present level B recommendations that physicians can use one of the many clinical decision rules (modified Wells, Geneva, etc) or clinical gestalt to consider the diagnosis of PE, although none of the approaches are superior to another. Once identified as low risk for PE by 1 of the processes, use of the Pulmonary Embolism Rule-out Criteria (PERC) rule can effectively exclude the diagnosis of PE (Level B). By combining the first and second diagnostic questions, a patient with a low pretest probability and a negative PERC rule requires no further diagnostic testing. This approach may limit further diagnostic testing but failure to present this direction as level A will result in skepticism and insecurity from a malpractice point of view.

EPs may then be motivated to add further testing, specifically a D-dimer. The ACEP guidelines present the only level A recommendation here, stating that a negative D-dimer is adequate to rule out PE and no further testing is required. The EP must confirm that the D-dimer is the quantitative variety. If a patient has intermediate risk, as defined by the modified Wells criteria, the negative D-dimer may be used to exclude PE.

The guidelines also speak to additional testing and testing results. Essentially, the authors present recommendations that computed tomography angiography is adequate to exclude PE in the low-risk patient (level B), but more testing (V/Q scan, D-dimer, lower extremity venous Doppler) may be necessary in the moderate- to high-risk patients. The lower extremity venous Doppler is only helpful if positive.

Lastly, the authors suggest that aggressive thrombolytic therapy may be beneficial in the critically ill patient with the confirmed PE, but risks, benefits, and alternatives must be considered.

E. C. Bruno, MD

Effectiveness and Acceptability of a Computerized Decision Support System Using Modified Wells Criteria for Evaluation of Suspected Pulmonary Embolism

Drescher FS, Chandrika S, Weir ID, et al (Veterans Affairs Med Ctr, White River Junction, VT; Norwalk Hosp, CT; et al)
Ann Emerg Med 57:613-621, 2011

Study Objective.—Ready availability of computed tomography (CT) angiography for evaluation of pulmonary embolism in emergency departments (EDs) is associated with a dramatic increase in the number of CT angiography tests. The aims of this study are to determine whether a validated prediction algorithm embedded in a computerized decision support system improves the positive yield rate of CT angiography for pulmonary embolism and is acceptable to emergency physicians.

Methods.—This study was conducted as a prospective interventional study with a retrospective preinterventional comparison group.

Results.—The implementation of the computerized physician order entry—based computerized decision support system was associated with an overall increase in the positivity rate of from 8.3% (95% confidence interval [CI] 4.9% to 12.9%) preintervention to 12.7% (95% CI 8.6% to 17.7%) postintervention, with a difference of 4.4% (95% CI −1.4% to 10.1%). A total of 404 patients were eligible for inclusion. Physician nonadherence to the computerized decision support system occurred in 105 (26.7%) cases. Fifteen patients underwent CT angiography despite low Wells score and negative D-dimer result, all of whose results were negative for pulmonary embolism. Emergency physicians did not order

CT angiography for 44 patients despite high pretest probability, with one receiving a diagnosis of pulmonary embolism on a subsequent visit and another, of DVT. When emergency physicians adhered to the computerized decision support system for the evaluation of suspected pulmonary embolism, a higher yield of CT angiography for pulmonary embolism occurred, with 28 positive results of 168 CT angiography tests (16.7%; 95% CI 11.4% to 23.2%) and a difference compared with preintervention of 8.4% (95% CI 1.7% to 15.4%). Physicians cited the time required to apply the computerized decision support system and a preference for intuitive judgment as reasons for not adhering to the computerized decision support system.

Conclusion.—Use of an evidence-based computerized physician order entry—based computerized decision support system for the evaluation of suspected pulmonary embolism was associated with a higher yield of CT angiography for pulmonary embolism. The computerized decision support system, however, was poorly accepted by emergency physicians (partly because of increased computer time), leading to possibly selective use, reducing the effect on overall yield, and leading to removal of the computerized decision support system from the computer order entry. These findings emphasize the importance of facilitation of rule-based decisionmaking in the ED and attentiveness to the complex demands placed on emergency physicians.

▶ The authors of this interventional study assessed whether a computerized decision support system focused around the modified Wells criteria for pulmonary embolism (PE) would affect the use of diagnostic testing in the emergency department. Excluding pregnant women and clinically unstable patients, the authors asked emergency physicians (EPs) to complete a computer-based system of the modified Wells criteria to guide decisions. If the calculated score predicted low risk, the EP was encouraged to order a D-dimer assay first rather than proceeding directly to computerized tomographic angiography (CTA) in the search for a PE. After the intervention, the authors demonstrated an increased percentage of positive CTAs for PEs, but they also found positive D-dimer assays with negative CTAs (53.7%) and a negative D-dimer assay with a positive CTA (1 patient). These results reinforce the elusive nature of the diagnosis of PE. Ultimately, EPs will continue to use physical examination, clinical decision tools (modified Wells criteria, PERC, etc), and overall gestalt to steer their practice in the quest to find a suspected PE.

E. C. Bruno, MD

12 Abdominal Pain

Racial disparity in analgesic treatment for ED patients with abdominal or back pain
Mills AM, Shofer FS, Boulis AK, et al (Univ of Pennsylvania, Philadelphia)
Am J Emerg Med 29:752-756, 2011

Objective.—Research on how race affects access to analgesia in the emergency department (ED) has yielded conflicting results. We assessed whether patient race affects analgesia administration for patients presenting with back or abdominal pain.

Methods.—This is a retrospective cohort study of adults who presented to 2 urban EDs with back or abdominal pain for a 4-year period. To assess differences in analgesia administration and time to analgesia between races, Fisher exact and Wilcoxon rank sum test were used, respectively. Relative risk regression was used to adjust for potential confounders.

Results.—Of 20 125 patients included (mean age, 42 years; 64% female; 75% black; mean pain score, 7.5), 6218 (31%) had back pain and 13 907 (69%) abdominal pain. Overall, 12 109 patients (60%) received any analgesia and 8475 (42%) received opiates. Comparing nonwhite (77 %) to white patients (23%), nonwhites were more likely to report severe pain (pain score, 9-10) (42% vs 36%; $P < .0001$) yet less likely to receive any analgesia (59% vs 66%; $P < .0001$) and less likely to receive an opiate (39% vs 51%; $P < .0001$). After controlling for age, sex, presenting complaint, triage class, admission, and severe pain, white patients were still 10% more likely to receive opiates (relative risk, 1.10; 95% confidence interval, 1.06-1.13). Of patients who received analgesia, nonwhites waited longer for opiate analgesia (median time, 98 vs 90 minutes; $P = .004$).

Conclusions.—After controlling for potential confounders, nonwhite patients who presented to the ED for abdominal or back pain were less likely than whites to receive analgesia and waited longer for their opiate medication (Table 2).

▶ Taken at face value, the results of this study are quite disturbing. The topic of oligoanalgesia, or the undertreatment of pain, has been well studied in the emergency medicine literature. Many proposed factors contribute to oligoanalgesia, including a preoccupation with the diagnosis and treatment of the underlying medical problem, concerns about masking symptoms, fears about contributing to or causing addiction, caregiver underestimation of pain experience by the patient, cultural difference in pain expression, poor communication, reluctance

TABLE 2.—Racial Differences in Patient Characteristics

Characteristic	Whites, n = 4681 (23%)	Nonwhites, n = 15 444 (77%)	P
Age, y (mean ± SD)	43 ± 17	42 ± 17	.0008
Sex			<.0001
Female	2612 (56)	10 296 (67)	
Male	2069 (44)	5148 (33)	
Presenting complaint			.0002
Abdominal pain	3339 (71)	10 568 (68)	
Back pain	1342 (29)	4876 (32)	
Triage class			<.0001
1 (emergent)	130 (3)	124 (1)	
2	1902 (41)	2953 (19)	
3	2136 (46)	9639 (62)	
4 (nonemergent)	508 (11)	2724 (18)	
Pain score (mean ± SD)	7.2 ± 2.4	7.5 ± 2.3	<.0001
0-8	3002 (64)	9006 (58)	
9-10	1679 (36)	6438 (42)	
Received any analgesia	3067 (66)	9042 (59)	<.0001
Opiate	2382 (51)	6093 (39)	
Nonopiate	685 (15)	2949 (19)	
Disposition			<.0001
Admission	1582 (20)	2714 (37)	
Discharge	3099 (80)	12 730 (63)	

of patients to demand pain treatment, and inadequate training in the recognition and management of pain.

On the topic of oligoanalgesia in nonwhites versus whites, several studies of emergency department patients with long bone fractures have been done and show conflicting results. Three studies showed that white patients were more likely to receive analgesia than nonwhites, and 2 studies showed no difference in analgesia administration. While there are some limitations to this study that I will discuss later, the results add to the disturbing trend of less analgesic medication, less opioid medication, and greater delay in giving medication to nonwhite patients.

There are many limitations to this study. First, it was retrospective; therefore, potential reasons for failure to treat or delays in analgesic treatment couldn't be studied. Reassessments of pain scores and patient desire for analgesia were not available. The authors did not assess other potential agents used for analgesia, including proton pump inhibitors, H2-receptor antagonists, gastrointestinal cocktails for abdominal pain, or muscle relaxants for back pain. Finally, the authors did not include discharge prescriptions for analgesics in this study.

What I found most shocking in this study was that the admission rate was almost twice as high in the nonwhite group—37% admission versus 20% in the white group. This presumably means that nonwhites had final diagnoses that were more concerning, ie, they were sicker.

Obviously, further studies on this topic need to be done, but the results from this study and trends of others should alert emergency physicians to do better in the management of pain. More specifically, emergency physicians need to make a concerted effort to be more proactive in treating pain in nonwhite patients.

D. K. Mullin, MD

13 Toxicology

Antidotes and Treatment

A dosing regimen for immediate N-acetylcysteine treatment for acute paracetamol overdose

Shen F, Coulter CV, Isbister GK, et al (Univ of Otago, Dunedin, New Zealand; Calvary Mater Newcastle Hosp, Australia)
Clin Toxicol 49:643-647, 2011

Context.—Current treatment of paracetamol (acetaminophen) poisoning involves initiating a 3-phase N-acetylcysteine (NAC) infusion after comparing a plasma concentration, taken ≥4 h post-overdose, to a nomogram. This may result in dosing errors, a delay in treatment, or possibly more adverse effects − due to the use of a high dose rate for the first infusion when treatment is initiated.

Objective.—Our aim was to investigate a novel dosing regimen for the immediate administration of NAC on admission at a lower infusion rate.

Methods.—We used a published population pharmacokinetic model of NAC to simulate a scenario where a patient presents to the hospital 2 h post-overdose. The conventional regimen is commenced 6 h post-overdose when the 4-h plasma paracetamol concentration is available. We investigated an NAC infusion using a lower dosing rate initiated immediately on presentation. We determined a dosing rate that gave an area under the curve (AUC) of the concentration-time curve that was the same or greater than that from the conventional regimen on 90% of occasions.

Results.—Lower dosing rates of NAC initiated immediately resulted in a similar exposure to NAC. An infusion of 110 mg/kg over the first 5 h (22 mg/kg/h) followed by the last two phases of the conventional regimen, or 200 mg/kg over 9 h (22.6 mg/kg/h) followed by the last phase of the conventional regimen could be used.

Conclusion.—The novel dosing regimen allowed immediate treatment of a patient using a lower dosing rate. This greatly simplifies the current dosing regimen and may reduce NAC adverse effects while ensuring the same amount of NAC is delivered.

▶ Although this pharmacokinetic model is fascinating and it appears that the suggested regimen would work, I am not certain it is that much easier to administer than the US Food and Drug Administration—approved method. I agree

285

with the authors that the approved administration schedule is complex and has resulted in errors. However, this could easily be overcome by human factor studies by the manufacturer and the hospital pharmacy, for example, discrete labeling of infusions and which order they are to be administered and for how long.

R. J. Hamilton, MD

A prospective, randomized, trial of phenobarbital versus benzodiazepines for acute alcohol withdrawal
Hendey GW, Dery RA, Barnes RL, et al (Community Regional Med Ctr, Fresno, CA)
Am J Emerg Med 29:382-385, 2011

Objective.—The aim of this study was to compare phenobarbital (PB) versus lorazepam (LZ) in the treatment of alcohol withdrawal in the emergency department (ED) and at 48 hours.

Methods.—Prospectively, randomized, consenting patients were assessed using a modified Clinical Institute Withdrawal Assessment (CIWA) score and given intravenous PB (mean, 509 mg) or LZ (mean, 4.2 mg). At discharge, LZ patients received chlordiazepoxide (Librium), and PB patients received placebo.

Results.—Of 44 patients, 25 received PB, and 19 LZ. Both PB and LZ reduced CIWA scores from baseline to discharge (15.0-5.4 and 16.8-4.2, $P < .0001$). There were no differences between PB and LZ in baseline CIWA scores ($P = .3$), discharge scores ($P = .4$), ED length of stay (267 versus 256 minutes, $P = .8$), admissions (12% versus 16%, $P = .8$), or 48-hour follow-up CIWA scores (5.8 versus 7.2, $P = .6$).

Conclusion.—Phenobarbital and LZ were similarly effective in the treatment of mild/moderate alcohol withdrawal in the ED and at 48 hours.

▶ Acute alcohol withdrawal is an emergent condition requiring aggressive sedation and supportive care. After the patient stabilizes and discharge is planned, a decision regarding outpatient sedative medications must be made. The authors of this study suggest that the use of phenobarbital would obviate the need for prescriptions for subsequent sedation. Phenobarbital was compared with lorazepam in the management of acute alcohol withdrawal. They were unable to demonstrate any significant difference between the compared medications in terms of sedation, length of stay, or hospital admission rates. One area of difference was the number of doses needed. Patients receiving phenobarbital needed more doses than those receiving lorazepam, although this was not statistically significant. These additional doses of phenobarbital translates to more nursing time and resources dedicated to these patients, which might be better used elsewhere. Treating physicians can consider the medication's dosing regimen in terms of cost-effectiveness and resource use when initiating medications.

E. C. Bruno, MD

Acetaminophen psi parameter: A useful tool to quantify hepatotoxicity risk in acute acetaminophen overdose

Chomchai S, Chomchai C, Anusornsuwan T (Mahidol Univ, Bangkok, Thailand; Mahidol Univ International College, Nakorn Pathom, Thailand; Sungnoen Hosp, Nakhonratchasima, Thailand)
Clin Toxicol (Phila) 49:664-667, 2011

Context.—The risk of hepatotoxicity secondary to acute acetaminophen overdose is related to serum acetaminophen concentration and lag time from ingestion to N-acetylcysteine (NAC) therapy. Psi (Greek letter ψ) is a toxicokinetic parameter that takes the acetaminophen level at 4 h post-ingestion ($[APAP]_{4h}$) and the time-to-initiation of NAC (tNAC) into account and was found to be significantly predictive of hepatotoxicity in Canadian patients with acetaminophen overdose treated with intravenous NAC.

Objective.—We report the relationship of psi and hepatotoxicity in a Thai population with acute acetaminophen overdose.

Methods.—This is a retrospective study of patients with acute paracetamol overdose during January 2004 to June 2009 at Siriraj Hospital. Patients were treated with the standard 21-h intravenous NAC regimen. Univariate analyses were performed with logistic regression to assess the relationships of psi, $[APAP]_{4h}$, and tNAC, and hepatotoxicity.

Results.—A total of 127 patients were enrolled. The median (interquartile range; IQR) of $[APAP]_{4h}$ was 267.8 (196.0–380.0) mg/L. The median (IQR) of tNAC was 8.5 (6.2–12.0) h. Thirteen patients (10.2%) developed hepatotoxicity. Univariate analysis revealed $[APAP]_{4h}$, tNAC, and psi as statistically significant predictors of hepatotoxicity.

Discussion and Conclusion.—The psi parameter is a reliable prognostic tool to predict hepatotoxicity secondary to acute acetaminophen overdose treated with intravenous NAC. Our evidence shows that psi may be a

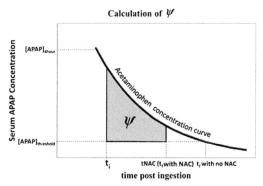

FIGURE 1.—Calculation of psi (ψ) parameter (shaded area). t_i = no-effect lag time, t_f = ending time, tNAC = lag time before N-acetylcysteine, $[APAP]_{4\,h}$ = equivalent acetaminophen level at 4h, $[APAP]_{threshold}$ = no-effect threshold acetaminophen level (see colour version of this figure online). (Reprinted from Chomchai S, Chomchai C, Anusornsuwan T. Acetaminophen psi parameter: a useful tool to quantify hepatotoxicity risk in acute acetaminophen overdose. *Clin Toxicol (Phila)*. 2011;49:664-667, reprinted with permission from Taylor & Francis, Ltd.)

TABLE 1.—Comparisons of Parameters Between the Non-Hepatotoxicity and Hepatotoxicity Groups

Parameter (Units) Median (IQR)	Non-Hepatotoxicity (n = 114)	Hepatotoxicity (n = 13)	p Value
Acetaminophen dose (mg)	15 000 (10 000–20 000)	15 000 (10 000–25 000)	0.49
tNAC (h)	8.3 (6.0–11.3)	12.00 (9.1–14.6)	<0.01
[APAP]$_{4h}$ (mg/L)	252.2 (191.3–343.3)	413.5 (378.5–478.5)	<0.01
{[APAP]$_{4h}$ (μmol/L)}	{1668.6 (1265.6–2271.3)}	{2735.7 (2504.2–3165.8)}	
Psi$_2$ (mmol/L × h)	6.5 (4.1–11.1)	14.3 (12.4–19.0)	<0.01
Psi$_4$ (mmol/L × h)	3.2 (1.7–6.6)	8.9 (6.7–12.2)	<0.01
Psi$_6$ (mmol/L × h)	1.3 (0.0–3.4)	4.9 (3.4–7.5)	<0.01

IQR: interquartile range; tNAC: lag time before N-acetylcysteine therapy; [APAP]$_{4h}$: equivalent acetaminophen level at 4 h; psi$_2$: psi parameter using t$_i$ of 2; psi$_4$: psi parameter using t$_i$ of 4; psi$_6$: psi parameter using t$_i$ of 6.

more superior tool than either acetaminophen level or time-to-initiation of NAC at predicting hepatotoxicity (Fig 1, Table 1).

▶ This research article is another investigation of a fascinating study originally done in Canada that created the acetaminophen psi parameter. This calculation basically uses the time from overdose to acetaminophen level and the time from acetaminophen level to N-acetylcysteine (NAC) treatment to predict who will get hepatotoxicity. It does this accurately and is a fascinating tool. However, if you examine the value of doing this calculation on a case-by-case basis, you are disappointed to find that it does not provide the clinician with any more information than they currently have: start NAC as soon as possible and within 8 hours of the overdose if at all possible. You can appreciate this by looking at Table 1, which shows the hepatotoxic group receiving NAC on average 12 hours after overdose (range: 9.0–14.6) and the nonhepatotoxic group receiving it on average 8.3 hours after overdose (range: 6.0–11.3). Nonetheless, the accuracy of the APAP psi parameter seems to be quite good.

R. J. Hamilton, MD

Acute cholestatic liver injury caused by polyhexamethyleneguanidine hydrochloride admixed to ethyl alcohol
Ostapenko YN, Brusin KM, Zobnin YV, et al (Res and Applied Toxicology Ctr of the Federal Med-Biological Agency, Moscow, Russia; Ural State Med Academy, Ekaterinburg, Russia; Irkutsk State Med Univ; et al)
Clin Toxicol 49:471-477, 2011

Introduction.—Polyhexamethyleneguanidine hydrochloride (PHMG) is an antimicrobial biocide of the guanidine family. In the period from August 2006 to May 2007, more than 12500 patients were admitted to hospital with a history of drinking illegal cheap "vodka" in 44 different regions in Russia, of whom 9.4% died. In reality, the "vodka" was an antiseptic liquid composed of ethanol ($\approx 93\%$), diethyl phthalate, and 0.1–0.14% PHMG (brand name "Extrasept-1").

Material and Methods.—We performed an analysis of the clinical features and outcome in four poisoning treatment centers in the cities of Perm, Ekaterinburg, Irkutsk, and Khabarovsk. A total of 579 patients (215 females and 364 males) with similar symptoms were included.

Results.—The main symptoms on admission included jaundice (99.7%), skin itch (78.4%), weakness (96%), anorexia (65.8%), dizziness (65.3%), nausea (54.8%), vomiting (22.6%), stomach ache (52.7%), diarrhea (32%), and fever (50%). Mild symptoms were found in 2.5% of cases, moderate in 63%, and severe in 34.5%. Laboratory results were (mean ± SD): total bilirubin 249 ± 158 μmol/L, direct bilirubin 166 ± 97 μmol/L, cholesterol 14 ± 8 mmol/L, alanine aminotransferase 207 ± 174 IU/L, aspartate aminotransferase 174 ± 230 IU/L, alkaline phosphatase 742 ± 751 IU/L, and gamma-glutamyltranspeptidase 1199 ± 1095 IU/L. Patients generally recovered over a period of 1–5 months, although high levels of alkaline phosphatase and gamma-glutamyltranspeptidase were still found in all patients examined after 6 months. Sixty-one patients (10.5%) died between 23 and 150 days after poisoning. Local cholestasis, inflammatory infiltration, and fibrosis developing into cirrhosis were found by liver biopsy.

Conclusion.—Acute liver injury caused by PHMG-hydrochloride or PHMG in combination with either ethanol or diethyl phthalate can be characterized as cholestatic hepatitis with a severe inflammatory component causing high mortality.

▶ The scope of this catastrophe is stunning. The mechanism of cholestatic liver injury is not clear, but hopefully investigators will look more closely at the issue. Often, in the case of these epidemics, further spread of the problem is limited by good public health work, and the pathophysiology of the poison is identified with good basic science.

R. J. Hamilton, MD

Acute Ethanol Intoxication and the Trauma Patient: Hemodynamic Pitfalls
Bilello J, McCray V, Davis J, et al (Univ of California San Francisco - Fresno Campus)
World J Surg 35:2149-2153, 2011

Many trauma patients are acutely intoxicated with alcohol. Animal studies have demonstrated that acute alcohol intoxication inhibits the normal release of epinephrine, norepinephrine, and vasopressin in response to acute hemorrhage. Ethanol also increases nitric oxide release and inhibits antidiuretic hormone secretion. This article studies the effects of alcohol intoxication (measured by blood alcohol level, BAL) on the presentation and resuscitation of trauma patients with blunt hepatic injuries. A retrospective registry and chart review was conducted of all patients who presented with blunt liver injuries at an ACS-verified, level I trauma center. Data collected included admission BAL, systolic blood pressure, hematocrit, International Normalized Ratio (INR), liver injury grade, Injury Severity Score (ISS), intravenous fluid and blood product requirements, base deficit, and mortality. From September 2002 to May 2008, 723 patients were admitted with blunt hepatic injuries. Admission BAL was obtained in 569 patients, with 149 having levels >0.08%. Intoxicated patients were more likely to be hypotensive on admission ($p = 0.01$) despite a lower liver injury grade and no significant difference in ISS. There was no significant difference in the percent of intoxicated patients requiring blood transfusion. However, when blood was given, intoxicated patients required significantly more units of packed red blood cells (PRBC) than their nonintoxicated counterparts ($p = 0.01$). Intoxicated patients also required more intravenous fluid during their resuscitation ($p = 0.002$). Alcohol intoxication may impair the ability of blunt trauma patients to compensate for acute blood loss, making them more likely to be hypotensive on admission and increasing their PRBC and intravenous fluid requirements. All trauma patients should have BAL drawn upon admission and their resuscitation should be performed with an understanding of the physiologic alterations associated with acute alcohol intoxication.

▶ Many trauma centers have stopped the routine ordering of serum ethanol measurements because they often force them to provide testimony in criminal or civil cases related to an accident. This is unfortunate because knowledge of the patient's ethanol level can be helpful in dealing with the subtleties in clinical management.

R. J. Hamilton, MD

Amanita Poisoning and Liver Transplantation: Do We Have the Right Decision Criteria?

Garcia de la Fuente I, McLin VA, Rimensberger PC, et al (Univ Hosp Geneva, Switzerland)
J Pediatr Gastroenterol Nutr 53:459-462, 2011

Background.—Most of the cases of mushroom poisoning that produce acute liver failure (ALF) are caused by *Amanita phalloides*. If liver transplantation is not done, the survival rate is between 10% and 30%, with mortality from ALF especially high in young children. Several sets of criteria for emergency transplantation have been proposed, but their relevance to cases of amanita poisoning in young children is unknown. A case of amanita intoxication and ALF in a young child who recovered without transplantation was reported.

Case Report.—Boy, 17 months, was diagnosed with ALF after amanita poisoning and seemed unlikely to survive without liver transplantation. Factors considered included his age, factor V levels

(<10%), prothrombin time (PT; >100 ms), and etiology. The King's College and Clichy criteria for urgent liver transplantation were clearly met, but within 72 hours of ingestion the patient showed signs of spontaneous recovery and regained normal liver function within days without liver transplantation.

Analysis.—Managing children with ALF is challenging for several reasons. For example, encephalopathy can be a late event in the course of ALF and delay the decision to transplant beyond a clinically reasonable point. In addition, most series that assess prognostic factors in childhood ALF do not include cases of amanita poisoning. A study in adults indicated that fatal outcome after amanita poisoning was best predicted by a PT less than 25% and serum creatinine level less than 106 µmol/L 3 or more days after ingestion. A second study found fatal outcome correlated best with PT under 10% 4 or more days after ingestion and an interval shorter than 8 hours between ingestion and diarrhea. In the absence of these findings, one can predict the patient will likely survive without liver transplantation.

Conclusions.—The optimal course for managing children with amanita poisoning has not yet been determined. However, although observations indicate that extreme caution should be exercised when managing young children with amanita-induced ALF, criteria related to various clinical parameters 3 to 4 days after ingestion of mushrooms have proved predictive of survival.

▶ I am abstracting the conclusions from the article as a summary in my commentary. I have been amazed at the degree of liver damage that some Amanita-poisoned patients recover from.

Liver transplantation should rapidly be considered in children with *Amanita phalloides* poisoning. Because of the absence of clear standardized criteria for urgent transplantation and the chance of spontaneous recovery, however, the need for liver transplantation must be continuously reassessed. Liver function should be closely monitored with serial factor V measurements until transplantation because of possible spontaneous recovery even in those cases fulfilling established transplantation criteria. Given our observation in a toddler and the reported experience in adult patients, it may be important to consider postponing transplantation until 3 to 4 days after ingestion because of the potential for recovery. Commonly accepted transplantation criteria for acute liver failure may need to be optimized for the assessment and management of Amanita-induced liver failure.

R. J. Hamilton, MD

Fatal poisoning in children: Acute Colchicine intoxication and new treatment approaches

Ozdemir R, Bayrakci B, Teksam O (Zekai Tahir Burak Maternity Teaching Hosp, Ankara, Turkey; Ihsan Dogramaci Children's Hosp, Ankara, Turkey)
Clin Toxicol 49:739-743, 2011

Background.—Colchicine poisoning is potentially life-threatening. Deaths generally result from hypovolemic shock and cardiovascular collapse or secondary to rapidly progressive multiorgan failure.

Objective.—The purpose of this study is to discuss the clinical effects, treatments and outcomes of pediatric colchicine poisoning and highlight the possible benefits of urgent plasma and whole blood exchange therapy for those patients who were believed to ingest potentially lethal doses of the drug.

Methods.—Current study was designed as an observational case series study. The medical records of children aged 0–16 years who were hospitalized for colchicine poisoning at the Pediatric Intensive Care Unit of, between November 1985 and March 2011 were retrospectively evaluated.

Results.—We present twenty-three children with colchicine poisoning. Nausea and vomiting were the most common presenting complaint, in 70% of patients. Sixteen of the 23 cases presented after ingesting subtoxic doses of colchicine (<0.5 mg/kg), whereas 3 patients had consumed toxic doses of the drug (0.5–0.8 mg/kg). The remaining 4 patients were hospitalized after taking colchicine at a lethal dose (>0.8 mg/kg). Three patients (13%) died.

Conclusions.—Any patient suspected of ingesting high doses of colchicine should prompt immediate fluid and electrolyte resuscitation and invasive hemodynamic monitorization in a pediatric intensive care unit. Although there is lack of strong evidence, early initiation of either whole blood or plasma exchange may be considered in patients presenting with lethal-dose colchicine intoxication. These reported experience of us put forth further research for consideration.

▶ Colchicine is one of the deadliest of drugs with a narrow therapeutic window. The old rule of thumb still applies that a subtoxic dose is 0.5 mg/kg, a toxic dose is 0.5 to 0.8 mg/kg, and a lethal dose is 0.8 mg/kg. I agree with the authors' conclusions, and if I suspect a toxic dose of colchicine ingestion, I am going to recommend early plasmapheresis.

R. J. Hamilton, MD

Improved survival in severe paraquat poisoning with repeated pulse therapy of cyclophosphamide and steroids

Lin J-L, Lin-Tan D-T, Chen K-H, et al (Chang Gung Memorial Hosp, Taipei, Taiwan)

Intensive Care Med 37:1006-1013, 2011

Purpose.—To clarify the efficacy of repeated methylprednisolone (MP) and cyclophosphamide (CP) pulse therapy and daily dexamethasone (DEX) therapy in patients with severe paraquat (PQ) poisoning.

Methods.—A total of 111 patients with severe PQ poisoning and dark-blue color in urine tests within 24 h of intoxication were included prospectively. The control group consisted of 52 patients who were admitted between 1998 and 2001 and who received high doses of CP (2 mg/kg per day) and DEX (5 mg every 6 h) for 14 days. The study group consisted of 59 patients who were admitted from 2002 to 2007 and who received initial MP (1 g) for 3 days and CP (15 mg/kg per day) for 2 days, followed by DEX (5 mg every 6 h) until a PaO_2 of >80 mmHg had been achieved, or treated with repeated 1 g MP for 3 days and 1 g CP for 1 day if the PaO_2 was <60 mmHg.

Results.—There were no differences between the two groups with regard to baseline data and plasma PQ levels. The study group patients had a lower mortality rate (39/59, 66%) than the control group patients (48/52, 92%; $P = 0.003$, log-rank test). Multivariate Cox regression analysis revealed that the repeated pulse therapy was correlated with decreased hazard ratios (HR) for all-cause mortality (HR = 0.50, 95% CI 0.31−0.80; $P = 0.004$) and death from lung fibrosis-related hypoxemia (HR = 0.10, 95% CI 0.04−0.25; $P < 0.001$) in severely PQ-intoxicated patients.

Conclusion.—Repeated pulses of CP and MP, rather than high doses of CP and DEX, may result in a lower mortality rate in patients with severe PQ poisoning.

▶ The outcome of this approach is very promising. I look forward to seeing more reports from this group as well as the results of others.

R. J. Hamilton, MD

Increase of paradoxical excitement response during propofol-induced sedation in hazardous and harmful alcohol drinkers

Jeong S, Lee HG, Kim WM, et al (Chonnam Natl Univ Med School and Hosp, Jebongro Dong-gu, Gwangju, Republic of Korea)

Br J Anaesth 107:930-933, 2011

Background.—Paradoxical excitement response during sedation consists of loss of affective control and abnormal movements. Chronic alcohol abuse has been proposed as a predisposing factor despite lack of supporting evidence. Because alcohol and propofol have a common site of action, we postulated that paradoxical excitement responses during propofol-induced sedation occur more frequently in hazardous and harmful alcohol drinkers than in social or non-drinkers.

Methods.—One hundred and ninety patients undergoing orthopaedic knee joint surgery were enrolled in this prospective and observational study. Subjects were divided into Group HD (hazardous and harmful drinkers) or Group NHD (no hazardous drinkers) according to the alcohol use disorder identification test (AUDIT). In study 1, propofol infusion was adjusted to achieve the bispectral index at 70—80 using target-controlled infusion. In study 2, the target concentration of propofol was fixed at 0.8 (study 2/Low) or 1.4 $\mu g \, ml^{-1}$ (study 2/High). Paradoxical excitement responses were categorized by intensity into mild, moderate, or severe.

Results.—The overall incidence of paradoxical excitement response was higher in Group HD than in Group NHD in study 1 (71.4% *vs* 43.8%; $P=0.022$) and study 2/High (70.0% *vs* 34.5%; $P=0.006$) but not in study 2/Low. The incidence of moderate-to-severe response was significantly higher in Group HD of study 1 (28.6% *vs* 3.1%; $P=0.0005$) and study 2/High (23.3% *vs* 3.4%; $P=0.029$) with no difference in study 2/Low. Severe excitement response occurred only in Group HD of study 1 and study 2/High.

Conclusions.—Paradoxical excitement occurred more frequently and severely in hazardous and harmful alcohol drinkers than in social drinkers during propofol-induced moderate-to-deep sedation, but not during light sedation.

▶ The authors used the following measure of paradoxical excitement. "Paradoxical excitement responses were categorized with modification of cooperation score as follows: 0, none (no excitement response); 1, mild (increased talkativeness, irrational talking, or brief spontaneous movement with position remaining); 2, moderate (restlessness, loss of cooperation, or spontaneous movements requiring repositioning with no need of restraint); 3, severe (agitation and spontaneous movements with a need to restrain the patient). The response was observed for 30 minutes and scored every 5 minutes by one of the authors who was blind to the patient's Alcohol Use Disorder Identification Test score, and the highest score was used for statistical analysis. The observation period was limited to 30 minutes in both studies to eliminate a confounding factor caused by a different sedation time.

The authors' findings that "hazardous and harmful" alcohol drinkers had an increase in paradoxical excitement might best be explained as a version of the paradoxical excitement that occurs at low dose—that is, the normal dose of propofol may be low for a hazardous and harmful drinker. In simple terms, low doses may be enough to antagonize the gamma-aminobutyric acid receptor and create excitement; high doses are required to stimulate the receptor and cause sedation. The explanation is merely speculative, because the phenomenon is not completely explained.

R. J. Hamilton, MD

Ketamine With and Without Midazolam for Emergency Department Sedation in Adults: A Randomized Controlled Trial

Sener S, Eken C, Schultz CH, et al (Acıbadem Univ School of Medicine, Bursa, Turkey; Akdeniz Univ Hosp, Antalya, Turkey; UC Irvine School of Medicine, Orange, CA; et al)
Ann Emerg Med 57:109-114, 2011

Study Objective.—We assess whether midazolam reduces recovery agitation after ketamine administration in adult emergency department (ED) patients and also compared the incidence of adverse events (recovery agitation, respiratory, and nausea/vomiting) by the intravenous (IV) versus intramuscular (IM) route.

Methods.—This prospective, double-blind, placebo—controlled, 2×2 factorial trial randomized consecutive ED patients aged 18 to 50 years to 4 groups: receiving either 0.03 mg/kg IV midazolam or placebo, and with ketamine administered either 1.5 mg/kg IV or 4 mg/kg IM. Adverse events and sedation characteristics were recorded.

Results.—Of the 182 subjects, recovery agitation was less common in the midazolam cohorts (8% versus 25%; difference 17%; 95% confidence interval [CI] 6% to 28%; number needed to treat 6). When IV versus IM routes were compared, the incidences of adverse events were similar (recovery agitation 13% versus 17%, difference 4%, 95% CI −8% to 16%; respiratory events 0% versus 0%, difference 0%, 95% CI −2% to 2%; nausea/vomiting 28% versus 34%, difference 6%, 95% CI −8% to 20%).

Conclusion.—Coadministered midazolam significantly reduces the incidence of recovery agitation after ketamine procedural sedation and analgesia in ED adults (number needed to treat 6). Adverse events occur at similar frequency by the IV or IM routes.

▶ Emergency physicians may be resistant to use ketamine for procedural sedation because of concerns related to emergence phenomenon. If treating physicians could decrease or even prevent the adverse psychiatric circumstances, the use of ketamine may increase. In this prospective, randomized, double-blind, placebo-controlled trial, the authors endeavored to determine whether the addition of midazolam to ketamine decreased the incidence of the emergence phenomenon when sedating adults. Patients receiving the midazolam-ketamine cocktail were less likely, with statistical significance, to experience recovery agitation or gastrointestinal events, when compared with the ketamine alone cohort. They present a number needed to treat of 6. The authors used a dichotomous approach (agitation or not) to assess the midazolam response, and therefore any additional graduated improvement is lost in the details. One lost outcome of the study is that no patient in either group experienced a respiratory adverse event (apnea, laryngospasm, or oxygen desaturation), further testifying to the safety of ketamine.

E. C. Bruno, MD

Management of intentional superwarfarin poisoning with long-term vitamin K and brodifacoum levels

Gunja N, Coggins A, Bidny S (The Children's Hosp at Westmead, Sydney, Australia; Westmead Hosp, Sydney, Australia; Division of Analytical Laboratories, Sydney, Australia)
Clin Toxicol 49:385-390, 2011

Context.—Brodifacoum is a widely available superwarfarin used as a commercial rodenticide. Toxicity from long-acting anticoagulant rodenticides, primarily from uncontrolled bleeding, has been reported. Very little published toxicokinetic data are available for human brodifacoum poisoning. Management is also contentious with uncertainty over the dose, frequency, and duration of antidote treatment with vitamin K. The role of brodifacoum levels in guiding management is not entirely established.

Methods.—A novel, highly sensitive method was developed for measuring all commercially available rodenticide-hydroxycoumarin anti-coagulants. Monthly brodifacoum levels were performed in two patients to determine half-life and expected time for levels to fall below 10 μL.

Results.—We report two concurrent cases at our clinical toxicology service that required prolonged treatment with oral vitamin K to achieve normalisation of coagulation studies. Brodifacoum elimination appears to follow first-order kinetics. Case 1 had a brodifacoum elimination half-life of 33 days and was treated with vitamin K (100 mg) for 6 months. Case 2 was treated with vitamin K (100 mg) for 3 months with a half-life of 15 days.

Discussion.—Our cases illustrate the positive experience in the utility of brodifacoum levels to confirm diagnosis and aid in directing antidote therapy. Large ingestions of brodifacoum-containing rodenticides are likely to require high-dose oral vitamin K administered daily. A brodifacoum level below 10 μL was associated with a normal coagulation profile following completion of vitamin K_1 therapy in our cases; this level may prove to be a safe treatment cessation threshold.

▶ A patient overdoses on a long-acting anticoagulant, and you prevent or treat toxicity with vitamin K. But when do you stop the vitamin K? You would not want to risk allowing the patient to become anticoagulant again. This article provides some valuable guidance in managing these cases and is valuable to keep in your reference library.

R. J. Hamilton, MD

Serum concentrations in three children with unintentional tetrahydrozoline overdose
Lowry JA, Garg U (Univ of Missouri School of Medicine, Kansas City)
Clin Toxicol 49:434-435, 2011

Background.—Major symptoms can occur from tetrahydrozoline (THZ) overdoses in young children, requiring intensive care management. We report three cases that presented with CNS depression and cardiovascular effects where serum concentrations were performed.

Case Report.—Case 1 ingested an unknown amount of eye drops containing THZ, resulting in altered mental status, bradycardia, hypothermia, and hypotension. Cases 2 and 3 ingested 7.5 mL of eye drops containing THZ. Case 2 presented to the emergency department (ED) without symptoms but became lethargic and bradycardic 90 min after ingestion. By contrast, Case 3 became lethargic 15 min after ingestion and required intubation on arrival to the ED. All children were admitted to ICU for observation and improved within 24 h of ingestion. Urine obtained for drug screening was positive for THZ. Blood was obtained to assess level using gas-chromatography mass-spectrometry (GC-MS).

Case Discussion.—Case 1 had plasma levels of 51.4 and 23.6 ng/mL at 7 and 12 h, respectively, after ingestion, revealing a half-life of 4.4 h. Numerous case reports have been published documenting the dangers of ingesting these topical over-the-counter (OTC) products. However, human PK data are not available to help in our understanding of THZ toxicokinetics and disposition in humans after ingestion.

Conclusion.—We report three pediatric cases after ingestion of THZ where plasma concentrations were obtained with a calculated half-life of 4.4 h in one case.

▶ Note the typical pattern of hypertension and bradycardia, which is specific for only a few overdoses, baclofen overdose being the other common one. The forensic data are useful in confirming ingestion and also in predicting the length of time required for improvement.

R. J. Hamilton, MD

Serum uric acid level as a marker for mortality and acute kidney injury in patients with acute paraquat intoxication
Kim J-H, Gil H-W, Yang J-O, et al (Soonchunhyang Univ Cheonan Hosp, Korea)
Nephrol Dial Transplant 26:1846-1852, 2011

Background.—Paraquat (PQ) is a non-selective herbicide that generates reactive oxygen species (ROS) *in vivo*. Uric acid emerged as a marker of oxidative stress and may enhance ROS-mediated injury in acute PQ intoxication. Therefore, we investigated the association between uric acid levels and mortality and acute kidney injury (AKI) in the present study.

Methods.—From January 2007 to December 2008, patients who arrived at our hospital with acute PQ intoxication ($n = 513$) were included in the study. Patients were divided into two groups (hyperuricaemia *vs* non-hyperuricaemia) based on uric acid levels. Mortality and AKI were analysed in reference to uric acid level.

Results.—Patient mortality was higher in the hyperuricaemia group than the non-hyperuricaemia group (68.4% *vs* 38.3%, $P < 0.05$). The incidence of AKI and kidney failure was 64% and 43.3%, respectively. Hyperuricaemia increased the risk of mortality and kidney failure to 3.7- and 3.3-fold after adjustments for age, sex and the estimated amounts of PQ ingestion. Mean serum uric acid level was higher in death group than survival group and higher in kidney failure group than non-AKI group and non-failure group.

Conclusions.—Baseline serum uric acid level might be a good clinical marker for patients at risk of mortality and AKI after acute PQ intoxication.

▶ Predicting outcome in paraquat exposure is difficult. Paraquat does have a nomogram, but most US hospitals cannot turn a level around quickly. This approach has promise for providing quick surrogate marker information.

R. J. Hamilton, MD

Severe acute cardiomyopathy associated with venlafaxine overdose and possible role of CYP2D6 and CYP2C19 polymorphisms
Vinetti M, Haufroid V, Capron A, et al (Université catholique de Louvain, Brussels, Belgium; et al)
Clin Toxicol (Phila) 49:865-869, 2011

Introduction.—Venlafaxine (VEN) is a serotonin-norepinephrine-dopamine reuptake inhibitor that causes usually a mild cardiotoxicity when ingested in overdose. We report a patient who developed acute heart failure following overdose. As the toxicokinetic data suggested a prolonged metabolism, genetic polymorphisms for cytochrome P450 isoenzymes CYP2D6 and CYP2C19 were also investigated.

Case Report.—A 34-year-old woman was admitted to the hospital 10 hours after the ingestion of an 11.25 g overdose of VEN. She was comatose and suffered two self-limited seizures. The electrocardiogram showed diffuse ST segment depression, but normal QRS and QTc duration. The plasma levels on admission were 18015 and 3846 ng/ml for VEN and the metabolite O-desmethylvenlafaxine (ODV), respectively. The patient developed severe cardiodepression. The left ventricular shortening fraction was only 9% on echocardiography. The patient was oliguric and required continuous venovenous hemofiltration. The administration of milrinone was required for 12 days, and norepinephrine for 10 days. Left ventricular function recovered. The calculated elimination half-life was 30.8 and 72.2 hours for VEN and ODV, respectively. The patient genotype was CYP2D6*1/*5, the *5 allele corresponding to a complete deletion of CYP2D6 gene.

Conclusions.—Severe and sustained cardiotoxicity following VEN overdose may be related to the amount ingested, as well as to the genetic polymorphism for CYP2D6 leading to a delayed elimination of active metabolite (Fig3).

▶ Venlafaxine is a serotonin-norepinephrine-dopamine reuptake inhibitor that usually results in sedation that resolves with supportive care. Rarely do we see cardiovascular effects. This drug is extensively metabolized by the liver mainly through the cytochrome P450-2D6 and -2C19 isoenzymes (CYP2D6 and CYP2C19) to form its major pharmacologically active metabolite, O-desmethyl-venlafaxine (ODV); a minor metabolite, N-desmethylvenlafaxine, is also formed

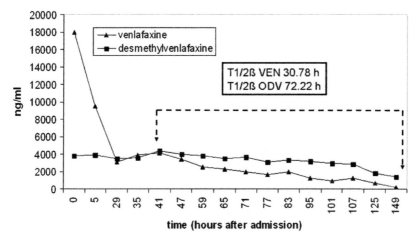

FIGURE 3.—Tokicokinetic data with elimination half-life of venlafaxine (VEN) and O-desmethylven-lafaxine (ODV) calculated from the 41st hour after admission. (Reprinted from Vinetti M, Haufroid V, Capron A, et al. Severe acute cardiomyopathy associated with venlafaxine overdose and possible role of CYP2D6 and CYP2C19 polymorphisms. *Clin Toxicol (Phila).* 2011;49:865-869, reprinted with permission from Taylor & Francis, Ltd.)

by CYP3A4 and possibly CYP2C19. In this case, CYP2D6 and CYP2C19 genetic polymorphism lead to severe toxicity from altered toxicokinetics and toxicodynamics. This is a fascinating article and opens up the concept of toxicogenetics in acute overdose—how do you predict the patient who might have a severe reaction? In this case, the patient presented with the toxicity, so there was no need to discover it, but the genetic polymorphism explains the clinical course. We know this issue is present in other overdoses—the rate of alcohol metabolism being one of them. It is an intriguing issue.

R. J. Hamilton, MD

Studies on ethylene glycol poisoning: One patient – 154 admissions
Hovda KE, Julsrud J, Øvrebø S, et al (Oslo Univ Hosp, Ullevaal, Norway; Univ of Tromsø, Norway; Natl Inst of Occupational Health, Oslo, Norway)
Clin Toxicol 49:478-484, 2011

Objective.—Fomepizole is the antidote of choice in toxic alcohol poisonings. Potential side effects from frequent use of fomepizole were studied in a patient admitted 154 times with ethylene glycol (EG) poisoning. The intra-individual correlation between the serum-ethylene glycol (serum-EG) and the osmolal gap (OG) EG-kinetics, and other laboratory parameters were also studied.

Methods.—Combined pro- and retrospective collection of material from three different hospitals, and results from autopsy.

Results.—A 26-year-old female with a dissociative disorder was admitted with EG poisoning a total of 154 times. Her admission data revealed a median pH of 7.31 (range 6.87−7.49), pCO$_2$: 4.2 kPa (1.26.7) (32 mmHg [950]), HCO$_3^-$: 15 mmol/L (42−6) (15 mEq/L [42−6]), base deficit (BD): 10 mmol/L (−4 to 27) (10 mEq/L [−4 to 27]), serum-creatinine 65 μmol/L (40−133) (0.74 mg/dL [0.45−1.51]), OG 81 mOsm/kgH$_2$O (25−132), and serum-EG 44 mmol/L (4−112) (250 mg/dL [25−700]). She was treated with fomepizole 99 times, ethanol 60 times (with a combination of both six times), and dialysis 73 times. The correlation between serum-EG and OG was good (r^2 = 0.76). She was finally found dead outside hospital with an EG blood concentration of 81 mmol/L (506 mg/dL). An autopsy revealed calcium oxalate crystals in the kidneys, slight liver steatosis, and slight edema of the lungs.

Discussion.—The frequent use of fomepizole in this young patient was not associated with any detectable side effects; neither on clinical examination and lab screening, nor on the later autopsy. Regarding the sequelae from the repetitive EG-poisoning episodes, her kidney function seemed to normalize after each overdose. She was treated with buffer and antidote without hemodialysis 81 times without complications, supporting the safety of this approach in selected cases.

▶ This report amazed me: 154 episodes of ethylene glycol toxicity and the use of fomepizole—enough said!

R. J. Hamilton, MD

Tricyclic Antidepressant Overdose in a Toddler Treated With Intravenous Lipid Emulsion
Hendron D, Menagh G, Sandilands EA, et al (Craigavon Area Hosp, Portadown, Northern Ireland; Royal Belfast Hosp for Sick Children, Northern Ireland; Royal Infirmary of Edinburgh, Scotland)
Pediatrics 128:e1628-e1632, 2011

We report a case that involves the use of intravenous lipid emulsion as an antidote for a drug overdose involving a 20-month-old girl who had ingested a potentially lethal amount of the tricyclic antidepressant (TCA) dothiepin. The patient's condition continued to deteriorate despite implementation of standard pediatric treatment recommendations for TCA toxicity. Administration of intravenous lipid emulsion in addition to standard therapy (including sodium bicarbonate) and direct-current cardioversion for ventricular arrhythmia led to a successful outcome. The case report is followed by a review of the current evidence underlying this novel therapy and the background on its use. TCA toxicity is addressed specifically.

▶ I include the dose used in this case to illustrate the nonstandardized approach that currently exists. This 10-kg patient received a bolus dose of 10 mL of intravenous lipid emulsion (1 mL/kg Intralipid 20% followed by an infusion of 150 mL/h [0.25 mL/kg per minute]). Although it is possible that the NaHCO3 had a delayed effect, the improvement in the patient does seem to correspond to the administration of Intralipid.

R. J. Hamilton, MD

Unrecognized fatalities related to colchicine in hospitalized patients
Mullins M, Cannarozzi AA, Bailey TC, et al (Washington Univ, St Louis, MO)
Clin Toxicol 49:648-652, 2011

Background.—Colchicine is commonly used for the treatment of gout and occasionally for other inflammatory diseases. It has a narrow therapeutic index and the potential for severe or fatal toxicity.

Objectives.—We sought to determine (1) the frequency of colchicine toxicity among hospitalized patients taking colchicine who died during an admission, (2) the likelihood that colchicine contributed to death, (3) whether patients were taking interacting medications that could have contributed to toxicity, and (4) whether colchicine dosing among these patients adhered to established guidelines.

Methods.—We conducted an IRB-approved, retrospective chart review at an urban, tertiary care, 1228-bed, university hospital. Subjects included hospitalized patients who received colchicine and died in hospital between 1 January 2000 and 28 February 2007. We reviewed charts for signs and symptoms of colchicine toxicity. An expert panel reviewed each case and classified the likelihood of colchicine toxicity, the likelihood of a causal

---

TABLE 3.—Narrative Summaries of Patients With Colchicine Toxicity Classified as Certain

---

Patient A was a 69-year-old woman with no history of gout. She had taken amoxicillin/clavulanate for sinusitis for 10 days before hospital admission for pleuritic chest pain. Her estimated CrCl was 74 mL/min. She received IV ceftriaxone and oral azithromycin in the ED for possible pneumonia before a chest CT scan and echocardiogram showed pleural and pericardial effusion. Her pericardial fluid had abundant neutrophils, but no growth on the culture. She was treated with oral colchicine 0.6 mg twice daily for the pericarditis and oral amiodarone 400 mg three times daily for atrial fibrillation. She developed nausea, vomiting, diarrhea with negative stool cultures, and early leukocytosis followed by leukopenia. Colchicine was continued, and she was started on amiodarone IV infusion. Colchicine was stopped after 10 days as she progressed to multi-system organ failure. She developed cardiogenic shock, which was refractory to dobutamine, norepinephrine, phenylephrine, and vasopressin, and died of cardiac arrest. Her serum colchicine concentration in blood obtained 65 h after her last dose was 3.3 ng/mL (National Medical Laboratories, Willow Grove, PA), which is in the range expected for the peak concentration after 1 mg orally.
Patient B was a 68-year-old man with multiple medical problems prior to admission. His estimated CrCl was 53 mL/min. He was taking amiodarone 400 mg three times daily. He began having knee pain in hospital and received 1 mg IV followed by 1.2 mg orally every 2—4 h with a total dose of 11.8 mg over 17 h. He developed acute renal failure and thrombocytopenia. He died of cardiac arrest the next day.
Patient C was a 75-year-old man with a prior history of gout. His estimated CrCl was 70 mL/min. He received colchicine 1.2 mg orally every 2—4 h and received a total of 12.2 mg over 30 h. He developed acute renal failure, hypotension, and cardiac arrest with pulseless electrical activity.
Patient D was an 86-year-old man admitted for non-operative care after a femur fracture. His estimated creatinine clearance was 30 mL/min. He was unable to take oral colchicine, so he received an IV loading dose of 2 mg followed by 0.5 mg IV every 6 h with a total of 5 mg within 36 h. He developed acute renal failure, diarrhea with negative stool studies, and cardiac arrest.

---

role of colchicine in the death using the WHO classification system, and the appropriateness of colchicine dosing.

Results.—Thirty-seven hospitalized patients who died during the 86-month study period received colchicine. Toxicity was unlikely in 20/37, possible in 8/37, likely in 5/37, and certain in 4/37. A contributing role for colchicine in causing death was unlikely in 24/37, possible in 7/37, likely in 3/37, and certain in 3/37. Colchicine doses (based on creatinine clearance) exceeded the accepted range for 12 patients, including 10 of 17 cases of toxicity and 8 of 13 cases of death classified as possible or higher. Seventeen patients received interacting medications, including 8 of 17 cases of toxicity and 8 of 13 cases of death classified as possible or higher.

Conclusion.—Colchicine toxicity was frequent in this cohort and may have contributed to about one-third of the deaths. Inappropriate dosing of colchicine occurred frequently and was related to toxicity and death (Table 3).

▶ When I was a student in pharmacology class, I was taught about the concept of therapeutic window—that range of drug exposure that is therapeutic and safe. Above this amount, the drug becomes toxic. Colchicine has a narrow therapeutic window. The physician should never prescribe this drug without a heightened sense of concern.

R. J. Hamilton, MD

The effects of intravenous calcium in patients with digoxin toxicity

Levine M, Nikkanen H, Pallin DJ (Banner Good Samaritan Med Ctr, Phoenix, AZ; Brigham and Women's Hosp, Boston, MA)

J Emerg Med 40:41-46, 2011

Background.—Digoxin is an inhibitor of the sodium-potassium ATPase. In overdose, hyperkalemia is common. Although hyperkalemia is often treated with intravenous calcium, it is traditionally contraindicated in digoxin toxicity.

Objectives.—To analyze records from patients treated with intravenous calcium while digoxin-toxic.

Methods.—We reviewed the charts of all adult patients diagnosed with digoxin toxicity in a large teaching hospital over 17.5 years. The main outcome measures were frequency of life-threatening dysrhythmia within 1 h of calcium administration, and mortality rate in patients who did vs. patients who did not receive intravenous calcium. We use multivariate logistic regression to ensure that no relationship was overlooked due to negative confounders (controlling for age, creatinine, systolic blood pressure, peak serum potassium, time of development of digoxin toxicity, and digoxin concentration).

Results.—We identified 161 patients diagnosed with digoxin toxicity, and were able to retrieve 159 records. Of these, 23 patients received calcium. No life-threatening dysrhythmias occurred within 1 h of calcium administration. Mortality was similar among those who did not receive calcium (27/136, 20%) compared to those who did (5/23, 22%). In the multivariate analysis, calcium was non-significantly associated with decreased odds of death (odds ratio 0.76; 95% confidence interval [CI] 0.24—2.5). Each 1 mEq/L rise in serum potassium concentration was associated with an increased mortality odds ratio of 1.5 (95% CI 1.0—2.3).

Conclusion.—Among digoxin-intoxicated humans, intravenous calcium does not seem to cause malignant dysrhythmias or increase mortality. We found no support for the historical belief that calcium administration is contraindicated in digoxin-toxic patients.

▶ In this retrospective review, the authors attempted (and failed) to find an association between the development of a lethal arrhythmia and the administration of intravenous calcium in patients with digoxin-induced hyperkalemia. Residency training programs perpetuate the dogma that this practice is associated with the "stone heart" phenomenon. This medical myth is based on pre-World War II literature regarding concurrent use of cardiac glycosides and intravenous calcium. The referenced articles from the 1920s and 1930s were predominantly canine studies that demonstrated the potency of rapid calcium infusions to induce life-threatening ventricular arrhythmias, rather than the lethality of the cardiac glycoside - calcium combination. The landmark study that vilified the digoxin-calcium combination is based on 2 patients, and the referenced autopsy of 1 patient describes a "flabby heart," not a rigid one.[1] "Stone heart" is actually a pediatric cardiothoracic surgery term, first described by Cooley in 1972.[2]

The authors found an overall mortality rate of 20% in patients with digoxin toxicity, but the rates were similar among patients who received calcium and those who did not. The only variable that correlated with increased mortality was the serum potassium concentration. Based on the results of this retrospective review, the challenge now falls to the national and international toxicology organizations to present a position statement endorsing the appropriate management of hyperkalemia, regardless of digoxin's potential involvement.

E. C. Bruno, MD

References

1. Bower JO, Mengle HAK. The additive effect of calcium and digitalis: a warning, with a report of two deaths. *JAMA.* 1936;106:1511-1553.
2. Cooley DA, Reul GJ, Wukasch DC. Ischemic contracture of the heart: "stone heart". *Am J Cardiol.* 1972;29:575-577.

Drugs of Abuse

Identification of Recent Cannabis Use: Whole-Blood and Plasma Free and Glucuronidated Cannabinoid Pharmacokinetics following Controlled Smoked Cannabis Administration

Schwope DM, Karschner EL, Gorelick DA, et al (Natl Inst on Drug Abuse, Baltimore, MD)
Clin Chem 57:1406-1414, 2011

Background.—Δ^9-Tetrahydrocannabinol (THC) is the most frequently observed illicit drug in investigations of accidents and driving under the influence of drugs. THC-glucuronide has been suggested as a marker of recent cannabis use, but there are no blood data following controlled THC administration to test this hypothesis. Furthermore, there are no studies directly examining whole-blood cannabinoid pharmacokinetics, although this matrix is often the only available specimen.

Methods.—Participants (9 men, 1 woman) resided on a closed research unit and smoked one 6.8% THC cannabis cigarette ad libitum. We quantified THC, 11-hydroxy-THC (11-OH-THC), 11-nor-9-carboxy-THC (THCCOOH), cannabidiol (CBD), cannabinol (CBN), THC-glucuronide and THCCOOH-glucuronide directly in whole blood and plasma by liquid chromatography/tandem mass spectrometry within 24 h of collection to obviate stability issues.

Results.—Median whole blood (plasma) observed maximum concentrations (C_{max}) were 50 (76), 6.4 (10), 41 (67), 1.3 (2.0), 2.4 (3.6), 89 (190), and 0.7 (1.4) μg/L 0.25 h after starting smoking for THC, 11-OH-THC, THCCOOH, CBD, CBN, and THCCOOH-glucuronide, respectively, and 0.5 h for THC-glucuronide. At observed C_{max}, whole-blood (plasma) detection rates were 60% (80%), 80% (90%), and 50% (80%) for CBD, CBN, and THC-glucuronide, respectively. CBD and CBN were not detectable after 1 h in either matrix (LOQ 1.0 μg/L).

Conclusions.—Human whole-blood cannabinoid data following cannabis smoking will assist whole blood and plasma cannabinoid interpretation, while furthering identification of recent cannabis intake.

▶ This article is valuable for individuals who may do review of forensic specimens. Fig 6 in the original article alone is an excellent guide to understanding how metabolites rise and fall after marijuana use. However, it does not appear the authors have identified a tell-all metabolite.

R. J. Hamilton, MD

Myocardial Infarction Associated With Use of the Synthetic Cannabinoid K2

Mir A, Obafemi A, Young A, et al (UT Southwestern Med Ctr, Dallas, TX)
Pediatrics 128:e1622-e1627, 2011

Designer drugs have been problematic over the years. Products such as K2 and Spice, which contain synthetic cannabinoids, are marketed as incense and are widely available on the Internet and at various specialty shops. The effects are reported as cannabis-like after smoking them. In addition, use of these synthetic cannabinoids will not appear on a routine urine toxicology screen. Recently, K2 became a popular alternative to marijuana among youths. Health implications of these designer drugs are not completely understood. Little has been reported about the harmful effects of K2. We report here the first (to our knowledge) cases of myocardial infarction (MI) after smoking K2. Three patients presented separately to the emergency department complaining of chest pain within days after the use of K2. Acute MI was diagnosed in each case on the basis of electrocardiogram changes and elevated troponin levels. Coronary angiography was performed, and the results were normal for the first 2 patients. The incidence of STelevation MI is low among teenagers, and association with drug use should be suspected. Public education and awareness need to be heightened about the possible health implications of K2.

▶ Definitely keep a look out for this drug, as it has exploded in its abuse. Measures are currently underway to remove it from shelves and make it unavailable, which will decrease the incidence but not eliminate it. The mechanism on how this synthetic cannabinoid causes myocardial ischemia is completely unclear. Note the delay onset in chest pain after smoking K2 by about a day and the presence of normal coronary arteries at catheterization.

R. J. Hamilton, MD

Treatment of cocaine overdose with lipid emulsion

Jakkala-Saibaba R, Morgan PG, Morton GL (East Surrey Hosp, Redhill, UK)
Anaesthesia 66:1168-1170, 2011

We describe the management and recovery of a 28-year-old man following a history of overdose by nasal inhalation of cocaine. The patient was presented in a comatose state suffering from seizures and marked cardiovascularly instability. Intravenous lipid emulsion was administered following initial resuscitation and tracheal intubation, as a means of treating persistent cardiac arrhythmias and profound hypotension. Following lipid emulsion therapy, the patient's life-threatening cardiovascular parameters rapidly improved and he recovered well without any side effects, thus being discharged within 2 days.

▶ Note the dose used here was a 20% lipid emulsion (Intralipid) administered intravenously as an initial bolus dose of 1.5 mL/kg (120 mL), followed by an infusion of 15 mL/kg (380 mL) over 20 minutes. This adds to the growing body of knowledge about the use of lipid emulsion. So far, sporadic case reports are encouraging, but, of course, no one is reporting their failures.

R. J. Hamilton, MD

Environmental and Occupational

Carbon monoxide poisoning associated with water pipe smoking

Türkmen S, Eryigit U, Sahin A, et al (Karadeniz Technical Univ, Trabzon, Turkey)
Clin Toxicol 49:697-698, 2011

The water pipe is a means of tobacco consumption widespread in Turkey and Arab countries. We present two patients brought to our emergency department due to a syncopal attack secondary to carbon monoxide toxicity following water pipe use. This rare form of poisoning should be borne in mind by emergency physicians as a differential diagnosis in water pipe smokers. Water pipes should be used where there is adequate ventilation.

▶ "Normal" carboxyhemoglobin (COHb) levels are less than 2% from the catabolism of hemoglobin. In a smoker, the expected COHb levels are 5% to 6%, and for a water-pipe smoker, the expected level is 10%. The case reports here had levels of 26% and 27%. Water-pipe smoking is not common in the United States, but add this to the list of things to which an ED physician must maintain a heightened awareness.

R. J. Hamilton, MD

Residential Carbon Monoxide Detector Failure Rates in the United States
Ryan TJ, Arnold KJ (Ohio Univ, Athens)
Am J Public Health 101:e15-e17, 2011

There are more than 38 million residential carbon monoxide detectors installed in the United States. We tested 30 detectors in use and found that more than half failed to function properly, alarming too early or too late. Forty percent of detectors failed to alarm in hazardous concentrations, despite outward indications that they were operating as intended. Public health professionals should consider community education concerning detector use and should work with stakeholders to improve the reliability and accuracy of these devices.

▶ I think this is an important article for emergency department physicians for a number of reasons. First, do not assume that because the CO detector did not go off that there was no CO exposure, especially if the detector has been in place for several years. In addition, emergency medical services and fire departments should remind individuals to replace batteries and check to determine whether the unit needs replacement according to manufacturer recommendations twice a year.

R. J. Hamilton, MD

Solid organ procurement from donors with carbon monoxide poisoning and/or burn - a systematic review
Busche MN, Knobloch K, Herold C, et al (Hannover Med School, Germany)
Burns 37:814-822, 2011

Introduction.—Traditionally, carbon monoxide poisoning and/or burn are considered contra-indications to organ procurement. Previously reported cases have shown mixed results and many have been redundantly reported in the literature.

Methods.—We performed a systematic review of all reported cases of organ transplantation procured from donors with carbon monoxide poisoning and/ or burn to investigate whether these patients are suitable donors for solid organ transplantations.

Results.—Organ survival rates of reported organs were high (86%). All organs procured from donors with carbon monoxide poisoning and burn survived during follow-up. Mean donors' peak carbon monoxide levels were comparable for organs surviving or failing during follow-up (31 ± 2.7 vs. 29 ± 26.8; $p = 0.95$). Eighty-seven per cent of organs procured from donors supported with inotropes or vasopressors prior to organ procurement and 91% of organs procured from donors who were cardiopulmonary resuscitated prior to organ procurement survived during follow-up.

Conclusions.—Burn, carbon monoxide poisoning, high peak carbon monoxide-levels, use of inotropes or vasopressors or cardiopulmonary resuscitation prior to procurement are not contraindications for organ procurement and transplantation. New guidelines for burn units defining the special requirements for organ procurement from donors with carbon monoxide poisoning and/or burn are needed to raise the awareness for potential organ donors and to ultimately increase the donor pool and save patients' lives.

▶ I include this article to remind emergency medicine physicians and toxicologists that carbon monoxide—poisoned patients are potential organ donors.

R. J. Hamilton, MD

Natural Toxins and Envenomation

"Spider Bite" Lesions are Usually Diagnosed as Skin and Soft-Tissue Infections

Suchard JR (Univ of California, Orange)
J Emerg Med 41:473-481, 2011

Background.—Many people seek medical attention for skin lesions and other conditions they attribute to spider bites. Prior experience suggests that many of these lesions have alternate causes, especially infections with community-acquired methicillin-resistant *Staphylococcus aureus* (CA-MRSA).

Objectives.—This study determined the percentage of emergency department (ED) patients reporting a "spider bite" who received a clinical diagnosis of spider bite by their physician vs. other etiologies, and if the diagnoses correlated with demographic risk factors for developing CA-MRSA infections.

Methods.—ED patients who reported that their condition was caused by a "spider bite" were prospectively enrolled in an anonymous, voluntary survey regarding details of their illness and demographic information. Discharge diagnoses were also collected and categorized as: spider bite, bite from other animal (including unknown arthropod), infection, or other diagnosis.

Results.—There were 182 patients enrolled over 23 months. Seven patients (3.8%) were diagnosed with actual spider bites, 9 patients (4.9%) with bites from other animals, 156 patients (85.7%) with infections, and 6 patients (3.3%) were given other diagnoses. Four patients were given concurrent diagnoses in two categories, and 8 (4.4%) did not have the diagnosis recorded on the data collection instrument. No statistically significant associations were found between the patients' diagnostic categories and the demographic risk factors for CA-MRSA assessed.

Conclusion.—ED patients reporting a "spider bite" were most frequently diagnosed with skin and soft-tissue infections. Clinically confirmed spider bites were rare, and were caused by black widow spiders when the species could be identified.

▶ This study took place in Orange, California. The results would have been different in areas of the country where necrotic spider species are more prevalent. Nonetheless, the point is well made: the presentation of a spider bite is the same presentation as a rapidly progressing community-acquired methicillin-resistant *Staphylococcus aureus* skin infection. In areas where recluse and widow spiders are rare to nonexistent, there is no need to challenge the patient's assertion that the lesion was caused by a spider. It is probably more important to prescribed antimicrobials as indicated and follow up the wound to make sure that is improving appropriately.

R. J. Hamilton, MD

A heteromeric Texas coral snake toxin targets acid-sensing ion channels to produce pain
Bohlen CJ, Chesler AT, Sharif-Naeini R, et al (Univ of California, San Francisco; et al)
Nature 479:410-414, 2011

Natural products that elicit discomfort or pain represent invaluable tools for probing molecular mechanisms underlying pain sensation. Plant-derived irritants have predominated in this regard, but animal venoms have also evolved to avert predators by targeting neurons and receptors whose activation produces noxious sensations. As such, venoms provide a rich and varied source of small molecule and protein pharmacophores that can be exploited to characterize and manipulate key components of the pain-signalling pathway. With this in mind, here we perform an unbiased *in vitro* screen to identify snake venoms capable of activating somatosensory neurons. Venom from the Texas coral snake (*Micrurus tener tener*), whose bite produces intense and unremitting pain, excites a large cohort of sensory neurons. The purified active species (MitTx) consists of a heteromeric complex between Kunitz- and phospholipase-A2-like proteins that together function as a potent, persistent and selective agonist for acid-sensing ion channels (ASICs), showing equal or greater efficacy compared with acidic pH. MitTx is highly selective for the ASIC1 subtype at neutral pH; under more acidic conditions (pH < 6.5), MitTx massively potentiates (>100-fold) proton-evoked activation of ASIC2a channels. These observations raise the possibility that ASIC channels function as coincidence detectors for extracellular protons and other, as yet unidentified, endogenous factors. Purified MitTx elicits robust pain-related behaviour in mice by activation of ASIC1 channels on capsaicin-sensitive nerve fibres. These findings reveal a mechanism whereby snake venoms produce pain, and highlight an unexpected contribution of ASIC1 channels to nociception.

▶ Acid sensing ion channels (ASICs) are a family of cation channels expressed principally in neurons and that are activated by hydrogen ions, thus making them the important receptors responsible for the perception of the pain of acidosis. It's very interesting that coral snake venom triggers these channels, but it may turn out that the value of this information is in further elucidating the role of ASIC channels in nociception.

R. J. Hamilton, MD

Acute Generalized Exanthematous Pustulosis and Coombs-Positive Hemolytic Anemia in a Child Following *Loxosceles reclusa* Envenomation

Lane L, McCoppin HH, Dyer J (Univ of Missouri, Columbia)
Pediatr Dermatol 28:685-688, 2011

Previously reported cases of acute generalized exanthematous pustulosis secondary to brown recluse spider bite have been questioned due to lack of identification of the spider or because of the concomitant administration of antibiotics. We report a 9-year-old boy who arrived at the emergency department with a confirmed *Loxosceles reclusa* bite to the neck. On the third day of hospitalization, he developed hundreds of monomorphous, sterile pustules, initially in intertriginous areas. The eruption disseminated and was followed by pinpoint desquamation typical for acute generalized exanthematous pustulosis. During this he also developed late onset Coombs-positive hemolytic anemia and systemic loxoscelism. Sphingomyelinase in *Loxosceles* venom induces the production of interleukin-8 and granulocyte-macrophage colony-stimulating factor, cytokines involved in the pathogenesis of acute generalized exanthematous pustulosis, providing a mechanism by which

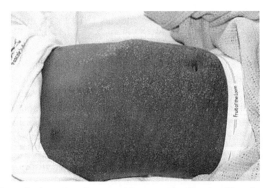

FIGURE 2.—Generalized eruption of monomorphous pustules. (Reprinted from Lane L, McCoppin HH, Dyer J. Acute generalized exanthematous pustulosis and coombs-positive hemolytic anemia in a child following *Loxosceles reclusa* envenomation. *Pediatr Dermatol.* 2011;28:685-688, with permission from Wiley-Blackwell.)

Loxosceles reclusa bite may trigger acute generalized exanthematous pustulosis. We suggest that this case adds *Loxosceles* envenomation to the spectrum of agents that can trigger acute generalized exanthematous pustulosis (Fig 2).

▶ Since very few of the spider bites I see in the Northeast United States are actually *Loxosceles reclusa*, the first thing I look for is the positive identification of the species, the correct habitat in the region of the United States, and an appropriately evolving lesion. This case report meets all those requirements, so I agree with the author's conclusion of attributing this reaction to loxoscelism.

R. J. Hamilton, MD

Cardiac abnormalities in severe acute dichlorvos poisoning
He X, Li C, Wei D, et al (Capital Med Univ, Beijing, China)
Crit Care Med 39:1906-1912, 2011

Objective.—Patients with organophosphorus poisoning sometimes die suddenly during rigorous treatment, possibly from myocardial injury. This study sought to elucidate the mechanisms underlying organophosphorus poisoning-induced cardiotoxicity.

Design.—Prospective observational study.

Setting.—Urban, tertiary teaching hospital emergency intensive care unit with 10 beds.

Patients.—Forty-one patients with severe acute dichlorvos poisoning were consecutively enrolled (n = 92) at emergency intensive care unit and followed for 3 months.

Measurements and Main Results.—Levels of serum creatine kinase isoenzyme myocardium, cardiac troponin I, acetylcholinesterase, acetylcholine, epinephrine, and norepinephrine were tested on hospital days 1, 3, and 5 and on discharge day. Electrocardiography was recorded on admission and then every other day. Transthoracic echocardiography was performed at admission, in the acute phase, before discharge, and during follow-up. Technetium 99m-sestamibi myocardial single photon emission computed tomography was conducted in four patients. Thirty-seven (90.2%) patients survived and four (9.8%) patients died during treatment. We observed sinus tachycardia in 37 (90.2%) patients and ST-T changes in 33 (80.4%) patients. Creatine kinase isoenzyme myocardium and cardiac troponin I levels peaked at day 3 postadmission and then decreased to normal levels. Serum acetylcholine, epinephrine, and norepinephrine peaked at day 1 after admission and then decreased. Echocardiography revealed marked decreases in wall motion of the interventricular septum and left ventricle in the acute phase but returned to normal in the recovery phase. The left ventricular ejection fraction improved significantly from 42 ± 5% to 59 ± 4% (*p* = .001). Single photon emission computed tomography showed abnormal left ventricle perfusion.

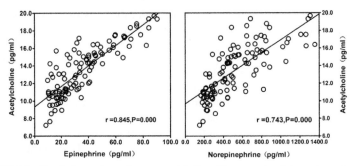

FIGURE 6.—Correlation analyses of serum acetylcholine with serum epinephrine and norepinephrine. Correlation coefficients (*r*) were analyzed with a Pearson's correlation test. (Reprinted from He X, Li C, Wei D, et al. Cardiac abnormalities in severe acute dichlorvos poisoning. *Crit Care Med.* 2011;39:1906-1912, with permission from the Society of Critical Care Medicine and Lippincott Williams & Wilkins.)

Conclusion.—Severe acute dichlorvos poisoning is associated with reversible myocardial dysfunction, possibly through an increase in catecholamine levels (Fig 6).

▶ The authors present evidence that the myocardial dysfunction seen in severe acute dichlorvos poisoning is directly related to the elevated catecholamine levels. One wonders if there is a subsegment of the population that displays this particular relationship. Further elaboration of this mechanism will be revealing.

R. J. Hamilton, MD

Evaluation of the Test-mate ChE (Cholinesterase) Field Kit in Acute Organophosphorus Poisoning

Rajapakse BN, Thiermann H, Eyer P, et al (South Asian Clinical Toxicology Res Collaboration, Peradeniya, Sri Lanka; Bundeswehr Inst of Pharmacology and Toxicology, Munich, Germany; Ludwig-Maximilians Univ, Munich, Germany; et al)
Ann Emerg Med 58:559-564, 2011

Study Objective.—Measurement of acetylcholinesterase (AChE) is recommended in the management of organophosphorus poisoning, which results in 200,000 deaths worldwide annually. The Test-mate ChE 400 is a portable field kit designed for detecting occupational organophosphorus exposure that measures RBC AChE and plasma cholinesterase (PChE) within 4 minutes. We evaluate Test-mate against a reference laboratory test in patients with acute organophosphorus self-poisoning.

Methods.—This was a cross-sectional comparison study of 14 patients with acute organophosphorus poisoning between May 2007 and June 2008. RBC AChE and PChE were measured in 96 and 91 samples, respectively, with the Test-mate ChE field kit and compared with a reference laboratory, using the limits of agreement method (Bland and Altman), κ statistics, and Spearman's correlation coefficients.

Results.—There was good agreement between the Test-mate ChE and the reference laboratory for RBC AChE. The mean difference (Test-mate—reference) was -0.62 U/g hemoglobin, 95% limits of agreement -10.84 to 9.59 U/g hemoglobin. Good agreement was also observed between the categories of mild, moderate, and severe RBC AChE inhibition (weighted κ 0.85; 95% confidence interval [CI] 0.83 to 0.87). Measurement of PChE also showed good agreement, with a mean difference (Test-mate—reference) of +0.06 U/mL blood, 95% limits of agreement -0.41 to 0.53 U/mL blood. Spearman's correlation coefficients were 0.87 (95% CI 0.81 to 0.91) for RBC AChE and 0.76 (95% CI 0.66 to 0.84) for PChE. Analysis for within-subject correlation of subjects did not change the limits of agreement.

Conclusion.—The Test-mate ChE field kit reliably provides rapid measurement of RBC AChE in acute organophosphorus poisoning.

▶ This is a very interesting article that supports the quality of this test. However, it has been my experience with field and office testing that the accuracy of the kit is related to the training of the individual using it and the frequency with which he or she uses it. This product seems to be for areas of the world where organophosphorus poisoning is common and decisions need to be made in the field to determine severity.

R. J. Hamilton, MD

Is there a role for fasciotomy in *Crotalinae* envenomations in North America?
Cumpston KL (Virginia Commonwealth Univ, Richmond)
Clin Toxicol 49:351-365, 2011

Context.—The local effects of Crotalinae envenomation can cause significant tissue destruction, pain, paresthesias, and deformity of the limb, which mimic findings of compartment syndrome, despite rare subfascial penetration of the fangs. Complicating this are the various techniques and ideas about what determines compartment syndrome combined with the fact that elevated intracompartmental pressures have been documented after Crotalinae envenomation, without clear evidence of compartment syndrome or tissue hypoperfusion.

Objective.—The purpose of this review is to evaluate the North American literature to provide an evidenced-based conclusion about the indications for fasciotomy in Crotalinae envenomations.

Methods.—The search was conducted with studies published only in the English language. The search included all human and animal publications, regardless of the format of study. The Cochrane Central Register, MEDLINE/Pub Med, Scopus, and Biological Science databases were searched. Citations from all the articles were also cross-referenced if they were pertinent to the review. Major toxicology and emergency medicine and surgical textbooks were also referenced. Abstracts from the North American Congress of Clinical Toxicology, Poisonidex®, and personal articles were also scanned to complete the process, resulting in a total of 640 sources. Papers were excluded if they were duplicates, non-North American, involved excisional therapy, or did not discuss fasciotomy. This left 99 publications applicable to our study.

Findings.—No randomized controlled trials, 8 animal experiments, 1 human prospective observational study, 24 retrospective reviews, 32 review articles, 10 case reports, 15 textbooks references, 2 abstracts, and 7 editorials were included in the analysis. Controlled animal experiments show that crotaline Fab antivenin reduces intracompartmental pressure and increases tissue perfusion, while fasciotomy either has no beneficial effect or worsens myonecrosis. The case reports and opinions supporting fasciotomy come from the surgical literature and precede the modern crotaline Fab antivenin.

Conclusion.—The current evidence does not support the use of fasciotomy or dermotomy following Crotalinae envenomation with elevated intracompartmental pressures. At present, early and adequate administration of crotaline Fab antivenin is the treatment of choice. Fasciotomy cannot be recommended until further well-designed investigations are completed.

▶ Traditionally, snake envenomations were admitted to surgical services because of the possible need for fasciotomy due to compartment syndrome. This article questions this practice in general, and this topic is worth discussing ahead of time so that guidelines for when a fasciotomy is a must and when further observation is worthwhile can be agreed upon by the treating team.

R. J. Hamilton, MD

Pressure bandaging for North American snake bite? No!
Seifert S, White J, Currie BJ (Univ of New Mexico Health Sciences Ctr, Albuquerque; Women's and Children's Hosp, North Adelaide, South Australia, Australia; Charles Darwin Univ, Northern Territory, Australia)
Clin Toxicol 49:883-885, 2011

This issue of Clinical Toxicology includes a Position Statement regarding the use of pressure immobilization for the pre-hospital treatment of North American Crotalinae envenomation. This Commentary discusses the background behind the creation of the Position Statement and explores the issues involved in applying science to real world public health recommendations and practice.

▶ Here's the bottom line—no tourniquet, no freezing, no cutting, no sucking, no wrapping, no electricity, no elevation, and no dependency. Just take jewelry off the injured extremity and go to the emergency room!

R. J. Hamilton, MD

Miscellaneous

Acute leukoencephalopathy after buprenorphine intoxication in a 2-year-old child

Bellot B, Michel F, Thomachot L, et al (Centre Hospitalier Universitaire Nord, Marseille, Cedex, France; et al)
Eur J Paediatr Neurol 15:368-371, 2011

Leukoencephalopathies have been reported after heroin inhalation or ingestion, and buprenorphine injection, but the physiopathology remains unclear. We report here the first case of leukoencephalopathy caused by buprenorphine ingestion in a 2-year-old child who was admitted for coma and fever. Due to technical problems, the toxicology screen was delayed, and infectious disease was first suspected. A brain MRI found bilateral and symmetric white matter damages in the cerebral hemispheres and the cerebellum. Rapid recovery and positive toxicology screen for buprenorphine on day 4 confirmed the diagnosis of acute intoxication.

▶ Leukoencephalopathy from heroin is a well-known phenomenon and was first described as "chasing the dragon." Heroin or a pure opioid pill is heated on a foil, and the smoke is sucked into the lungs through a straw. It is necessary to allow the pill or heroin to slide down the aluminum foil so it heats the drug to evaporation. For years it has been thought that the aluminum foil itself was the origin of a toxin that caused leukoencephalopathy, but I think this case report on buprenorphine is our first clue that it is the opioid. This is a syndrome waiting for an explanation; perhaps some great disease mechanism will be uncovered once it is understood.

R. J. Hamilton, MD

Cefixime-Induced Oculogyric Crisis

Bayram E, Bayram MT, Hiz S, et al (Dokuz Eylul Univ, Izmir, Turkey)
Pediatr Emerg Care 28:55-56, 2012

Oculogyric crisis is a neurologic adverse event characterized by bilateral dystonic, usually upward, conjugate eye deviations. Cefixime is a third-generation cephalosporin and is widely used in clinical practice in childhood. Confusion, encephalopathy, coma, myoclonus, nonconvulsive status epilepticus, and seizures have been described with the use of cephalosporins. We presented a cefixime-induced oculogyric crisis in a 7-year-old boy during the treatment of urinary tract infection, and this is the first case of cefixime-induced oculogyric crisis whose ocular symptoms gradually disappeared within 48 hours after the drug was discontinued.

▶ The proof of cause and effect came 2 weeks later in this patient when cefixime was started again for a respiratory infection and the same oculogyric crisis recurred. The mechanism is speculative, but it is worthwhile to include this drug on the list of causes.

R. J. Hamilton, MD

Falsely Normal Anion Gap in Severe Salicylate Poisoning Caused by Laboratory Interference
Jacob J, Lavonas EJ (Denver Health and Hosp Authority, CO; Univ of Colorado, Aurora)
Ann Emerg Med 58:280-281, 2011

Severe salicylate poisoning is classically associated with an anion gap metabolic acidosis. However, high serum salicylate levels can cause false increase of laboratory chloride results on some analyzers. We present 2 cases of life-threatening salicylate poisoning with an apparently normal anion gap caused by an important laboratory interference. These cases highlight that the diagnosis of severe salicylism must be considered in all patients presenting with metabolic acidosis, even in the absence of an increased anion gap.

▶ This is another article that provides readers with a little known fact. A false-normal anion gap was in fact the result of a falsely elevated chloride level. According to the authors, the presence of high concentrations of salicylate can interfere with some ion-selective electrodes. In addition, there is some competition between salicylate and chloride ions to bind to albumin, resulting in hyperchloremia. Watch out for this one!

R. J. Hamilton, MD

First-Onset Seizure After Use of 5-hour ENERGY
Babu KM, Zuckerman MD, Cherkes JK, et al (Warren Alpert Med School of Brown Univ, Providence, RI; Rhode Island Hosp Toxicology Laboratory, Providence)
Pediatr Emerg Care 27:539-540, 2011

The health consequences of energy drink use in adolescents are unknown. We discuss an adverse event in an adolescent who presented to the emergency department with his first-ever seizure after consumption of 5-Hour Energy. We review the typical presentation of caffeine toxicity, as well as the importance of screening for energy drink use in adolescents with appropriate clinical findings. We pay particular attention to the identification of energy drink—related adverse events in the emergency department and the need for subsequent reporting to the Food and Drug Administration. To our knowledge, this is the first reported case of an adolescent presenting with a new-onset seizure associated with energy drink use.

▶ There are a number of stimulants in 5-Hour Energy, but this patient's presentation was sufficiently consistent with caffeine toxicity to attribute the effects to that ingredient. Prior studies have shown that drug screens are useful in the workup of new onset neurologic problems in children. Perhaps a caffeine screen might prove to be a useful addition.

R. J. Hamilton, MD

Massive acetylcysteine overdose associated with cerebral edema and seizures
Heard K, Schaeffer TH (Rocky Mountain Poison and Drug Ctr, Denver, CO; Univ of Colorado School of Medicine, Aurora)
Clin Toxicol 49:423-425, 2011

Context.—Acetylcysteine is a safe and effective treatment for the prevention of hepatic injury due to acetaminophen poisoning. While dosing errors are common, in most cases, overdoses produce minimal clinical effects.

Case Report.—We describe a patient who received 150 g of IV acetylcysteine over 32 h when the clinician ordered the infusion doses be administered as an hourly dose (100 mg/kg/h) rather than administered over the infusion duration (100 mg/kg over 16 h). After approximately 28 h of receiving 100 mg/kg/h, the patient developed delirium, and seizures that progressed to cerebral edema, uncal herniation, and ultimately severe brain injury. No other cause for her symptoms was identified during an extensive workup.

Discussion.—This case suggests that massive IV acetylcysteine overdose can cause cerebral dysfunction and life-threatening effects.

▶ Here is another article from this year that discusses the relative complexity of the Acetadote dosing and the increased probability of medication errors as a result. This is a good example of this problem and suggests that dosing intravenous acetylcysteine should be done with great care. Computer order entry might have averted this particular case report, but even those systems need human validation at the pharmacy.

R. J. Hamilton, MD

Methanol and ethylene glycol acute poisonings — predictors of mortality
Coulter CV, Farquhar SE, McSherry CM, et al (Univ of Otago, Dunedin, New Zealand; et al)
Clin Toxicol (Phila) 49:900-906, 2011

Context.—Methanol and ethylene glycol cause significant mortality post-ingestion. Predicting prognosis based on the biomarkers osmolal gap, anion gap and pH is beneficial.

Objective.—To evaluate the relationship between biomarkers, measured post-methanol and ethylene glycol exposure, and clinical outcomes.

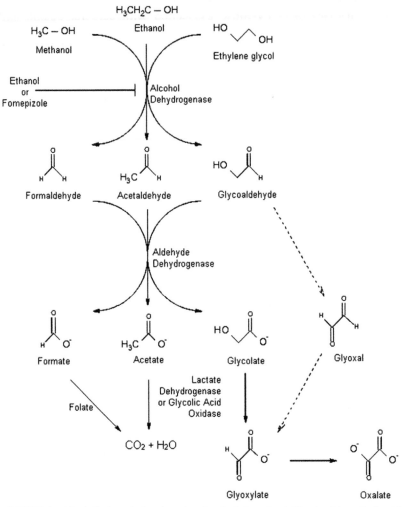

FIGURE 1.—Metabolic fate of ethanol, methanol and ethylene glycol. (Reprinted from Coulter CV, Farquhar SE, McSherry CM, et al. Methanol and ethylene glycol acute poisonings — predictors of mortality. *Clin Toxicol (Phila)*. 2011;49:900-906, reprinted with permission from Taylor & Francis, Ltd.)

Methods.—A review of the literature identified cases where methanol or ethylene glycol had been ingested and clinical outcomes were recorded. Biomarkers were extracted including osmolal gap, anion gap and pH, with clinical outcomes categorised as recovered, recovered with adverse sequelae and death. Biomarkers were analysed using the Mann—Whitney test for two samples; sensitivity and specificity were evaluated using receiver operating characteristic (ROC) curves.

Results.—In total, 119 cases of methanol and 88 of ethylene glycol poisoning were identified; 21 methanol and 19 ethylene glycol patients died. For methanol ingestion the mean values, for survival compared to

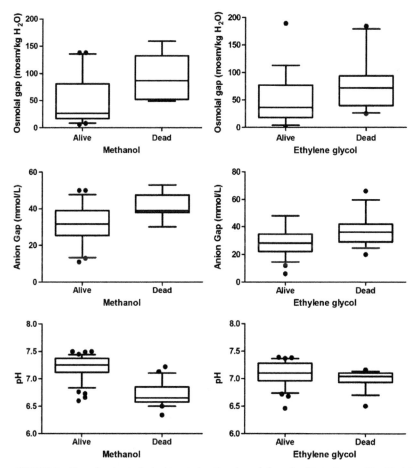

FIGURE 2.—Fate of patients who had ingested methanol or ethylene glycol in toxic quantities. The left panels show methanol survival and mortality while the right panels show that for ethylene glycol. The upper panels show osmolal gap, the middle panels show anion gap and the bottom panels show pH. The box shows the median value and the interquartile range (25th and 75th percentiles) and the whiskers mark the 5th and 95th percentiles while dots show the values that fall beyond these. (Reprinted from Coulter CV, Farquhar SE, McSherry CM, et al. Methanol and ethylene glycol acute poisonings – predictors of mortality. *Clin Toxicol (Phila).* 2011;49:900-906, reprinted with permission from Taylor & Francis, Ltd.)

death, were 48 (range: 61–38) and 90 (range: 49–159) mOsm/kg water for osmolal gap (p = 0.0052), 31 (range: 11–50) and 41 (range: 30–53) mmol/L for anion gap (p = 0.0065) and 7.21 (range: 6.60–7.50) and 6.70 (range: 6.34–7.22) for arterial pH (p < 0.0001). The area under the ROC curve was highest for arterial pH, 0.94 (95% CI: 0.89–0.99). For ethylene glycol, these were 49 (range: 0–189) and 79 (range: 25–184) mOsm/kg water for osmolal gap (p = 0.050), 28 (range: 6–48) and 38 (range: 20–66) mmol/L for anion gap (p = 0.0037) and 7.08 (range: 6.46–7.39) and 6.98 (range: 6.50–7.16) for pH (p = 0.072), for survival compared to death. The area under the ROC curve was highest for anion gap, 0.73 (95% CI: 0.60–0.87).

Conclusion.—Post-methanol ingestion a large osmolal gap, anion gap and low pH (<7.22) were associated with increased mortality; and pH has the highest predictive value. Post-ethylene glycol ingestion, both osmolal gap and anion gap were associated with increased mortality (Figs 1 and 2).

▶ On a first read, this article seemed to state the obvious because higher osmolal gaps imply more toxin, but after looking at the data closely, I feel that it does provide some useful insights. First, it affirms the practice of checking an osmolal gap and, of course, an anion gap in all these patients. Second, because patients often will not appear ill when their osmolal gap is elevated in the course of their illness, it properly alerts the emergency department physician to a patient whose condition may deteriorate.

R. J. Hamilton, MD

Nicotine, Carbon Monoxide, and Carcinogen Exposure after a Single Use of a Water Pipe

Jacob P III, Abu Raddaha AH, Dempsey D, et al (Univ of California, San Francisco)
Cancer Epidemiol Biomarkers Prev 20:2345-2353, 2011

Background.—Smoking tobacco preparations in a water pipe (hookah) is widespread in many places of the world, including the United States, where it is especially popular among young people. Many perceive water pipe smoking to be less hazardous than cigarette smoking. We studied systemic absorption of nicotine, carbon monoxide, and carcinogens from one water pipe smoking session.

Methods.—Sixteen subjects smoked a water pipe on a clinical research ward. Expired carbon monoxide and carboxyhemoglobin were measured, plasma samples were analyzed for nicotine concentrations, and urine samples were analyzed for the tobacco-specific nitrosamine 4-(methylnitrosamino)-1-(3-pyridyl)-1- butanol (NNAL) and polycyclic aromatic hydrocarbon (PAH) metabolite biomarker concentrations.

Results.—We found substantial increases in plasma nicotine concentrations, comparable to cigarette smoking, and increases in carbon monoxide levels that are much higher than those typically observed from cigarette smoking, as previously published. Urinary excretion of NNAL and PAH biomarkers increased significantly following water pipe smoking.

Conclusions.—Absorption of nicotine in amounts comparable to cigarette smoking indicates a potential for addiction, and absorption of significant amounts of carcinogens raise concerns of cancer risk in people who smoke tobacco products in water pipes.

Impact.—Our data contribute to an understanding of the health impact of water pipe use.

▶ We have 2 articles demonstrating that hookah smoking will cause substantial increases in carboxyhemoglobin levels. This study shows that it is not safer than cigarettes from a carcinogenic standpoint as well.

R. J. Hamilton, MD

Quail consumption can be harmful

Korkmaz I, Güven FMK, Eren ŞH, et al (Cumhuriyet Univ, Sivas, Turkey)

J Emerg Med 41:499-502, 2011

Background.—Intoxication due to quail consumption is rarely seen. Such a toxicological syndrome (also called coturnism) occurs during the migration of quails from north to south, when they consume hemlock seeds. The clinical symptoms and laboratory results are indicative of acute rhabdomyolysis.

Objectives.—Acute rhabdomyolysis has a wide range of etiologies. Coturnism is a rare cause of acute rhabdomyolysis that can be lethal due to renal failure and shock. To avoid severe complications, coturnism may be considered if the history is appropriate.

> *Case Report.*—We report four cases of coturnism from quail consumption; the patients were admitted with some combination of symptoms including muscle tenderness, extremity pain, nausea, and vomiting. They were treated with vigorous isotonic crystalloid hydration and urine alkalinization. Consequently, the laboratory results returned to normal ranges and the clinical symptoms disappeared.

Conclusion.—Although coturnism is a rarely seen toxicological syndrome that causes rhabdomyolysis, we present this case to increase awareness that it may present with symptoms of muscle tenderness, extremity pain, nausea, and vomiting after quail consumption.

▶ I like this article because now I will get the following question correct on my board recertification: What is coturnism, and what toxin causes it? Coturnism is rhabdomyolysis caused by ingestion of quail who have eaten hemlock seeds that have concentrated the toxic alkaloid conine. According to the authors, all of the following plants could contribute to this condition because they are consumed by the quail: *Ballota nigra*, *Galeopsis* spp, *Hyoscyamus niger*, *Lathyrus* spp, *Lolium* spp, and *Stachys annua*.

R. J. Hamilton, MD

The rising incidence of intentional ingestion of ethanol-containing hand sanitizers

Gormley NJ, Bronstein AC, Rasimas JJ, et al (Clinical Ctr, Bethesda, MD; Univ of Colorado School of Medicine, Denver; Natl Inst of Mental Health, Bethesda, MD; et al)
Crit Care Med 40:290-294, 2012

Objective.—To describe a case of intentional ingestion of hand sanitizer in our hospital and to review published cases and those reported to the American Association of Poison Control Centers' National Poison Data System.

Design.—A case report, a literature review of published cases, and a query of the National Poison Data System.

Setting.—Medical intensive care unit.

Patient.—Seventeen-yr-old male 37-kg with an intentional ingestion of a hand sanitizer product into his gastrostomy tube.

Interventions.—Intubation, ventilation, and hemodialysis.

Measurements and Main Results.—Incidence and outcome of reported cases of unintentional and intentional ethanol containing-hand sanitizer ingestion in the United States from 2005 through 2009. A literature search found 14 detailed case reports of intentional alcohol-based hand sanitizer ingestions with one death. From 2005 to 2009, the National Poison Data System received reports of 68,712 exposures to 96 ethanol-based hand sanitizers. The number of new cases increased by an average of 1,894 (95% confidence interval [CI] 1266–2521) cases per year ($p = .002$). In 2005, the rate of exposures, per year, per million U.S. residents was 33.7 (95% CI 28.4–39.1); from 2005 to 2009, this rate increased on average by 5.87 per year (95% CI 3.70–8.04; $p = .003$). In 2005, the rate of intentional exposures, per year, per million U.S. residents, was 0.68 (95% CI 0.17–1.20); from 2005 to 2009, this rate increased on average by 0.32 per year (95% CI 0.11–0.53; $p = .02$).

Conclusions.—The number of new cases per year of intentional hand sanitizer ingestion significantly increased during this 5-yr period. Although the majority of cases of hand sanitizer ingestion have a favorable outcome, 288 moderate and 12 major medical outcomes were reported in this National Poison Data System cohort. Increased awareness of the risks associated with intentional ingestion is warranted, particularly among

TABLE 1.—Case Reports of Intentional Alcohol-Based Hand Sanitizer Ingestions

Case No.	Reference	Age, Yrs, Sex	Psychiatric Illness	Hospital Admission Diagnosis	Stated Ingestion Intent	Location of Ingestion (Number of Acute Attempts)	Hand Sanitizer Alcohol Concentration	Blood Concentration of Alcohols, mg/dL	Therapeutic Interventions	Outcome
1	(3)	49, M	Alcoholism	Alcohol intoxication	NS	Hospital	85% ethanol	Ethanol 335	Gastric lavage, intubation	Recovery
2	(4)	38, M	Alcoholism	Suspected intoxication	NS	Hospital	Not specified	Ethanol >500	Intubation	Recovery
3	(5)	38, F	Chronic psychosis	Pancreatic duct stone	Suicide attempt	Hospital	51% isopropanol, 34% propanol-1	isopropanol 37, acetone 227, propanol-1 <10	Fomepizole	Recovery
4	(6)	27, M	Polysubstance abuse, depression	Pancreatitis	Suicide attempt	Emergency department (2 episodes within 2 months)	63% isopropanol	Elevated isopropanol levels	Intubation	Recovery
5	(7)	NS, F	Alcoholism	Alcohol withdrawal	Intoxication	Hospital	65% to 75% ethanol	Ethanol 700	Intubation	Recovery
6	(8)	81, F	NS	Cardiac rehabilitation	Suicide attempt	Cardiac rehabilitation	85% ethanol	Ethanol 228	Supportive care	Recovery
7	(9)	43, M	Alcoholism	Chest pain	Intoxication	Hospital	63% isopropanol	Isopropanol 13.6, acetone 269	Supportive care Vasopressors Fluid repletion	Recovery
8	(10)	49, M	NS	Acute intoxication	NS	Correctional facility	62% ethanol	Ethanol 335		Recovery
9	(11)	37, M	NS	Hospital visitor	NS	Hospital	27.6% 1-propanol, 36.1% 2-propanol	NS	Gastric lavage, activated charcoal, intubation	Recovery
10	(12)	53, M	Alcoholism	Acute intoxication	Intoxication	Outpatient and hospital	Isopropanol with first ingestion episode and second episode 61% ethanol	Isopropanol 100 acetone 207 both from first episode, ethanol 376, second episode	Intensive care admission	Recovery
11	(13)	46, M	Bipolar disorder, alcoholism	Acute intoxication	Intoxication	Outpatient and in hospital	62% ethanol	NS	Observation	Recovery

(Continued)

TABLE 1.—*(Continued)*

Case No.	Reference	Age, Yrs, Sex	Psychiatric Illness	Hospital Admission Diagnosis	Stated Ingestion Intent	Location of Ingestion (Number of Acute Attempts)	Hand Sanitizer Alcohol Concentration	Blood Concentration of Alcohols, mg/dL	Therapeutic Interventions	Outcome
12	(14)	NS	Borderline personality syndrome	NS	NS	Correctional facility	Isopropanol,	Isopropanol 195, acetone 128	Intubation hemodialysis	Recovery
13	(15)	71, M	Alcoholism	Hyponatremia	NS	Hospital, 2 episodes	70% alcohol first episode 48% 2-propanol and 32% 1-propanol, second episode	1st episode ethanol 180 2nd episode 1-propanol 850, 2-propanol 1600, acetone 55	Intensive care	Death
14	(16)	33, F	Depression alcoholism	Depression	Suicide attempt	Psychiatric ward	43% ethanol	Ethanol 414	Intubation	Recovery

M, male; F, female; NS, not specified.
Editor's Note: Please refer to original journal article for full references.

healthcare providers caring for persons with a history of substance abuse, risk-taking behavior, or suicidal ideation (Table 1).

▶ Whenever ethanol is mixed with another substance, it becomes a potential target for abuse—from mouthwash to hand sanitizer. The table included also shows that isopropanol toxicity must also be considered because the 2 alcohols are often mixed.

R. J. Hamilton, MD

Article Index

Chapter 1: Trauma

Chapter 2: Resuscitation

Chapter 3: Cardiovascular

Chapter 4: Gastrointestinal

Chapter 5: Neurology

Chapter 6: Infections and Immunologic Disorders

Chapter 7: Pediatric Emergency Medicine

Chapter 8: Emergency Medical Service Systems

Chapter 9: Emergency Center Activities

Chapter 10: Respiratory Distress

Chapter 11: Pulmonary

Chapter 12: Abdominal Pain

Chapter 13: Toxicology

Author Index

Printed and bound by CPI Group (UK) Ltd, Croydon, CR0 4YY

08/05/2025

01864678-0009